# IN ARTHUR'S SHADOW

# IN ARTHUR'S SHADOW

## Daily Musings on Exercise:
### A TRIBUTE TO NAUTILUS INVENTOR ARTHUR JONES

Gary Bannister, B.A., B.P.E., M.Ed.

**Authors Choice Press**

New York   Bloomington   Shanghai

**IN ARTHUR'S SHADOW**
**Daily Musings on Exercise:**
**A TRIBUTE TO NAUTILUS INVENTOR ARTHUR JONES**

Copyright © 2005, 2008 by Dick Dadamo

Authors Choice Press
an imprint of iUniverse, Inc.

iUniverse books may be ordered through booksellers or by contacting:

iUniverse
1663 Liberty Drive
Bloomington, IN 47403
www.iuniverse.com
1-800-Authors (1-800-288-4677)

Because of the dynamic nature of the Internet, any Web addresses or links contained in this book may have changed since publication and may no longer be valid.

You should not undertake any diet/exercise regimen recommended in this book before consulting your personal physician. Neither the author nor the publisher shall be responsible or liable for any loss or damage allegedly arising as a consequence of your use or application of any information or suggestions contained in this book.

Originally published by Cork Hill Press

Arthur Jones articles by permission from Arthur Jones, *Ironman Magazine* and MedX®

ISBN: 978-0-595-48915-2

Printed in the United States of America

To Jack and Beverly Bannister who provided the genes
. . . and so much more.


To Arthur Jones who provided the content
. . . and so much more.


To Judy Barre who provided the support
. . . and so much more.


To physical trainers who can and should provide
. . . so much more.

# TABLE OF CONTENTS
**\* indicates accompanying chart(s)**

## JANUARY

# FEBRUARY

# MARCH

# APRIL

# MAY

# JUNE

# JULY

# AUGUST

# SEPTEMBER

# OCTOBER

# NOVEMBER

# DECEMBER

# TABLE OF CONTENTS – CHARTS and DIAGRAMS

# ACKNOWLEDGEMENTS

Celeste Ulrich, Ph.D., University of North Carolina at Greensboro, who provided the awareness that I possessed a talent for writing.

Digby Sale, Ph.D., McMaster University (Hamilton, Ontario), who stirred my interest in exercise physiology and first introduced me to a Nautilus® machine.

Michael Fulton, M.D., orthopedic representative for Nautilus and MedX®, who believed that proper strength training was a step in the right direction, if not the solution to most medical problems, as well as the window to effective heart exercise - and who believed in me.

Ellington Darden, Ph.D., the voice of Nautilus through his writing, who provided plenty of research and ideas to keep my gym members strong and healthy.

John Balik, publisher of *Ironman*, who allowed me to reprint sections from Arthur Jones' series that appeared in his magazine (1970's and 1990's).

Jim Flanagan, General Manager of Nautilus (and later MedX), who often went "beyond the call of duty" and introduced me to the medical lectures of Arthur Jones, from which part of the book's content is derived.

Arthur Jones, the supreme educator, who taught everyone who crossed his path to think, allowed me to "hang around" long after the welcome mat was worn, and who allowed the reproduction of quotes, charts and graphs from his writings.

Judy Barre, more than a friend, who provided the support to complete the project by tolerating and correcting the frequent reading of articles.

The cast of characters in the book who had a positive influence on my life and the cast of characters in my life who had a positive influence on the book.

# FORWARD

I first heard the name "Nautilus" in the office of exercise physiology professor, Digby Sale at McMaster University (Hamilton, Ontario) in the spring of 1971. Two years later, I used the equipment (and system) for three months in Danville, Virginia. It made my workout look like a picnic. At the same time, I purchased a glimpse into the mind of its inventor, Arthur Jones - *Nautilus Training Principles: Bulletin No. 2* - but put it aside after a few pages. What did animals and airplanes have to do with exercise?

It wasn't until I spotted Jones at Nautilus headquarters in Lake Helen, Florida (1976) and opened a gym in Caracas, Venezuela (1980) that I dusted it off. That dusting changed the direction of my life.

I bought and read everything I could and, thanks to a special invitation, took it a step beyond. "If you think his articles are interesting," said General Manager Jim Flanagan, "you've got to hear him speak. He's ten times better."

Jim was on the money.

I attended a week of daily medical seminars and wasn't the only one who didn't understand everything said. Jones wasn't comfortable to be around - he could bite with or without warning - but he was passionate, honest and made sense.

In 1996, I began writing a weekly fitness column in *The Forum*, a Wellington, Florida newspaper. The column was limited to 600 words - one 8½" X 11" page - and featured the ideas of Jones. Years later, I moved to Jupiter, Florida and continued to write, vowing one day to put my efforts under one cover.

Like Jones, writers are rarely satisfied with their final product. My attempt to capture the essence of his character and philosophy is no exception. First, the majority of the exercise information comes from his writing and my interpretation of it. Second, many of the stories stem from one of two sources: (1) memory of the brief time I spent with him, a memory faded by time; and (2) favorite moments of others who spent more time with him. The accuracy of the tales over time may be skewed. Third, although I had Jones' autobiography during the final stages of my work, I chose not to read it, not to have it influence my effort - a decision that may or may not have been prudent.

With apologies to Arthur, a stickler for accuracy, *In Arthur's Shadow* is an attempt to re-introduce the concepts of proper strength training and muscle testing to those unaware of their existence. Not a "How To" book, it says more about what to avoid than what to do. And, other than a few obvious groupings and a vague time-line (Nautilus first, MedX last), the daily readings have no logical beginning or end. Each can be plucked from the text to stand on its own.

On one visit to MedX, I stopped at a Po' Folks® restaurant in Ocala. The place was emptier than a Scottish pay-toilet, so I picked a table in the middle of the room. Within minutes, I realized that one of the two men in the booth at the far end was Arthur Jones. He didn't know me from Adam at the time, but he sure owned the ear of the man with him. He talked and gestured and talked, all the while drawing on a napkin. I never heard a word, but you could cut the passion with a knife. It was a picture worth a thousand words. It was Jones at his best.

Arthur was about education; his style, entertaining. *In Arthur's Shadow* is a bit of both - education and entertainment.

Daily Musings on Exercise. Enjoy.

# JANUARY

"How fast one moves while performing exercises for the purpose of building strength has absolutely nothing to do with how fast one can move while using the strength of those same muscles."

Arthur Jones

## Faster Airplanes, Bigger Crocodiles and Younger Women

Only the Bank that stood before the right turn leading to the heart of town looked familiar. Only the Bank had the sense to distance itself from the unkempt shacks, spooky mansions and craggy trees that smothered the landscape in Spanish moss, like something from a movie.

Amid the chaos stood an item common to every tract - a mailbox that flaunted the name and vocation of its resident. From clairvoyant and palmreader to psychic and fortune-teller, Lake Helen, Florida could have laid claim to "Witch Capital of the World" - even after the arrival of its newest inhabitant.

Despite a growing national presence, Nautilus Sports/Medical Industries® blended in without raising a brow. It began with a dilapidated sign on the main building at the end of the street - "*Nautilus Time Machines*" - and ended with two sturdy pens, each home to a large crocodile, 20 feet from the reception desk. There was not a magazine in sight.

Things were different inside.

Steps beyond the reptilian gates was a spacious foyer featuring a three-story photo of the inventor's wife and the entrance to "The World's Largest Television Studio," its corridors lined with massive cameras. The studio boasted a capacity larger than that of ABC®, NBC® and CBS® combined - and there were eight more in progress. In another section, a pitch-black room housed five salt-water aquariums of chambered Nautilus crustaceans brought in from the coast of Japan. The adjacent room was the future site of the "Crocodile Lounge," a glassed-in parlor that would electronically lower into a man-made lake full of crocodiles and provide the setting for debates with 'experts' in the field of exercise.

Once the tour was complete, I crossed the street to the refuge of the company's medical facility. But it wasn't long before a man sporting a long-sleeve shirt and sunk in a posh chair behind a desk appeared on the wide-screen TV in the waiting room. His message was loud and clear: "There are only three things of value in life: faster airplanes, bigger crocodiles and younger women."

It was my first glimpse of Nautilus inventor, Arthur Jones.

Years later, I visited his getaway - "JumboLair" - on the outskirts of Ocala, Florida. Horse country was now home to more than 100 African elephants, an

African lowland gorilla, three white rhinoceroses, the world's largest collection of poisonous snakes and 1,400 crocodiles (all 24 species, including a 17½-foot Australian brute).

Jones didn't fool around with airplanes either. On the largest private jetport in the world, he showcased a Boeing® 747, three 707's and 14 other planes he used to fly medical doctors to his home to educate a group that "knew nothing about exercise, rehabilitation or nutrition."

In addition, he rented a Concord® so that his fifth wife could assault the around-the-world speed record. Jones had a penchant for youth but didn't snatch all of his wives from the womb and divorce them at 21, as reported. "The age of a woman is irrelevant," he said, "as long as she falls somewhere between a mature 13 and a well-preserved 16."

Someone once said, "You never get a second chance to make a first impression." Arthur didn't give a damn about either. The most brilliant mind in the field of exercise lived on his terms and his terms only.

Perhaps that's all anyone can ask of life.


## JANUARY 2

---

### The Evolution of an Exercise Philosophy

The exercise philosophy of Arthur Jones formally emerged with the introduction of his equipment and book, *Nautilus Training Principles, Bulletin No. 1*, in 1970. The Second World War had provided some unexpected lessons.

In 1948, Jones was training in the crude gym of a Tulsa, Oklahoma YMCA where he experienced a frustration common to many - some body parts grew, while others didn't. The workouts were long, the room hot and his bodyweight stuck at 172 pounds. He needed change. After 10 years in which he "tried literally 'everything'" to progress, Jones heeded the conclusion of several large-scale experiments conducted during World War II: "There is a definite limit to the 'amount' of exercise that will produce beneficial results - carried beyond that point, exercise will reverse its own previous results, leading to losses in weight, condition and stamina."

He reduced his efforts to "three weekly workouts of exactly one hour and 20 minutes each" and performed "exactly the same exercises in exactly the same way, reducing only the number of 'sets' of each exercise (from four to two)." It paid.

"I started to grow again," he said, "added a full half inch to the size of my upper arms, added 10 pounds to my bodyweight, and greatly increased my strength, and all of these gains were produced within a period of only a week as a result of three workouts."

After that week, Jones stopped training for more than a year (travel commitments) but didn't stop thinking. "If cutting my workouts by half produced that kind of results," he speculated, "what would happen if I cut my workouts even more?" When he resumed, he performed "only two sets of eight basic exercises: standing barbell press, behind-neck chin-up, bench press with a barbell, regular grip chin-up, dip on a parallel bar, barbell curl, behind-neck triceps curl with a pulley, and squat with a barbell and safety rack."

In seven weeks (20 sessions), he "reached levels of both muscular size and strength that were far above anything previously produced." Again, he was forced to quit for a year. When he resumed, he recovered his previous seven-week gains (using 16 total sets as before) and then reduced his training for six more weeks. At 5'7½," he peaked at a lean bodyweight of 205 pounds with a cold upper-arm of 17 1/8".

In the process, Jones attempted to determine the ideal training time for others and concluded: "In almost all cases, best results from heavy exercise will be produced by the practice of a very limited number of compound exercises that involve the major muscular masses of the body, and such training should be limited to not more than five hours of weekly training in any case and to about four hours in most cases." (1970)

His recommendation: perform 4-6 compound movements chosen from squats, stiff-legged deadlifts, standing presses, barbell curls, pullovers, chin-ups and dips; and "Not more than two sets of each exercise...three times weekly."

By 1971, Jones reduced the 'amount' of required training for bodybuilders to three 25-minute sessions per week and later to one set of 10-12 exercises when his equipment line was complete. All along, he used *less* exercise to surpass training plateaus.

In 1986, he developed tools that isolated muscle function and accurately measured strength, fatigue and recovery rates, advocating even less exercise for some individuals.

The approach echoed what he concluded in 1998 about his own progress: "Thirty-odd years later, I firmly believe that my results would have been even better if I had used only one set of exercise and if I had trained only twice each week."

# JANUARY 3

---

## When More is Less

In today's 'more-is-better' society, gym trainees measure the value of a workout by how long they stay - two hours is better than one. When they fail to produce the desired result, they increase the amount of exercise, a step that leads to the question, "How much can I tolerate?" If they focused, instead, on the minimum stimulation required for the production of best results from exercise, the answer to the same question for many would be a shocking, "Not much."

Muscles have thresholds of stimulation. In strength training, intensity of work below those thresholds does little or nothing to stimulate change; reaching them sends a signal to adapt. Physiologists agree that the level of intensity required to stimulate change may vary from muscle to muscle, but remains some high percentage (if not 100) of a maximum contraction. You must work 'hard' to get stronger.

Common sense and experience as an athlete, physical educator and coach have led me to believe that the relationship between the intensity and duration of physical endeavors is one of mutual exclusivity. If you have one, you cannot have the other. You can run 100 meters full out, but you must lower the intensity to run five miles. In the gym, if your workout is 'hard,' it will never last long; if it is long, it can't be hard. Since a high level of intensity is a prerequisite for producing best results from strength training, workouts, by definition, *must be brief.*

A session should last no more than 20-25 minutes with exercise machines and no longer than 45 minutes with free weights. To ensure a high level of intensity, try the following:

- Continue each exercise to the point of 'momentary muscle failure,' where a 100% effort no longer produces a complete repetition. Properly performed, one set of each exercise is all that's required. In a recent study at the University of Florida in Gainesville, one set of leg extensions and one set of leg curls taken to failure produced the same strength gains as three sets to failure. In general, best results are produced when muscle failure occurs between 60-90 seconds (8-15 repetitions).
- Move slowly during the performance of each repetition, using a speed that allows you to 'feel' the weight being lifted through the

entire range of motion. Slower movements ensure better form, a higher potential level of intensity and a greater margin of safety.

- Move as quickly as possible from one exercise to another. A series of exercises completed in 20 minutes is more intense than the same series performed in 30 minutes.

In a similar way, the heart has a threshold of stimulation commonly known as the "target heart-rate zone." Depending on age, the heart rate must be elevated to a certain minimum and sustained for at least 15 minutes to produce a benefit. Dr. Kenneth Cooper, Director of The Aerobic Institute in Dallas, Texas (and long an advocate of 'more is better') recently wrote in the *Wall Street Journal*: "If anyone does more than one hour of weekly cardiovascular activity, they are not doing it for physiological reasons." The heart muscle needs exercise, but again, "Not much."

Train more efficiently and effectively by using a 'harder-slower-briefer' approach, and enjoy the time you save and an increase in health.

JANUARY 4

---

### It's Time for Physiology

A few months after I inaugurated Venezuela's first Nautilus® gym in 1980, a member asked, "Why don't you set up a juice bar in the corner by the reception and sell health drinks, sandwiches and salads? It would provide a service to the members and an additional source of profit."

"Well," I replied, "I won't put a juice bar here for the same reason that, when I go to my favorite restaurant in town, I can't find a Nautilus machine."

This was a gym, and the equipment came with a philosophy born of a brilliant mind (that of Arthur Jones), a philosophy based on physiology and logic. I was aware of the success of the system in the United States and of the fact that I was the only one in town, both minor factors. If I was going to do it, I was going to do it right. I was also aware that people don't like to have things (food or exercise) jammed down their throats, but I was willing to take the chance.

The place was meager, yet clean, controlled and supervised. To some, the 12-machine circuit resembled 'boot camp,' to others, an oasis from the stress of city life or of belonging elsewhere. There was no air-conditioning, personal training, free-weights, aerobics, women's locker room or choice of cardiovascular equipment. But there was energy and, to those who joined, one guarantee - when you crossed the line, you had better tighten your shorts.

I was determined to make the statement Jones had a decade before - that brief, high-intensity training was the most efficient and effective way to get from A to B.

Labor was cheap. I hired as many as 15 instructors during peak hours and kept 'bodybuilders' to a minimum by offering metal without rust, letters (A,B,C) instead of numbers on weight stacks, and by making it clear from the beginning that certain things were not allowed. Nonetheless, 30 gorillas showed up the first year. Most had never seen a Nautilus machine, were unaware that physiology played a role in 'Fisico Culturismo' and failed to comprehend one set, 8-12 repetitions, 12 exercises, three sessions per week. And most had never seen the floor during a workout.

I may have been the only one prepared.

The sequence was brutal and non-stop: Leg Press, Leg Extension, Leg Curl, Hip and Back, Overhead Press, Negative Chin-Ups, Chest Press, Pullover, Negative Dips, Behind-Neck Torso Arm, Triceps and Biceps. One candidate, a young man who claimed he trained 'hard' two hours a day, six days a week, disappeared after four exercises. I was attending several clients at the time and eventually found his pale face staring at the lights from a bench in the locker room.

"You OK?" I asked.

"Yeah, just need some air," he gasped. "When are we going to do chest and biceps?"

"Don't worry. We'll get around to them. Take all the air you need."

The young man vanished four times during a 20-minute workout that took 90. When he arrived at the final station, he announced what Arnold Schwartzenegger had from the same position - the floor - after four minutes of exercise with Jones in 1971.

"This isn't exercise, this is torture." He crawled out the door.

Exercise was as social then as it is today, and things aren't likely to change.

Looking back, I don't know whether I would do it over again, but one thing is certain: there would be *no* juice bar.

## JANUARY 5

---

### A Perfect Form of Exercise

In the late 1930's, Arthur Jones judged the value of exercise by two factors: the quality of the resistance and the quantity of movement. Frustrated by arm curls with a barbell because they felt "easy" at both ends, he welded a chain to the bar to pick up additional weight at the start and end of each movement. It worked. In 1970, he introduced a series of exercise tools called "Nautilus® Time Machines" that incorporated ten (10) ingredients essential to what he called "full-range exercise," a concept that would revolutionize the field of strength training.

By 1948, Jones had identified the first (1) requirement, rotary resistance - resistance that rotated on a common axis with the body part that was directly moved by the muscle. He recognized that most joint systems were rotary, while gravity was linear - which explained why arm curls felt difficult only in the mid-range of motion (when forearms were parallel to the floor). In that position, the direction of movement exactly opposed the direction of gravity.

But rotary resistance was not enough. Muscles were not equally strong in all positions, and movement produced changes in the mechanical efficiency of the joint itself. The need for (2) a resistance that automatically varied to match the change in strength and leverage throughout the range of motion was resolved by creating a 'cam' specific to the potential strength curve of each movement.

The resistance then had to be (3) balanced according to the needs of the strength curve in all positions. This was accomplished by adding a counterweight to the movement-arm of each machine to balance its weight as the resistance varied.

Jones was frustrated with barbells in another way - they exhausted his arms before his torso, leaving him "the arms of a gorilla on the body of a spider monkey." To access the torso muscles, he (4) applied resistance directly to the body part moved by the muscle (for example, had the upper-arm push against a pad during exercise).

Full-range exercise required resistance in both (5) the lifting and (6) lowering phases - some tools allowed work only in the lifting phase, while 'bad form' generally ignored the lowering phase - and resistance at the start and end of each movement. Adequate resistance at the start of an exercise accommodated (7) 'stretching' and (8) 'pre-stretching.' Stretching occurs when a body part is pulled or pushed into a position that temporarily exceeds the existing range of joint, muscle or connective tissue motion. It increases flexibility. Pre-stretching occurs when a muscle is pulled into a position of increased tension just prior to the start of a contraction. Both pre-stretching and (9) adequate resistance in a position of full contraction trigger the recruitment of a greater percentage of muscle fibers, increasing the potential for strength.

The final ingredient was (10) "unrestricted speed of movement" based on the known limitations of constant-speed (isokinetic) exercise tools.

Despite the brilliance of his findings, the response to his concepts and equipment followed a pattern typical of new ideas in any field. They were first ignored, then ridiculed, then adopted, then copied and finally, stolen.

Throughout the process, Jones remained clear, "If anyone discovers an additional ingredient for a perfect form of exercise, we will immediately incorporate it into our equipment and give credit where credit is due."

No one has come up with anything yet.

## JANUARY 6

### Hangin' Around

I watched enough cowboy movies to know that in the old days punishment was swift, a matter of finding the nearest tree. The vigilantes tightened a 'noose' around the neck, frightened the horse away and thump, the deed was done. The neck was the direct way to the desired result; they didn't tie the rope to the bad guy's hair and expect the same.

But they do in the field of exercise.

Direct exercise, where resistance is applied directly to the involved muscle is more productive than indirect exercise. Yet, the attempt to strengthen major muscles by applying the resistance to smaller ones is all too common in gyms. In every case, the weak link fails in advance of its powerful allies.

The problem lies in the equipment, where the most popular choice is also the worst. With few exceptions, barbells do not provide direct resistance to any muscles.

Nautilus® inventor Arthur Jones was one of the few who understood the problem and the physics involved. "I knew," he said, "that most barbell exercises weren't quite 'right' when I first started using barbells." He set out to improve the situation.

Jones defined 'direct' exercise in two ways. First, "The resistance must be applied against the 'prime body-part,' against the body-part that is directly moved by the involved muscles." He accomplished this by placing pads on the movement arm of each machine. For the lower body, he positioned them against the lower-leg to work hamstrings and quadriceps; and against the upper-leg to work 'hip' muscles. For the torso (shoulder, chest and back), he applied pads to the upper-arm. A proper push into the pads eliminated failure from the small muscles.

Second, "The resistance must be directly opposed to the movement." Gravity pulls straight down, yet most human movement rotates around an axis. Therefore, during a barbell exercise, there is only *one* angle in the range of motion at which resistance is directly opposed to the movement. In *all* other angles, the resistance is less - and inappropriate to the muscle's requirements. In full contraction (where more fibers are available for work), for example, there is usually little or no resistance. Jones addressed this problem by attaching a 'cam' to the rotational axis of the machine. During exercise, the resistance exactly opposed the direction of the moving part *throughout* the movement and changed with the needs of the muscle.

Despite the brilliance of the new noose, there were plenty of vigilantes around to scare off the horse. One man altered a Nautilus machine to improve its safety and convenience, to which Jones replied, "Having spent more than twenty years of his life desperately searching for direct and 'actually proper' exercise, this man not only remained totally unaware of what he was really seeking but promptly ruined it when it was provided."

It reminded him of an incident in Africa when he gave a native a helicopter ride.

"I asked him if he thought he could fly the helicopter, and he said, '...oh, yes; I saw what you did, you turned that switch, and then you held onto that stick. I can do that, too.'... But the African, at least was innocent in his ignorance. He didn't remove the engine and rotor - replace them with a tree - and then complain that it wouldn't fly."

It's ironic that the only free-weight exercises to provide resistance in a position of full contraction - standing calf raises, wrist curls, and shoulder shrugs - are the very muscles trainees complain are hardest to develop. The next time Barbell Bob moans about slow calf growth, take him to the nearest tree and hang him by the hair.

## JANUARY 7

### Around and Around

I was no Roger, but I was a Bannister nonetheless. When I took the starting line for the high-school mile that day, I was prepared, favored and nervous.

At the gun, the field burst for position into the turn and jockeyed down the backstretch. I secured the inside lane early, a move that proved essential on a track that measured only 220 yards. My strategy was to maintain a brisk pace and grind them down. I had no finish, so I had to widen the gap. Round and round. Slowly, the moist breath on the back of my neck and the sound of pounding feet subsided. I was clear at the half-mile, but ran hard in fear of someone's break. One lap to go, the cheers heightened. I crossed in 5:25 with silent bliss behind.

A desire to better that time surfaced when I attended graduate school five years later. The plan was to supplant some 7-10 mile runs with interval training. If I ran 6-10 quarter miles in 75 seconds or less, with a descending break between, I could eventually put four of them together to reach the attainable goal of five minutes.

Oh, Roger, what I didn't know.

A good quarter-mile time (and I ran only those I had to) was in the neighborhood of 50-55 seconds. The distance, run with a best effort (by choice or by twisted arm), always left a degree of discomfort so severe during the final 100 yards that it caused even world-class runners to "tie up" down the stretch. The run was tough and the pain I didn't need, so I rationalized the following:

- If I ran a comfortable pace, say 65-70 seconds, I would derive most of the benefit without the discomfort.
- If I repeated my efforts 6-10 times with a rest between, the stimulation for change would eventually accumulate and exceed that of a single, all-out effort.

My reasoning was false. According to Nautilus® inventor Arthur Jones, no number of sub-maximal efforts will produce as great a result as one 100% effort. The full-out attempt forces the body to overcompensate and become stronger or better prepared for the next onslaught.

Jones applied the same analogy to strength training. If you continue to do something you can already do, your body falls into a comfort zone and provides no overcompensation. If you repeatedly force the body to try 'the impossible,' it will prepare for 'the impossible' - and then some.

He also recognized that hard exercise required supervision - a constant reminder to slow down, to relax uninvolved body parts, to breathe, to avoid excessive gripping and facial grimaces, and most important, to attempt the last repetition of each exercise.

He was right again.

The only free time I had that summer was early-to-mid afternoon when the heat and humidity of Greensboro, North Carolina stopped me in my tracks. The intensity of interval training (more work in less time) and the recovery required between sessions was more than I was used to. I eventually settled on my high-school time.

Five years later at a soccer clinic sponsored by Virginia Technical Institute in Blacksburg, coaches were invited to participate in a mile run, part of the certification process for referees. The gun went off early the next morning. Pushed by a rival coach, I finished in 5:34 with less silent bliss behind.

The aging process had already set in.

## JANUARY 8

### The Repetition

A year ago, our gym ordered one thousand 8½" x 11" workout cards. One side listed the major exercise machines in a logical sequence; the other left space for additional activities. Both featured columns to record repetitions performed and weight used. When the cards arrived, 'repetitions' was spelled 'repititions,' an error on the part of the printer - which proved to be the least of its worries.

Nautilus® inventor Arthur Jones often commented, "Ninety-five percent of the people in this country who perform progressive resistance training do not know how to lift or lower one repetition of any exercise." He then paused and spoke from the side of his mouth, "It's more like 99.9%."

If you stood in the doorway of most gyms for 30 minutes, you would not see many, if any, repetitions performed correctly. Seats are too high or low, weights too heavy or light, repetitions too fast, no pauses where there should be pauses, limbs locked-out where they shouldn't be locked. It's a mess.

A properly performed repetition should proceed as follows:
- Assume a safe and productive position or posture from which to work.
- Grasp the bar or handle, or contact the pad on the movement-arm (machine).
- SLOWLY apply force against the bar, movement-arm or pad until it begins to move. Maintain a constant pressure on the resistance so that it continues to move SLOWLY, without momentum, to the end of the range of motion. Feel the weight being lifted every inch of the way. When the resistance reaches the end of the range (a theoretical position of complete contraction), do ONE of the following TO KEEP TENSION ON THE MUSCLE:
1. If it is difficult to hold the weight in that position, pause for a second or two.

2. If it feels easy to hold the weight there, don't pause or fully extend your limbs. Exercises that push away from your body's center, such as chest, leg and shoulder presses, dips and squats, fall in this category. If it is difficult to tell, close your eyes and hold an extended pause. It won't take long to find out.

- After the pause/no-pause scenario, reduce the applied force and allow the weight to return SLOWLY to its original position without touching the weight stack.
- Repeat a smooth, controlled lifting and lowering exertion until the weight no longer moves using an all-out effort (and without throwing or jerking).

While the number of personal trainers has increased dramatically over the past decade, the correct performance of a repetition has not. The other day a young lady entered our gym with her boyfriend. As I demonstrated the features of the equipment, she asked, "Are you certified?" She was eager to talk about *her* qualifications. Later, during *her* workout, Miss Qualified proceeded to improperly perform *every* repetition of *everything* she did, and insisted that her boyfriend follow - grounds for divorce.

If the application from the panel of a Korn Flakes box and silicone implants are the modern-day requirements for certification, I'm not for it. I don't care about exercise philosophy - whether you stay all day, everyday; do one set or ten. I don't care about chest size. But I do care about the execution of a repetition - the core of a workout.

The certification of trainers has become little more than a racket that allows a chosen few to stand beside others and get fanned from the lousy reps they perform.

"Certified?" Sorry, I don't really like Korn Flakes.

JANUARY 9

---

**Human Growth and Potential**

The old sports adage, "The more you work, the better you get," is not necessarily true. Sometimes work that seems to bear little fruit, suddenly falls in line, just happens. I've shot some of my best golf when I didn't feel up to the task, and visa versa.

The same exists in strength training where the theory "The more you work, the more you improve," has often proved the opposite - the more you work, the less you improve. And the reason is clear. The human body is capable of tolerating any amount of exercise, but not capable of recovering from the same. Too little exercise and too much exercise can lead to similar ends - atrophy.

"The human muscular structure," declared Nautilus® inventor, Arthur Jones, "is capable of growing at an almost alarming rate, as has been clearly demonstrated in thousands of cases with beginning trainees." The rate, however, was rarely linear.

"It was recently noted in the scientific community," he added, "that growth occurs in very sudden spurts. A child may increase their height by as much as an inch overnight, literally in a few hours. I noticed the same thing in regard to gains in muscular size over 30 years ago; I have had my arms increase in size by a full inch from the time I went to bed at night until I got up the next morning, and while my increases in size have not always been that great, they have always been sudden, a matter of a few hours at most, and perhaps a matter of a few minutes. I was never able to determine just how much time was actually required for such spurts."

His novel exercise concepts provided immediate proof. "Starting from scratch, with a sixteen year-old, previously untrained boy," he said, "we built his lats to an unbelievable size in a period of less than eight weeks. With another subject, a man that had been in hard, constant training with weights for seventeen years, we increased his chest size by over three inches in a period of less than a month." It was only the start.

In 1975, he increased the strength of a group of conditioned football players by 60% in six weeks, while independent research with his MedX® Lumbar Extension machine in the 1980's produced increases of 100+%. He concluded, "If I ever produced only a 25% gain in strength from a 12-week program (as with the average study), I would probably go insane and kill all of the subjects."

Not only was Jones capable of producing outstanding results, he was certain that the rate of muscle growth could be sustained. "There is no slightest physical reason why such a fast rate of growth cannot be continued steadily right up to the point of individual potential."

Figure 1 shows a theoretical model of progress from stage one to ultimate potential, a process that Jones considered viable in 18 months. Note that to advance to the next stage requires less exercise - the reason, the limited supply of systemic energy for recovery. At higher strength levels, each workout takes a greater toll that can only be re-paid with time and rest. Yet, the concepts of less exercise and less frequency of training have been generally misunderstood, ignored or further complicated by the fact that many people are searching for results beyond their genetic realm.

How do you know your potential for strength and size? You don't. But because of the direct relationship between muscle strength and muscle size, the only way to find out is to make your muscles as strong as you can, so that they can grow as large as they will. Nothing else is even possible.

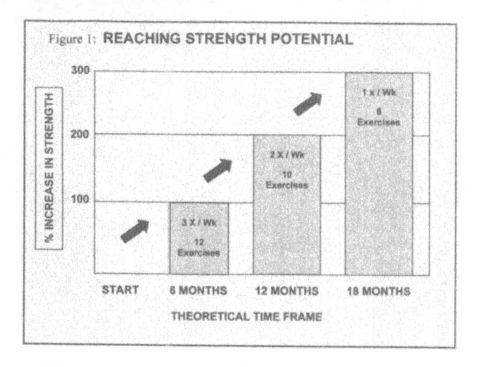

Figure 1: REACHING STRENGTH POTENTIAL

JANUARY 10

## Of Experts and Expectations

Nautilus® inventor Arthur Jones spent a lifetime criticizing self-proclaimed experts in the field of exercise. "There are no experts in any field," he claimed. "There are some people arrogant enough to call themselves experts and many people dumb enough to believe them. I quit school in grade four. I'm not an expert in anything."

Most of today's practical information on exercise comes from three sources: medicine, research and bodybuilding. As recently as 30 years ago, the subject of exercise was all but ignored by the medical community. Yet, it is common practice to recommend consulting a physician before initiating a program of exercise. According to Jones:

- Most doctors know little about the benefits associated with physical training.
- The majority of strength training research is unreliable due to poorly conducted studies, financial motivation and the use of inadequate measuring tools.
- The advice of successful bodybuilders is "worse than worthless" because it is misleading. Most have tried about everything, and can't honestly say what works or what doesn't. The recent merger of chemistry and exercise makes it all the more difficult to determine the outcome of any training regimen.

Things are further complicated by the fact that results are not immediate. In an era of 'instant' everything, it comes as no surprise to find a dropout rate above 90% among those starting an exercise program. Apparently, results do not live up to expectations.

In the early 1980's, I was approached by an 'expert' in a field I knew nothing about - beauty. The director of the Miss Venezuela Pageant, Osmael Sosa, asked if exercise would help the reigning Miss Venezuela, Barbara Palacios, become Miss Universe. Viewing a series of photos, he was quick to point out her shortcomings: thick ankles, excess fat on the back of her arms and the inside of her knees, disproportionate hip-to-shoulder width, and more. "As such," he declared, "she will not win Miss Universe."

"Has she ever exercised?" I asked.

"I don't think so," he replied, "but I don't care if she has to train 24 hours a day, seven days a week, we have to do something."

Poor Miss Palacios would not endure the training I had in mind, so I shifted the conversation to workout duration, general expectations and the time frame.

"One month and five days," he replied.

A degree in plastic surgery requires a little more time than that, I thought, and strongly hinted that it couldn't be done. He decided to bring her in.

The next morning, neither expensive after-shave nor a gym bustling with groomed instructors was enough. She didn't show.

People set themselves up for failure by trying to accomplish the impossible. The fact that someone once produced a 20-inch arm is no proof that everyone can. Exercise goals should be long-term and realistic: a decrease in body fat; an increase in heart-lung capacity, strength and flexibility; and a reduced risk of injury.

"Never train more than twice a week," suggested Jones. "Perform only one set of each exercise to a point where you can no longer continue the movement in good form, and move slowly by not throwing the weight up or dropping it down. If that fails, you may not have the potential for greater improvement."

Miss Palacios won Miss Universe a month later, which lent credence to Arthur's quote on expertise and her physical shape. As for Mr. Sosa...well, so much for experts.

# JANUARY 11

## Background Music

The short, balding and be-speckled man took center stage.

"Bring me ten Ph.D.'s from any university in the country and put them in the Oklahoma school system fifty years ago (when he went to school). Eight will be in grade two, one will be in grade three and the other *might* be a good student in grade one."

The crowd snickered. He continued.

"I don't have an affinity to music, but I could both read and write music in the first grade. You had to, to move on to the second."

More giggles.

"In grade four, there was a 16-year-old sitting across the aisle. They didn't just pass you on for 'showing up.' For all I know, he might still be there."

He went on about the decline of the education system in the United States as his guests doubled with laughter. In the end, he pointed to four members of the audience and asked, "Am I right?"

When they gathered their composure, one spoke up, "Well," he chuckled, "you're probably not far off."

The four represented the Florida State Department of Education and were there for "educational" reasons. Ironically, those reasons were satisfied by a man who dropped out of school in the fourth grade, Nautilus® inventor Arthur Jones. Jones could capture a crowd in seconds, not so much for what he said, but for how he said it. His delivery seemed prompted by monitors with inflection in *exactly* the right place.

Three steps to the right and every head followed; five to the left, and again. He kept in motion - sometimes up, sometimes back. He played with the volume - sometimes loud, sometimes soft - and kept the audience on their toes by calling them up to demonstrate things and to answer frequent questions. With Jones, everything and everyone was fair game. When sidetracked, his diverse background, eccentric nature and strong opinions (often backed by logic and statistics) pulled him through. It all pointed to one direction - Jones possessed a superior intellect.

Someone once commented that if he had applied his mind to science or mathematics, he would have been considered another Einstein.

To that, Jones replied, "Who'd want to be that dumb, anyhow?"

He ultimately devoted his genius to the field of exercise, a field inundated with everything but intellect. The splash was huge, but many thought a bit overboard.

"I used to believe that bodybuilders, as a group, were the dumbest people I had ever met; then, having worked with large numbers of them, I realized that coaches, as a group, are even dumber than bodybuilders; then, later yet, I worked with large numbers of scientists, and was finally forced to realize that they are even dumber, as a group, than coaches; most recently, I have been involved with large numbers of physical therapists, and don't yet know just which group is the dumber, the scientists or the therapists." He added doctors to the hierarchy when he entered the realm of rehabilitative medicine.

Both fields (exercise and medicine) ignored him and continued to shovel manure on their respective piles. They were relieved when he retired in 1998.

If you stumbled upon one of his lectures without knowing anything about the speaker, you'd think within minutes, 'This guy's not from this planet.'

Maybe he wasn't.


JANUARY 12

--------

### Avoiding and Preventing Injury Through Proper Exercise

Strength training should help prevent injury, not cause it; but it can do either. Properly performed, it can strengthen the muscles and joints of an athlete to the extent that the possibility of a sports-related injury is reduced. Improperly performed, it can cause an injury that might never have occurred.

The profile of injury is simple - if the amount of force applied to a muscle/joint system exceeds the breaking strength of that system, injury occurs. Prevention provides two options: reduce the applied force or increase the structural integrity. Improvements in protective equipment, rules and officiating have helped with the first on the field, but it's a different story in the weight room.

Thousands of athletes continue to train in a dangerous fashion - jerking and throwing weights - believing that it is safe. When a weight is moved suddenly, it is not being lifted - it is being thrown. In the process, the muscle generates a force 3-4 times greater than the weight itself at the start and then performs little or no work from then on due to the momentum created. In spite of the obvious, many athletes are taught to perform 'explosive' movements, and worse, activities that include exposure to impact. Both increase the potential for injury.

I once witnessed a 200-pound athlete register a force five times his body weight upon landing from a 4-inch jump on a force plate. Yet, 20 years later, *plyometrics* and jump squats are generally accepted as 'safe.' If the breaking strength of a muscle is unknown, explosive training becomes the equivalent of running athletes to the top of the stadium stairs and having them jump into the parking lot. Cross your fingers.

Despite belief in the value of strength training, many athletes remain convinced that hard exercise is dangerous exercise. As such, they often avoid the most productive part - the final repetitions - under the mistaken impression that they are avoiding injury. Yet, muscle overload and high levels of intensity do not necessarily imply high levels of force. And force is what causes injury...it doesn't matter how it 'feels.' It only matters what the force is in relation to the breaking strength of the system.

If an athlete has the ability to lift 150 pounds for one repetition, and does, he will be working as hard as he momentarily can - and produce a maximum-possible force in the process. If the breaking strength of his joint system is only 149 pounds, injury will occur. On the other hand, if he lifts 120 pounds slowly for the first several repetitions, he will probably not produce a force of more than 125 pounds and avoid injury. As such, the first repetitions would feel light - 120 pounds is well below the maximum strength level of the muscle - and then progressively heavier until the final repetition becomes impossible.

Danger? No.

The applied force is at its lowest during the final repetition because speed of movement, due to fatigue, is necessarily slow. Without speed, the muscle cannot produce a force high enough to result in injury, as long as jerking is avoided. If an injury is produced by exercise, it will usually occur during the first repetitions because the force is potentially highest at that point.

Avoid fast and jerky movements, maximum lifts and impact forces. The use of slow, smooth movements and high intensity is, by far, the safest and most productive way to increase strength. Some day strength training will go a long way in the direction of preventing injury...when the truth is applied.

## JANUARY 13

---

### Don't Hold Your Breath...

I learned a valuable lesson about 'holding your breath' on the way home from high school. The walk, about a mile up a hill through the local cemetery, usually followed an after-school sport, which meant I was tired and it was dark. On more occasions than I care to admit, I felt my heart and stride accelerate as I proceeded through the grounds. The rustling of the trees and other sounds launched my imagination and once, just once, I gave in to whistling.

So I learned, if you hold your breath a little, your physiology will race; if you hold your breath a lot, your physiology will stop, as demonstrated by the residents over whom I walked.

'Holding your breath' did not appear to have much value.

A reminder of its futility surfaces every time someone asks a trainer, "How should I breathe during strength training exercise?" The answer is simple, "Don't hold your breath," yet perhaps too simple for those awaiting the standard, "Exhale when you lift, and inhale when you lower."

If confessions like whistling are in order, I plead guilty to sharing such 'standard' advice with trainees and peers. In time, however, I have come to realize that it is only accurate in part. Which part? The first. The majority of grunts and groans heard in gyms amount to nothing more than a vocal expulsion of air during the lifting or exertion phase. If the resistance is a challenge, you will find yourself instinctively breathing out when you lift.

The second part, inhaling as you lower a weight, may be vital to life itself but is of little value to proper execution in strength training. In fact, if you are able to exhale once each time you lift and inhale once each time you lower a weight, then your exercise cadence is too fast or your resistance too light. Training with a weight that fails to challenge the respiratory system by allowing a one-breath-per-repetition pattern is not a productive way to increase strength.

On the other hand, working hard with a challenging weight will accelerate breathing to the point that one breath per repetition is totally inadequate. Research and logic suggest that moving weights with a fast cadence to accommodate the increased rate of breathing is neither safe nor productive.

If you exercise in a slow, controlled manner with a high level of intensity (as you should), breathing will take care of itself. The need to exhale vigorously as you lift and the need to 'catch up' with the demand as you lower will suddenly appear. Don't be surprised to find yourself breathing 6-8 times during the lowering phase of each repetition when the workload is heavy. Any attempt to control the rhythm at that point would be counterproductive. Forced breathing or 'holding your breath' for an extended length of time during training delays the return of blood to the heart (a phenomenon known as the Valsalva effect) and can result in dizziness or fainting.

A simple question deserves a simple answer, "Don't hold your breath. Let it happen." To those who insist on one breath per repetition, I can only say "good luck" in regard to results and survival.

And more.

Don't nourish the imagination of a high-school jock who'd prefer *not* to have reason to whistle.

## JANUARY 14

### "It's Not A Christmas Tree..."

Arthur Jones had an effective way of conveying a message - in your face - and this was no exception. He descended so quickly upon his prey that the after-shave and nicotine synonymous with his presence arrived well after the counsel. "It's not a (bleep...bleep) Christmas tree," he scowled. The Nautilus® inventor spent a lifetime assuring that every detail in the design of his equipment was functional. The victim had disregarded a seat belt, not a minor point.

The misuse of equipment in health clubs is common and on the rise. With ignored belts, fast repetitions, over-zealous weights, clanging movement arms and vacations between stations, it's no wonder trainees quit because they "don't see results." Much of their effort is wasted at best, dangerous at worst.

Progress is slow without sound fundamentals. The implementation of safe and effective guidelines for machine use in exercise is long overdue.

Try the following in your set-up:
- If the machine has a seat, place it at a height that will properly align your rotation point with that of the machine or that best isolates the muscle group in question. Most trainees place seats too high, which makes the majority of exercise too easy. Record its numerical height.
- If the machine has a seat belt, use it to stabilize body parts and to isolate the desired movement. It is essential to the production of best results.

- If the machine has handles that are not directly involved in the exercise, grip them lightly. Excessive gripping can elevate blood pressure to dangerous levels. If you require a firm hold during the lifting phase, relax as you lower.
- Select a resistance that allows the performance of at least eight, but no more than 12-15 repetitions. A weight too light will not stimulate a meaningful result regardless of how many repetitions are performed; while too heavy invites bad form, injury or both. Increase the resistance approximately 5% by using small side-weights to assure that progress is not at the expense of good form.

Try the following during execution:
- Use slow, controlled movements and 'feel' the muscle lifting the weight through every inch of the range of motion, with no momentum or jerking. If the movement arm bounces at the end of the lifting phase, the weight has been thrown, not lifted. Hold the resistance in the contracted position for a second or two, and lower it slowly. Repeat until no further movement is possible despite a full effort on your part. Slower movements provide better muscle isolation (less cheating), decrease the chance of injury and demand more of a working muscle.
- Contract and extend muscles through the entire range of motion provided by the machine on every repetition to maximize strength and flexibility gains.
- Train silently. Clanging weights indicates jerky movements - a waste of time and structural integrity. Reserve 'fast' movement for the time spent between exercises.

An exercise machine is *not* a Christmas tree, but it can decorate those who employ it wisely with festive results.

## JANUARY 15

### Speed of Movement During Exercise

More than 15 years ago, I witnessed a demonstration using a large platform scale (called a force plate) that recorded changes in force. The subject, a 6'4", 250-pound male, stood on the scale and performed an overhead press using a slow-to-increasingly-fast rhythm with a 60-pound barbell. At a slow speed (Figure 1), the signal on the attached oscilloscope moved in a smooth, steady motion and hovered close to 60 pounds. At maximum speed (Figure 2), however, the signal overshot the top and bottom of the screen. Freeze-frame analysis revealed that the barbell registered a force of over 200 pounds at the instant the repetition was initiated, and a force below zero for much of the remainder. The momentum of the barbell was lifting the subject's arms.

Multiplying the force to which you expose a muscle or joint system by moving a weight quickly, without knowing the 'breaking' tolerance of that system, is unsafe. In like fashion, strength training with a resistance that weighs little or nothing throughout most of its movement is unproductive. Yet, as undeniable as these principles are, they are not obvious to people involved in progressive-resistance exercise. Most trainees use 'fast' movements and wonder why their results are slow at best or why the result they produce is the only one that could have been produced - injury.

The same principles are equally ignored by those involved in the administration, sale and application of training programs - coaches, trainers and equipment manufacturers - who advocate methods that adhere to, or include, 'fast' movements against resistance such as power-lifting and plyometrics. At this level, it borders as much on criminal malpractice as it does plain ignorance.

Advocates of 'explosive' training rationalize their actions in two ways.

One, they believe that 'fast' movements trigger the brain to automatically select the stronger, more powerful fibers in the working muscles, precisely those required for athletic endeavors involving speed, strength and power. This theory has never been proven in studies involving humans. What research has demonstrated, however, is the orderly recruitment of muscle fibers according to the intensity of effort. When the intensity is low, as during the first repetitions of an exercise, the brain recruits the muscle's weakest fibers. As the exercise gets harder, a signal is sent for a higher order of fibers to assist. On the final 'impossible' repetitions, the strongest fibers join in. When they are working, all of the fibers are working.

Two, they believe that 'fast' movements in the gym result in 'fast' movements on the field, another idea yet to be proven. According to Nautilus® inventor Arthur Jones, "How fast one moves while performing exercises for the purpose of building strength has absolutely nothing to do with how fast one can move while using the strength of those same muscles." (1976)

In a recent issue of *Ironman* magazine (January, 1996) Jones reiterated, "Ignore this warning at your great peril; move fast during exercise and you will eventually hurt yourself...Train properly and you will probably never hurt yourself."

If there is a valid reason for lifting weights rapidly, it has eluded my attention. Whether using a barbell or a machine, safe and effective training begins and ends with 'slow' training. A slow speed of movement provides better isolation, a greater demand on the muscle and a safer alternative.

Its counterpart may one day prevent you from moving at all.

Figure 1: **SLOW MOVEMENT SPEED DURING EXERCISE**

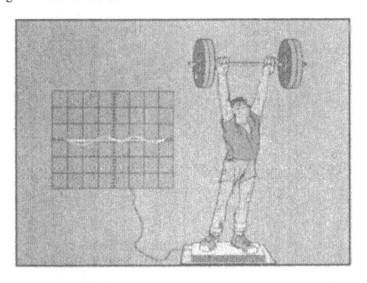

Figure 2: **FAST MOVEMENT SPEED DURING EXERCISE**

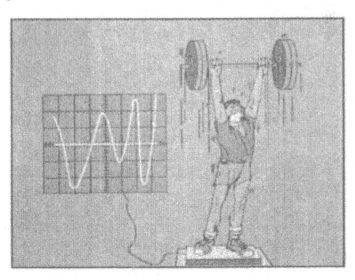

# JANUARY 16

---

## Progressive Resistance Equipment

Myth has it that progressive resistance exercise rose to new heights when Milo 'took the bull by the horns.' Soon after, stones, logs, weighted vests and growing animals were used as resistance in training regimens, which left a lot to be desired. It wasn't until 1902 that the issues of accurate measurement, practicality and progress were resolved with the introduction of the adjustable plate-loaded barbell.

Compared to what had gone before, the barbell was a miracle tool, yet attempts to improve it were on the horizon with the introduction of the Universal® gym in the early 1950's. Universal's self-contained, pin-selector weight stack allowed resistance to be altered by moving a peg from one hole to another instead of by adding or removing cumbersome plates. The idea improved the speed, convenience and safety of training, but did nothing to improve possible results from exercise. With few exceptions (leg extensions and curls), the 'new' exercises were copies of barbell movements - and subject to the same limitations.

In 1948, Nautilus® inventor Arthur Jones began designing tools that functioned according to the needs of the muscle and introduced his first device in 1970 at the Mr. America contest in Culver City, California. The huge (15' long X 6' wide X 8' high) multi-station, upper-back machine featured a pullover, a behind-neck, a pulldown and a rowing movement that took the industry by storm. At the same time through his training of athletes and bodybuilders, Jones slowly defined a philosophy of exercise that was as unique as his equipment.

He established a circuit of exercise with barbells, a Universal thigh-extension machine and with the four Nautilus tools available at the time. The thigh machine had a 150-pound weight stack that was attached to the movement arm by a re-directional cable. According to Jones, it went a long way toward ruining the function of the machine. The resistance was high in the starting position and decreased as the movement progressed - the reverse of what should have been.

"It is undoubtedly possible," he said, "to design a machine in such a manner that it would be WORSE, but you would be required to think about it first." Jones eventually attached a rod to the bottom of the movement arm to add barbell plates. The weight stack was inadequate for strong athletes.

One day, a trainee exerted a force against the movement arm that tore one of the pulley-brackets from the frame, rendering the primary source of resistance inoperable. Jones stuck it in the corner for repair but later realized that the breakdown was actually an improvement. The resistance curve of the secondary source of resistance - the barbell plates placed on the rod of the movement arm - "while certainly not perfect, was at least not backwards."

Universal continued to increase the number of exercise stations around each of their modules, while Jones focused on identifying the ingredients of what he called a "perfect form of exercise."

His comment on the competition? "How many people you can stuff in a phone booth is irrelevant. When you finally get them in and set the record, try using the phone." There was no regard to function, which eventually led to poor results, few sales, and now, no company.

And so it is with many of today's survivors, Milo - the only thing growing is the bull.

## JANUARY 17

---

### Exercise is Not Systemic?

Tell that to the ashen guy who, having barely completed three leg exercises, lies in shock on some carpeted gym floor. It's happened more than once, and provides a wonderful lesson.

During the first four years that Nautilus Sports/Medical Industries® existed (Lake Helen, Florida, 1970-74), thousands of athletes in excellent physical condition attempted the revolutionary one-set-to-failure, 12-exercise circuit its creator, Arthur Jones, had devised. No one came close to finishing. No one made it through the first few minutes. All were left gazing at the ceiling.

There were only four Nautilus machines available at the time, so Jones used barbells, Universal® machines and pulleys - but equipment was not the issue. The body's inability to make chemical changes quickly enough to meet the demand of working full-out with no rest between efforts (what Jones later called "metabolic conditioning") sent systems into shock.

The same occurred when I opened Venezuela's first Nautilus facility in 1980. Of the 30 bodybuilders who took the challenge that year, only one made it to the fifth machine. The others barely made it to the bathroom. When you ask muscles to work hard, regardless of how many are involved, the response is always 'systemic.' In this case, a few intense leg exercises threw trainees into shock.

The 'indirect effect of exercise' provides another example. When a muscle is stimulated, it sends a shock to its neighbors (the closer they are, the greater the effect). In the same way, a man who works only his torso will not reach his potential because the body does not take kindly to disproportionate growth. The moment he adds leg exercises, his torso will grow, even if his torso work-out remains the same.

I once trained for months without exercising arms. Yet, after each session, my arms felt 'pumped.' One day, I measured them before and after a workout in which I did nothing of biceps, triceps or gripping. Following an arm-cross (chest), a pullover (back) and a lateral raise (shoulders), none of which involved movement about the elbow, my arms were a half-inch larger - a systemic response to nearby, demanding exercise.

Strength training must be hard enough to stimulate a change without leaving the system's recovery ability in shambles. Too much can prevent a change from happening.

Need proof? Find out how much you can arm curl with a barbell for 10 repetitions. Let's say it is 100 pounds. Using 50% of that weight, perform 20 sets of 10 repetitions, three times a week for six months - and no other exercise. Test your strength again with 100 pounds. At best, you'll perform 11 repetitions; at worst, 8-9. In either case (a little stronger or weaker), you would have wasted six months.

On another occasion, take the 100 pounds and perform 20 sets of as many repetitions as possible (only the first sets will yield 10) three times a week for six months - with no other exercise. In the re-test, a notable loss will have occurred. The biceps cannot grow because the system is unable to recover from such a barrage.

Despite the obvious, the majority of hardcore trainees exercise almost every day by rotating muscle groups. Can their systems take it? Judging by the low levels of intensity apparent in most workouts (due to boredom and fatigue), I think not.

Millions of people for thousands of years believed that the world was flat. It turned out not to be.

## JANUARY 18

---

### Tails of Woe

In seconds and before the door closed behind, an eerie sound filled the room and escalated to levels that I hadn't heard since my last visit to Niagara Falls. This time, the deafening resonance of water rushing over the brink was replaced by the reverberating sound of 450 rattlesnakes protesting our intrusion. You couldn't talk or hear.

"The World's Largest Collection of Poisonous Snakes" was part of a tour of MedX® headquarters in Ocala, Florida. MedX was about exercise; its creator was into reptiles.

Arthur Jones learned about both through trial and error. He was bitten "hundreds of times," yet would often be found 'toying' with the most aggressive species. He also bred rattlers in hopes of one day reaching the eight-foot length others had claimed.

"We force fed one to the point he wouldn't take any more," he said. "We got him to about six and a half feet."

In the early 1950's, Jones claimed he could "read a snake's mind." He knew what it was going to do in advance of the action, despite having no idea of 'how' he knew. Half a million snakes later, he realized that the ability derived from observation and worked on a subconscious level. "Snakes," he claimed, "telegraph their punches... A rattlesnake does so with its tongue, a chickensnake with its upper lip, a boa constrictor with its neck." Jones made good use of this knowledge long before he was aware he possessed it.

He was equally astute in the field of exercise where he was cognizant of two common errors, "Some people think that intelligence is a substitute for experience - and some people think that experience is a substitute for intelligence."

"For the production of best-possible results from exercise," he theorized, "maximum-possible growth stimulation must be induced without disturbing the existing recovery ability any more than necessary." When asked the source, he tapped himself on the chest.

"It should be obvious that there will be no growth without growth-stimulation, and that maximum-possible stimulation is required for maximum-possible growth. It should be equally obvious that the muscular structures cannot grow if there is no recovery ability available to make such growth possible, and that a greater store of existing recovery ability will at least make a faster rate of growth possible... Logically, then, both factors are required for growth - and there must be a reasonable balance between them; the body WILL NOT grow without growth-stimulation, and CAN NOT grow without recovery ability. No amount of stimulation will produce growth if the body cannot supply the requirements for such growth - and the body cannot supply them if they are unavailable; unavailable perhaps because they are constantly being used up as fast as they are being produced in never-ceasing attempts to compensate for too much exercise."

With that, he wondered why so few bodybuilders questioned the fact that they always experienced such a rapid response after a prolonged layoff from training, but then quickly fell back into a rut where their progress was almost non-existent. It was obvious. During a layoff, the system rebuilt its recovery ability and existing reserves, which allowed it to meet the requirements for growth when training was resumed and growth stimulated.

Following the MedX tour, someone asked, "How do you force feed a rattle-snake?"

"Simple," replied Arthur. "Just tie the tail of one rat to the head of the next."

Common sense prevailed with Jones. "The signs are all there, in plain sight for anybody to see - but most bodybuilders choose not to look."

They're too busy shoving MORE down their throats.

## JANUARY 19

---

### Muscle Size vs Strength

"Dumbbells are for size and barbells are for strength," said one teen to another in the locker room. I hope I had a better grasp of things at that age, but maybe I didn't.

Innocence and ignorance are excusable, but statements about equipment and training methods that produce muscle size, shape and strength differences from people who should know better are not.

For example, the widespread belief that free weights are 'the only way to go' makes no sense. How you use a tool and how hard you work with that tool are far more important than the tool itself. Muscles can't distinguish between a barbell and a bale of hay and proof lies in the fact that the strongest back ever measured on a MedX® Lumbar Extension machine belonged to a man who never touched a barbell. He lifted hay. And the roundest muscles I've seen in a 25-year career belonged to a man who was towed by boats all day. Experience would lead me to believe that if you want strong muscles, lift hay; and if you want round muscles, water-ski.

The relationship between muscle size and strength has long been a source of confusion, yet the physiology is simple. Every textbook in the last half-century agrees that "the strength of a muscle is in direct proportion to its size," which means, a larger muscle is a stronger muscle; and a stronger muscle is a larger muscle. The confusion derives from comparing one person to another. Genetic advantages in leverage, bodily proportions, nervous system efficiency and body type (among other difficult-to-measure or yet-to-be-determined factors) greatly influence how much you can lift, resulting in the widespread belief that muscle size and strength are unrelated. If one person is considered, however, an increase in muscle size indicates an increase in strength; and an increase in strength results in an increase in size.

Research suggests that an untrained individual can increase his strength 30-60% in 6-12 months by progressive training. In the process, he might add a half-inch to his arm. Another person, with the same program and input, might add a millimeter. The difference is genetics. Exercise can only stimulate results; the body produces them - and bodies are different. While most people possess an average genetic potential and are likely to increase muscle size with proper training, some are 'duds' and will never produce much in the way of size or strength. Only a rare few can duplicate the results seen in bodybuilding magazines.

Most women are capable of producing a percentage increase in strength that rivals their male counterparts. Yet, according to Ellington Darden in *The Nautilus Bodybuilding Book* (1982), "99.9999% of American women cannot develop large muscles under any circumstances." Despite the fact that most females do not have the potential for size, many will go to their graves believing otherwise or squander the majority of their exercise time 'toning' and 'shaping.'

According to Nautilus® inventor Arthur Jones, "Hundreds of articles have been published on the subject of 'muscle-shaping' exercises and training routines. But the fact of the matter is that the shape of a muscle is entirely determined by heredity and by its existing degree of development in relation to the overall fat-tissue-to-muscle-tissue ratio. The people who write such trash have no slightest idea of the real facts - and any results they may have produced were done so almost literally in spite of their efforts."

Strengthen your muscles - leave their size and shape to the family tree.

## JANUARY 20

---

## You Don't Have To Live There

Super-sized carryalls with gloves, belts, gadgets, headgear, entertainment systems and water bottles are making a statement in today's gyms - "We're here for the long haul." And it shows. With plenty of time, rest and beverage at each station, there's a reluctance to leave, which makes it difficult to convince anyone that a better result can be produced by less, but harder exercise.

Compare the results of two genetically superior individuals, Arnold Schwartzenegger and Casey Viator. In 1973, Viator participated in a four-week experiment at Colorado State University. Prior to this, he had been hospitalized by a work-related accident and weighed 166 pounds, down from his top muscular weight of 212. Viator trained 14 times in 28 days (less than 30 minutes per session), regained 45 pounds of weight and lost 18 pounds of body fat, resulting in a net muscle gain of 63 pounds.

When Schwartzenegger began training for Mr. Olympia in 1975, he weighed 200 pounds, down from his competitive best of 232. He worked out twice a day, two hours per session, six days a week for four months. After approximately 288 hours of training, Arnold gained 25 pounds. When asked why he failed to reach his target weight, Schwartzenegger replied that he "did not have enough time to prepare." Since both men were accused of taking steroids at the time (although Jones would have nothing to do with drugs), the superior results of Viator's seven-hour input can be attributed, in part, to his training method.

Arnold watched one of Casey's high-intensity workouts at Nautilus® headquarters in Lake Helen, Florida (1971) and wrote, "...I never witnessed such ferocious, almost suicidal training in my life... If I had to do this every day, I'd opt for a hernia, go back to Austria and be a ski instructor." Arnold missed the point. It would be impossible to train with that intensity every day. So, like today's gym rats, he did something else.

Low-intensity training, regardless of how much, does little to stimulate an increase in strength. On the other hand, a large amount of high-intensity training can retard growth or result in losses. The only logical alternative is brief, high-intensity training, as advocated by Nautilus inventor, Arthur Jones. Jones often compared muscle stimulation to striking a stick of dynamite with a hammer, "You can tap it all day and nothing will happen. But hit it hard once..." Things happen.

They did with Oregon bodybuilder, Chuck Amato. Before 1971, Chuck performed up to 60 sets of arm curls each workout for more than two years with, in his own words, "no visible results." When he arrived at Nautilus, Amato rested four days and then trained 25 minutes every other day for 10 days. The 'arm' portion of each session was seven minutes (including biceps, triceps and forearm). After five workouts, he added 13/16ths of an inch to his arm by training harder and allowing time for recovery.

In a recent 14-week study at the University of Florida, one set each of leg extensions and leg curls, pushed to muscle failure, produced the same strength gains as three sets to failure. The tool that measured the result was Jones' MedX® knee machine that took 22 years to build at a cost of $120 million. As long as 'failure' was attained on the first set, additional exercise proved useless - which is what Jones said 30 years ago.

When 'a lot of nothing' fails to produce the desired result, instead of trying 'a lot *more* of nothing' - which only serves to decrease intensity, recovery and progress - perform less, but harder exercise. Camping in the gym may *prevent* the results you seek.


## JANUARY 21

---

### The Effect of the Exercise Cam

The horror of a visit to the dentist was always placated by the fact that, if we were good, there was a reward at the end of the tunnel. Dr. Ritz gave us a toy soldier.

Much the same exists in the field of strength training. Yet, the reasons why hardcore trainees avoid exercise machines are more physical than psychological. They like the feel of strapping their hands around something they can control and of the 'sticking point' that occurs during the movement, and of the effort required in overcoming it. They know where it will happen and prepare accordingly. Most of all, they enjoy the 'rest' they encounter - usually at the end of each repetition - a reward for a job well done.

When the Nautilus® inventor first came out with something different, he had a steep hill to climb. The majority of trainees didn't like the feel of the new equipment for several reasons. Few pieces gave them anything to hold on to and many, due to the tight security provided by seatbelts, felt the machine was in control of their destiny. There was no sticking point - no part of the movement that felt harder - to signal when a muscle might fail. There was no toy soldier at the end of each repetition...by design.

The Nautilus machine had a cam, an elliptical device that changed the resistance to meet the exact needs of the muscle as it moved through a complete range of motion. The result was what its inventor Arthur Jones called full-range strength - a complete activation of the muscle from stretch to contraction.

"As you move any part of your body from one position to another position in relation to other parts of the body," he said, "you change your strength, either become stronger or weaker; there is no movement of any part of the body wherein your strength remains constant throughout a full range of movement."

Jones used the standing biceps curl as an example. "If we have a full-range movement of 150 degrees, the resistance provided by a 100-pound barbell will be about as follows: ZERO at the start, 50 pounds after 30 degrees of movement, 70.7 pounds after 45 degrees of movement, 100 pounds after 90 degrees of movement, and LESS THAN ZERO during the last few degrees of full-range movement (the weight begins to move downward)."

The development of the cam was not a consensus of the existing strength curves of a large population. It was a calculation of the muscle's potential for strength throughout the range and incorporation of that information into the shape of the cam, specifically its radius. The process was complicated by the fact that muscle input was always less than output (due to friction and leverage) and that every muscle was unique.

Figure 1 shows the strength curve patterns (not the actual curves) of two movements. The bottom curve represents a biceps curl of the upper arm, a movement that rotates around a single axis, the elbow. The top curve is that of a squat, a movement that involves multiple muscle groups and rotation about several axes. Because of the simplicity of a single-axis movement and the magnitude of the required change in resistance, the construction of the bottom curve (and cam) took only 22 years - 12 less than that required for a compound-axis movement.

The effect of the cam is shown in Figure 2. The top curve (A) represents the ideal strength curve of the biceps (as dictated by *output* and provided by the cam of a Nautilus machine). The bottom curve (B) depicts the actual resistance provided by a barbell during a biceps curl. The area between the two curves (C) shows the difference between real and ideal, the additional benefit provided by the use of a machine with a proper cam.

The message is clear - to get it across is like pulling teeth.

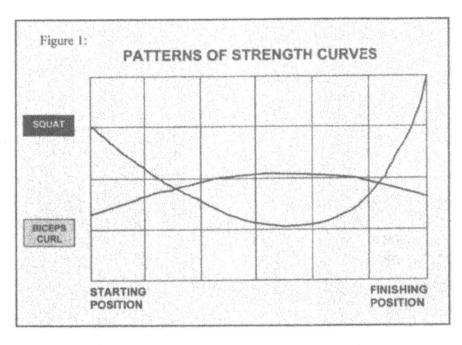

Figure 1:

PATTERNS OF STRENGTH CURVES

SQUAT

BICEPS CURL

STARTING POSITION

FINISHING POSITION

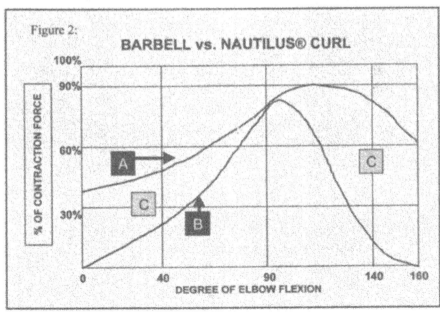

Figure 2:

BARBELL vs. NAUTILUS® CURL

% OF CONTRACTION FORCE

100%
90%
60%
30%

A

C

B

C

0    40    90    140    160

DEGREE OF ELBOW FLEXION

## JANUARY 22

---

## Of Rhinos and Cams

Arthur Jones awoke in the middle of a pitch-black African night with an idea he absolutely had to share. He was half-asleep when he grabbed the phone. "Get a sheet of paper and mark a spot three-and-a-half inches from the top left corner. Mark another spot two inches in and a quarter-inch down from the top right corner. From the center of the bottom edge of the sheet...," Arthur continued to describe the exact position of a series of dots that, connected, formed an odd-shaped sphere. "Build it and have it here in the morning."

The order was carried out.

According to Jones, the 'cam' installed in the prototype exercise machine that day "was a total, absolute, abysmal failure. But it failed so obviously that for the first time, I understood why."

He labored day and night to refine it and, despite the emergence of other problems, came up with what he described as "a thinking man's barbell." But the forerunner of the Nautilus® machine never came to fruition on the Dark Continent.

Jones was caught up in other interests - film-making (he hosted a TV show called *Wild Cargo*), thinning herds for preservation and capturing animals for export to zoos - that led to a greater, yet unexpected challenge. Rhino Hill near Salisbury, Rhodesia, was the site of the sale of hunting permits to tourists seeking 'trophy' animals, the government's solution to a reported overpopulation. Arthur knew better. He had the *real* count from frequent flights over the preserve.

When push came to shove, Jones received an ultimatum - leave the country. The government seized all of his assets: seven ground vehicles, two aircraft, a brand-new helicopter, 5,000,000 feet of film and two studios full of equipment, cameras, weapons, ammunition and machine prototypes. Even the personal items he left with a friend were sold off or kept.

Jones returned to Florida, broke, but the expulsion had a bright side - it provided time to re-examine exercise concepts and tools. In 1970, he launched his first product, a plate-loaded pullover with an elliptical sphere that provided a changing resistance through a full range-of-motion.

Despite its brilliance, the 'cam' was challenged from all sides. It was the wrong shape, wrong size, didn't fit everyone's strength potential, occupied too much space, etc.

I once met a gym owner in Miami, Florida who presented his Master's thesis - a critique of the cam - at an exercise conference in the early 1970's. He claimed its shape was incorrect and, during the question-answer phase of his performance, acknowledged a hand in the back of the room. A slight, be-speckled man stood up, bypassed the microphone in the aisle and headed straight for the stage. It was Jones, and there were only two things certain with Arthur: he was unpredictable, and generally carried a pistol.

You could hear a pin drop as he unzipped his jacket and reached deep. He slowly pulled out a small recorder and turned it to the microphone. Jones knew what 'they' were going to say and had his defense prepared in advance. When the tape finished, he shut off the recorder and returned to his seat without a word.

Among a barrage of insults, the message read the same as it had when he fled Africa, "Don't ask me to give you rational explanations for other people's insane actions."

It held equal weight on both sides of the Atlantic.

## JANUARY 23

---

### The Fireside Cam

There are two kinds of thieves: those who target specific items; and those who steal, just to steal. The thief who removed the #5-wood from my luggage on a recent trip to Canada was probably looking for a specific brand and shaft flex so that he could put it to good use. The thief who stole a 'cam' from the Nautilus® inventor in the early 1970's was probably thinking the same, until he got it home.

The 'cam' or spiral-like pulley that changes the resistance encountered during exercise lies at the heart of today's machines. While most remain hidden beneath shields, the first was large and in plain view on both sides of a contraption known as a 'pullover.'

The need was obvious.

The strength of a muscle increases as it moves from extension to contraction, while the resistance in most traditional exercises does not. To provide a superior overload, the resistance must match the potential strength curve so that a muscle encounters an exact and maximum load throughout its range of motion.

To understand the need, perform a bent-arm pullover with a dumbbell. Lie face-up at the end of a bench, press the weight upward and slowly lower it behind your head, paying close attention to the range of motion. The weight feels heavier as it lowers, heaviest when your upper arms are parallel to the floor and lightest when it returns to the start. Hard at the bottom (in an extended position) and easy at the top (in a contracted position) is exactly why your shoulders may 'hurt' for three months.

The change of resistance is the opposite of what it should be, as the inventor of the 'cam' suggested in a description of his new pullover device in 1970.

"In the starting position (arms fully stretched above the head)," he said, "the radius of the pulley is quite small and thus the resistance is low. Later in the movement, the radius of the pulley is greater and the resistance is increased in proportion. At the finishing position of the movement, the radius of the pulley is at its greatest, and the resistance has reached its highest point as well."

Arthur Jones was also aware of other facts:

- Although the strength of a muscle increased from the extended to contracted position, its *rate* of increase was not necessarily constant, and...
- "Changing positions bring about greater and lesser degrees of involvement of other muscular structures, and thus 'total' strength may be decreasing while the strength of a particular muscle is increasing."

In a pullover, help from muscles of the chest, shoulder, trapezoids and abdomen decreases the 'total' strength near the end of the movement, dictating a reduction in the radius of the cam, which modifies the 'feel' of the exercise.

According to Jones, "The resistance feels exactly the same in all positions. It is hard at the start of the movement, and remains hard throughout; but it is no harder, and no easier, at one point than it is at any other point... (but) it will not feel (that way) even to a man that has been training by conventional methods; at least not at first."

Function dictates design or as someone once said,

"There is only one way to build a wolf; and if it performs like a wolf, then it will look like a wolf."

Every muscle group has a unique strength curve, dictating a different cam in size and shape for each - enough to leave the best of thieves scratching his head.

With no wolf to show, there's likely a 'cam' on a wall high above a roaring fire.

## JANUARY 24

---

### Specificity of Training for Sports

As a young golfer, I was inspired by a man who had all the qualities I desired. A little man by golf standards, he was tenacious, disciplined and determined, and despite a hectic international tournament schedule and successful career, remained a gentleman both on and off the course. What proved most luring, however, was the stand he took on physical preparation for high-level competition. At a time it was considered taboo, Gary Player lifted weights to improve his performance in golf.

And so, with the hopes of a 14-year-old in head and *Gary Player's Positive Golf* in hand, I wore out the wood steps my father built to access the basement. Three times a week for 15 years I swung dumbbells and barbells like golf clubs and rhythmically pulled cables when I had the opportunity at college. Besides an overall approach to fitness, Player and I repeated the movements of the golf swing using resistance.

Years later, I met his antithesis - a gruff, chain-smoking non-golfer who earned my respect and admiration in a different way. Nautilus® inventor Arthur Jones hit home when he challenged the concept of specificity in sports training.

Jones believed that strength was general in nature (stronger triceps for golf meant an improved performance in all activities involving triceps) and that best results from strength training required a maximum overload (use of heavy weights). On the other hand, he believed that skill development relied on the practice of the movement itself with total specificity, using the same tool in exactly the same manner without an overload. For best results from both, he advocated their separation.

According to Jones, the more a strength exercise mirrored the movement found in a sport, the greater the possibility of interference with the skill. A talented basketball player, for example, will spend more money than he intends in an effort to win a 'teddy bear' at the circus free-throw booth. Something - the size, height or distance of the rim; the size or weight of the ball - is modified just enough to disorient his skill. When the change is minor (ounces or inches), confusion in the nervous system is heightened. The recruitment of muscle fibers, the timing of their contraction and the amount of force required for the task are so similar to the established patterns that the 'new' interferes with the 'old.' The result is short-term failure. When the change is major, the body cannot recognize the skill movement and develops a learning pattern that does not interfere with existing neural pathways.

As a teen, I often placed a three-pound, donut-shaped weight at the end of my golf club to warm-up and stretch muscles before play. On occasion, I swung the club in excess so that it would feel lighter when the weight was removed. It worked - but my golf bag also felt lighter when I couldn't find the balls. The slight increase in the weight of the club did very little to improve strength (wasn't heavy enough) and temporarily interfered with skill. In contrast, swinging a telephone pole would more likely have increased strength and, as a new experience, would not have hurt existing skill - unless it ruined my back in the process.

When training for strength in sports, identify the muscles involved and then build them in the most efficient and effective way possible *without* regard to duplicating the movements of the sport. Then learn to use the added strength to advantage in the only way possible - by practice of the skill itself.

Anything else will hurt far more than help.

JANUARY 25

---

### Training For Muscle Endurance

As rude as it seemed for a gym owner, I once stopped a man in the middle of a set of leg presses on a Nautilus® machine. His form, which originally caught my eye, was pitiful; and his weight, one my grandmother had mastered. There were others in line.

The night before, the man had watched a television program that revealed the 'secret' of world-class distance runner, Alberto Salazar, to improve the endurance of his legs - 200 repetitions with light weights. As I talked him from the scene of the crime, a phrase from the Nautilus inventor came to mind, "If you want to find out how to train a race horse, don't ask the race horse."

Muscle strength and muscle endurance are the same thing - training one will increase the other to the same degree.

Proof? Find how much you can bench press one time, a common (although dangerous) measure of strength. Let's assume you lift 100 pounds. Another day under 'fresh' conditions, lift the weight once, rest three minutes and perform as many repetitions as you can with 75% of the weight, a common measure of muscle endurance. Let's assume you complete 10 repetitions. Now, train for several months and re-test your strength. As before, perform the one-repetition lift, rest three minutes and attempt as many repetitions as possible with 75% of the new weight. You will perform exactly 10 repetitions, not 9 or 11, but 10 - proof that your muscle endurance and muscle strength increased at the same rate, and to the same degree. In a similar way, if you cease training and test again, both (strength and endurance) will decline equally.

If you know what you can lift once, you can determine what you can lift 10 times. Conversely, if you know how much you can lift 10 times, you can determine your maximum lift, as long as you have established the strength/ endurance ratio for that muscle. The ratio is determined by the fatigue characteristics of the muscle (its fiber-type), varies from one muscle to another and cannot alter through training.

The strength/endurance ratio is also determined by the efficiency of the nervous system, another genetic factor. If all of the fibers in a muscle are allowed to contract at once, such as when lightening strikes a person or when someone lifts a car to free a loved-one, bones break. To be safe, the nervous system allows a muscle to use only a small percentage (approximately 30%) of its capacity during a maximum effort. The remainder (70%) is held in reserve.

When a muscle gains strength, the performance of a known task becomes easier. Lifting the once-maximum 100 pounds with a stronger muscle, for example, demands a smaller percentage of the muscle's capacity. Instead of 30%, the muscle may require only 20% to lift 100 pounds, which means that it retains a greater percentage of its fibers (80%) in reserve for future efforts. More strength is logically more endurance.

This leads to two important applications:

- A one-repetition-maximum strength test is no longer necessary. Comparing one set of 8-12 repetitions with another over time will suffice, and save limbs.
- The benefits of muscle endurance can be realized by training for strength. The use of heavier weights, greater intensity and fewer repetitions will save time.

If my memory serves me well, and unless he quit the gym that day, the man increased the endurance of his legs by making them stronger. Without such a rude awakening and with all due respect, he and Alberto might still be there...

JANUARY 26

## Training for Definition

Many people waste time (and that of others) in what has become a health-club issue. Last week, I smoldered as I stood in front of a leg extension machine watching a lady 'define' her quadriceps by performing too many repetitions for my patience.

Definition, as it pertains to exercise, is a function of body fat. An excess of body fat rejects any attempt a muscle makes to surface; a low level displays bumps and ripples you never knew you had. Although genetically determined, body fat can be decreased by creating a negative calorie balance - ingesting fewer calories by eating less *or* expending more calories through exercise.

With intake, things are simple. Research shows that a calorie range of 1,400-1,500 for men and 1,200-1,400 for women (who weigh over 120 pounds) provides both adequate nutrition and a stimulus for change.

With output, things are not as simple. All forms of exercise burn calories before (in anticipation of), during and after, but some are more effective than others in reducing body fat. Aerobic activity, for example, results in 'indiscriminate' weight loss from fat, organ and muscle tissues. On the other hand, resistance exercise modifies the body's muscle-fat ratio by increasing muscle mass. For every pound of muscle it adds, the body burns 50-100 calories per day to maintain the new addition, a phenomenon known as the 'double-reducing effect.'

In a recent study at the University of Florida, one group of subjects cycled three times a week for 20 minutes while another performed resistance exercise with the same frequency and duration. Both groups ingested the same number of calories and had their exercise supervised and pushed. After six weeks, the cycling group lost an average of 3.2 pounds of body fat while the strength-training group lost an average of 10 pounds of fat. Three times the result is good reason to avoid the wait for a treadmill.

Yet, even among advocates of resistance exercise, many insist on a training method for definition. Their assumption is simple - 50 repetitions burn more calories than 10 - but hold on. Ten repetitions of a leg exercise carried to a point of muscle failure consume approximately 10-15 calories. Fifty repetitions at a lower intensity may burn more calories (2-3 per set) - or less, if the intensity is very low. Assuming it burns more, a 20-set workout would result in an added expenditure of 40-60 calories per session. At three times a week (and all other factors equal), it would take 5-6 months to burn the 3,500 calories needed to lose an extra pound of fat.

If you 'train for definition,' I send my condolences.

With heavier resistance, fewer repetitions (8-15) and higher levels of intensity, an average female can add three pounds of muscle to her body in six weeks; a male, 3-4 pounds in a month. Three pounds of muscle creates a surplus expenditure of up to 300 calories per day, the equivalent of a vigorous half-hour bike ride. Common sense suggests that it's easier to add muscle to your body and let it take care of fat stores than ride the bike every day.

Low-intensity, high-repetition exercise has little effect on changing muscle-mass-to-body-weight ratios. In excess, it can lead to a loss of lean tissue, as in the case of distance athletes. Brief, high-intensity strength training burns fat at a more efficient and effective rate.

It also leaves fewer trails of smoldering impatience.

## JANUARY 27

### Results With and Without Thinking

Not long ago, while putting on the practice green at the West Palm Beach Country Club in Florida, I came across a six-foot chalk line leading to one of the holes. The line had been set by a teaching professional or serious player to assist with alignment during short putts. Whenever I spot one, I take advantage of it - and this day would be no exception.

I placed the first ball on the line and sunk it. The second - in the middle of the hole; the third - the same; the fourth, fifth and sixth. By the 10th ball, I was soaring with confidence. The green was like a funnel. When I putted slightly to the left, the ball went in; pushed it a bit right, it curved back. Every putt ended in the bottom of the cup. Thirty-five, thirty-six; all I had to do was hit it far enough.

Suddenly, the 37th halted on the front lip of the cup.

With renewed focus, I sunk the next 51 in a row, missed the 89th, short again by half a turn, and finished at an even 100 attempts - 98 successful, two short. By repeating the same movement, I was led to believe that I couldn't miss. The line was fixed, regardless of execution. As long as I struck the ball with enough pace, enough effort, enough distance, the result was the same.

The laws of physics are such - a given set of circumstances invariably produces a given result. If the expected result is not forthcoming, then the only logical conclusion is that the circumstances were not those that were required.

Nautilus® inventor Arthur Jones experienced the same in a 15-year effort to increase his physical size and strength. In *The Nautilus Bodybuilding Book* (1982), he claimed that "a certain type and amount of exercise produced a particular result up to a point. Beyond that point, the same type and amount of exercise produced no apparent result at all."

The circumstances had changed, though it was not apparent at first.

Fortunately, Arthur was an insatiable thinker and eventually realized that what had changed was his system. It produced growth as long as it worked within the limits imposed by its recovery ability; but failed when the demands exceeded that ability, regardless of the stimulation provided. It became obvious that an increase in strength resulting from exercise was *not* paralleled by an increase in the system's ability to recover from exercise.

The potential for strength increase, he theorized, was approximately 300% (later modified to 100%), while the potential to increase the ability to recover from exercise was only 50%. As strength increased, the body worked closer to its limits and eventually reached a point where each workout consumed the system's recovery energy, leaving nothing for growth. If depleted recovery ability made growth impossible and recovery ability could not be increased (at that point), the only way to make progress was to limit the demand on the system.

Jones reduced his training regimen to two sets of exercise from four and gained 10 pounds of muscle in a week, passing a 15-year barrier of 172 pounds. He later discovered the same with bodybuilders and football players - that a reduction in the amount of exercise (from 12 to 10 exercises, from 10 to 8, from three days a week to two) allowed growth beyond plateaus.

Ultimate success in golf (and skill development) requires a non-thinking, automatic response. Success in strength training requires more thought than most display.

## JANUARY 28

### Close Your Eyes

"Copy the guy with the biggest arms" is generally poor and dangerous advice in any gym. But it wasn't when I witnessed the workout of Mike Chastain.

Mike puffed like a steam engine as he neared the sixth repetition of the first exercise. The weight was heavy. "Two more," I hollered. He barely made the next, then tried three partial reps, veins leaping from his neck. When movement was no longer possible, I helped him through another four. He grunted, "One more." Most trainees would have hit the floor, the water bottle or the shower, but not Chastain. He moved quickly to the next machine.

Throughout the workout, he mocked fatigue and my judgement of it. When I thought he had two left, he did eight; when I urged three, he tried seven. It was no ordinary performance. Yet, in a lifetime of overcoming obstacles, he treated this just as he had the others - with an all-out effort.

Mike lost sight in his right eye during a hunting accident at the age of five, and slowly developed glaucoma in the left. He was totally blind by 16, yet established himself as a top athlete in track and field, wrestling and football at Troy High School in Michigan. In his own words, "I wanted to be the toughest, strongest, quickest guy out there." According to his coaches, he was.

In addition to lettering in football his senior year (1971), Mike earned a special recognition award from the National Football League Players' Association at their annual dinner. That summer, he captured a gold medal at the World Junior Olympic Championships in Italy, wrestling in the 165-pound class.

Following a successful academic and wrestling career at Central Michigan University, Mike earned a spot as alternate on the Greco-Roman team at the United States Olympic trials in 1976. Four years later, he was a stronger candidate for the team, but the US boycotted the games. Chastain moved on.

With an exercise science degree in hand, he began working in the fitness industry until fate struck again. While demonstrating a piece of exercise equipment in 1986, he injured his back, which, together with a doctor's treatment, left him paralyzed from the chest down. Six weeks and a high-risk operation later, he regained only "slight feeling" in his legs and was told that his odds of ever walking again were 15%. That's all Chastain needed to hear. He eventually walked away without a scar.

I worked with Mike for three years, during which time he taught me far more than I could have taught him. We discussed ideas at length and found common ground on, among other things, the major ingredients for optimum results from strength training - good form and high intensity. Mike had both, and it showed.

Our friendship brought new meaning to an overworked gym phrase. In an effort to decrease speed of movement during exercise, I often reiterated, "Close your eyes and feel the weight being lifted through *every* part of the movement. Don't miss an inch." The advice instantly improves form, results and safety.

Mike had an advantage all along - built-in good form and a great work ethic. His aggressive spirit prompted a comment from Chicago Sun-Times' Jack Griffin before the NFL Award ceremony, "If the whole joint doesn't stand up and applaud this young man, then there is really something wrong with this world."

Close your eyes during strength training. There's a lesson to be learned.

## JANUARY 29

### Super-Seat or Super-Set?

The glaring, yawning, casual, music-filled wait for the next burst of activity seen in today's health clubs more resembles the stag line at a middle-school dance than a workout, with one exception - everyone's seated. No wonder my response to the question, "How much time should I spend between sets?" is a quick, "None."

I was schooled by a man who took 27 years to discover that two sets of exercise was better than four, and another 10 years to discover that one was better than two. Not only did a single set of 8-12 repetitions taken to a point of momentary muscle failure suffice for Nautilus® inventor Arthur Jones, it was effective with the majority of bodybuilders and athletes he trained. "If a man is capable of doing a second set," he'd growl, "he didn't do it right the first time." Arthur didn't have many friends (or trainees on their feet for that matter) when he concluded, "I didn't say it was easy. I just said it worked."

I learned early that good form and high levels of intensity were the major ingredients for optimum results from exercise. I also learned, as I gazed skyward on many gym floors, that, besides working harder on every movement, intensity could be increased by eliminating time between exercises.

One Saturday morning as I buckled into a leg-extension machine, I noticed a young man doing the same across the room in what appeared to be the start of his day. When I finished my whole-body workout and 25 minutes of cycling, he was still seated on the same machine...and might be there yet.

Work, rest, repeat, rest, repeat, rest and repeat may be a great workout for some, but it's a sad day for physiology. Results are better produced by performing 'super-sets' - *immediate* exercise involving complementary muscle groups - as follows:

- A single-joint exercise (rotation about the elbow, for example) followed by a compound movement (that involves both elbow and shoulder).
- A compound movement followed by a single-joint exercise.
- A single-joint exercise performed between two compound movements.

The first generation of Nautilus machines (Compound Leg, Double Shoulder, Double Chest, Pullover / Torso-Arm, Behind Neck / Torso Arm) offered two exercises from one seat to take advantage of the above, then called "pre-exhaustion." Because a fatigued muscle can recover more than 50% of its strength in less than three seconds, a trainee could work an exhausted muscle to greater fatigue with the immediate help of another group. Unfortunately, manufacturers no longer make dual-exercise tools, forcing trainees to prepare two machines for the same effect.

For best results from a two-exercise combination, reduce the weight on the second exercise by 20-40% and spend no time between movements. On sequences such as pullover / pull-down (upper back), chest fly / press (chest), lateral raise / overhead press (shoulders), biceps curl / chin-ups (biceps), and triceps extension / dips (triceps), perform the single-joint movement first. Reverse the order occasionally to vary the effect.

Three-exercise combinations - leg press / leg extension / squat (lower body), bench press / fly / dips (chest), pull-down / pullover / negative chin-ups (back), and upright row / lateral raise / overhead press (shoulders) - should be reserved for advanced trainees.

The key is intensity, and speed *between* exercises. If you stall to mourn the first, or save energy for the second, you might as well as Jones said, "Stay in the parking lot."

Try super-sets in your workout - or sit and hope for the best.

## JANUARY 30

---

### When Nothing's Better Than Something

When Arthur Jones requested a volunteer at one of his lectures, it was best to hide. The Nautilus® inventor demanded an all-out effort if the task was physical and an honest opinion if it was mental. Both left eager victims wobbling home.

Jones once called up a young man midway through a morning presentation. They had met briefly before the event and Jones pegged him as an 'ideal' candidate. Doug Weary, a bodybuilder and power-lifter from Florida, was familiar with Nautilus high-intensity training concepts.

"So, you're a weightlifter *and* a trainer," asked Arthur.

"Yes, Sir."

"If I gave you 20 untrained high-school students at random to prepare for a weight-lifting competition in eight weeks, how would you go about it?"

"Well, I'd start by..."

Doug went into a brief dissertation based on his experience, most of which reflected current trends in the sport.

"Fine," said Arthur. "Now, if I were to take 20 high-school students at random (for the same purpose) and had them do nothing, absolutely nothing, I bet my group would test stronger than yours at the end of eight weeks."

"You mean your group would do no weight training at all?" asked Doug.

"I said nothing, lie on the couch, and they'd be stronger than yours."

"I'd bet against that."

Arthur loved to provoke thought. His logic was simple. The proposed regimen would create such a high incidence of injury that, when final tests occurred, half the group would not be able to participate at all. Because of less-severe injury, another 25% would test lower than their original evaluation; and the remainder would be stronger. The trained group - as a whole - would be weaker than the untrained group.

Some of the current practices in the sport of weightlifting are dangerous and of no use. Many athletes are exposed to the basic techniques of power-lifting in an effort to increase strength and speed of movement in their sport. According to Jones, "Teaching a football player the clean and jerk is about as effective as teaching swimmers how to block and tackle." Danger without purpose is what he called 'stupidity.'

In 1972, Jones worked closely with Bill Bradford, coach of Deland High School's inaugural weight-lifting team (Deland, Florida). The approach was unique - build raw strength by performing slow, negative-only (lowering) exercise and then apply that strength to the practice of the lifting techniques.

Without a prior history of competition in the sport, Bradford established a record that is unprecedented in any sport. His team went untied and undefeated in more than 100 competitions over a seven-year span. Despite the success, the system went ignored: It was developed by an eccentric, and coaches were reluctant to buck tradition.

'Stupidity' reached new heights in a recent publication of a national organization that promotes weightlifting. The feature article was 'Power-Lifting for Children;' the cover, a child performing an Olympic lift. The organization should be shot on the spot, but they're too busy certifying personal trainers around the country.

Let's hope you don't get one.

## JANUARY 31

### Conditioning for Golf and Tiger Woods

Thirty years ago, I contended that professional golf would embrace strength training only when a Mr. Universe won the United States Open title. As dumb as it sounds, that's how popular lifting weights was at the time. With few exceptions, players went out of their way to avoid such 'nonsense.'

Therefore, when I read in a recent issue of a leading golf publication that today's professionals are engaged in serious exercise, I did so with a degree of skepticism. It took little time for the fear of strength training to emerge. The majority of players emphasized cardiovascular activity and stretching over strength training. They also talked about getting strong enough for golf without becoming too strong. Touring pro, Justin Leonard summed it up when he said, "We don't want to look like linebackers."

How strong do you need to be for golf?

The first piece of that puzzle smacked me in the face when I was 16. The fellow with whom I was paired in a junior tournament in Toronto ignored the fact that I had lifted weights for several years and consistently out-drove me by 60 yards - with arms the size of my wrists. The experience was a humbling example of the minor role strength plays in the sport of golf.

The importance of that role magnifies, however, when the facts are examined:

- Of all the components of fitness, muscle strength (the strength of muscle contraction) is the only factor that produces human movement. All other factors (cardiovascular, flexibility, balance, etc.) assist in the movement process.
- Increased muscle strength goes a long way in the direction of preventing injury.
- An athlete can never reach his potential without becoming as strong as possible.

Can you become 'too strong' for golf?

Nautilus® inventor Arthur Jones thinks not. "It has been clearly demonstrated hundreds of times, with no exception I would believe unless I saw it myself, that proper strength training will markedly improve the performance of any athlete in any sport. And the great athletes have the most to gain from strength training...and are the most unlikely to use it; having been falsely convinced that it will hurt them."

Tiger Woods and David Duval are out to prove Jones both right and wrong. The #1- and #2-ranked players in the world respectively take an aggressive approach to strength training. Duval performs plenty of hard upper-body exercise (a fear of most), while Woods has been bench pressing 300 pounds, a heavy weight for a man his size, since college. Both have discovered, like most, that they do not have the genetic potential to build muscles large enough to get in the way of a golf swing.

Now it's up to the rest of the field to wake up. A serious approach is long overdue.

For the past year, I have been involved in the design of exercise programs for PGA®, LPGA®, European, Buy.com and Golden Bear® Tour professionals. Without exception, the players have worked hard to improve their condition. I hope they don't wrongly perceive strength training, the new kid on the block, as the source of their problems in a moment of crisis. I've seen it before.

As for Tiger Woods, his contribution to golf may be far more than a major dent in the record-books. His focus on the conditioning required to maximize potential in a high-skill sport may make him the Mr. Universe the golf world has been waiting for.

# FEBRUARY

"No amount of exercise will produce worthwhile results if the 'intensity of effort' is too low; and if the 'amount' of exercise is too great then no exercise will produce any worthwhile result regardless of the other factors."

Arthur Jones

# FEBRUARY 1

## Homeostasis

I threw my body a curve during its third year of college by increasing its intake of protein. According to my physiology professor and the latest body-building magazines, protein was the way to gain muscle weight. So, at every meal I consumed four glasses of milk, drank a powdered version between, ate all the meat I could and cut my strength training to five sets of three basic exercises. In 10 weeks, I gained 17 pounds - but my body didn't appreciate the overload.

I could hear myself jog.

The body does one of two things with excess: stores it, or eliminates it. In the case of protein, the body eliminates it - which made the process attractive in the first place. The excess protein, however, provided excess calories and the body stores calories as fat. I was larger and stronger, but my body-fat had increased.

When exposed to too much or too little, the body goes to great lengths to reestablish the status quo, a state called 'homeostasis.' It continually strives for what it perceives as normal in regard to temperature control, body weight, blood flow, heart rate and chemical balance, and then establishes a reserve for emergency purposes. In the process, it is capable of anticipating needs with great accuracy.

To the chagrin of those who claim to train 'by instinct,' and to the delight of those who choose to do nothing, the body, if given a choice, would not select exercise. Exercise represents change. When any physical task is initiated, the body quickly recognizes the intrusion, strives to maintain a definite but unknown percentile of reserve and attempts to terminate the effort long before a point of exhaustion is reached. When the effort approaches the limits of the body's established reserves, the system rebels and tries to prevent further loss.

No wonder most of us quit well in advance of momentary muscle failure.

Arthur Jones, an advocate of high-intensity strength training, once stated, "There is an obvious limit beyond which you should not go, but this limit applies only to the actual 'amount' of exercise - not to the intensity of effort. Maximum intensity of effort is an absolute requirement for the greatest possible degree of growth stimulation - but it must be achieved without totally exhausting the body's recovery ability." He recognized that a body perpetually drained of its reserves due to excess training responds in a negative way.

In his quest to determine the amount of stimulation required to produce best results, Jones launched a high-intensity training philosophy that stirred controversy. Most found it "too brief, too hard." Others thought it was "dangerous."

Brief and hard it was, but dangerous it wasn't.

Jones recognized that, during an all-out effort (a maximum attempt to lift a heavy weight), the body controls the extent of its use. During such an event, the system allows the involved muscle to use only 30% of its available fibers (70% remain in reserve). Individuals with a superior nervous system can activate as much as 50% of this capacity; others only 10%.

The body abandons its status quo only when it senses an extraordinary threat such as the rescue of a loved-one pinned beneath a car. Yet, when the muscle is allowed to use 100% of its fibers in such cases, the result is always the same - bones break.

'Hard' training is 'safe' training. Your body wouldn't have it any other way.


## FEBRUARY 2

---

### The Early Thought Process

When Nautilus® inventor Arthur Jones showed up at Veterans Memorial Auditorium, Culver City, California for the Sr. National Weightlifting Championships on July 13, 1970, it was his first public step into the arena. Yet, his new creation - an exercise tool that looked like a spaceship and promised the moon - had been in the works for 30 years.

"Carefully controlled research with these machines," said *Ironman* editor Peary Rader, "indicates that you can develop maximum muscular size and power with about 10% of the usual time expended." The figure came from Jones, who left nothing to chance.

The same results in half the previously elapsed time meant a 100% (2X) increase in production; the same results in half as many workouts, another 100% (4X). Half the time per workout, another 100% (8X); and instead of the same results, a 25% increase in mass and strength. Ten times the results of conventional training.

"Impossible?" asked Jones. "No, expected."

His research led to the identification of "things that seem to be required for producing good results." Exercise, he claimed, should be brief, infrequent, fast, full-range, carried to failure against continuous and variable resistance, direct, balanced to a muscle's strength in all positions and performed in proper order in sets of 6-20 repetitions. When things were added, results failed to improve; when things were removed, results were less.

To activate the greatest quantity of muscle mass during exercise, Jones realized that a muscle had to be in a fully contracted position and pulling against a resistance heavy enough to signal activation. "But not too heavy," he warned, "because if it is too heavy then it will be impossible to move such a load into the required position."

With conventional exercise, there was no resistance in contracted positions, which meant only a small percentage of the muscle was 'worked.' Jones compared new to old by measuring the amount of oxygen demanded by the body and the amount of heat produced during exercise. He also looked at the production of horsepower (resistance, distance of vertical movement, and speed) and results (strength and mass increases, the latter by specific gravity tests). "It appears that conventional forms of exercise," he concluded, "involve only between 14 and 18 percent of the total number of individual muscle fibers even when the muscle is worked to the point of momentary failure."

At the same time, he recognized the need for rotary resistance: "While the muscles may work in a relatively straight-line fashion, the body parts (that they move) rotate." It wasn't enough - muscles were stronger near contraction and weaker near extension. They required a resistance that varied at the same rate that strength increased.

To determine that rate, Jones calculated strength curves for muscles free from the bias of exercise, using subjects in hospitals and old-folks homes. "A lack of any exercise will eventually result in a very low level of strength, but a perfectly balanced strength curve." He checked his results against a study of the muscle's cross-sectional area in different positions to determine the rate of strength increase, then added the contribution of other muscles (in compound movements) with regard to magnitude, extent and timing.

After all that, he still missed the mark. "I built a machine well over ten years ago," he said, "that had every single one of the required characteristics, and no faults; but, at the time, I not only failed to recognize the machine for what it really was, I then didn't even bother to test its result producing ability."

It wasn't the first or last of his mistakes.

## FEBRUARY 3

---

## The 'Split' Routine

If everyone wore white, I wore black. If they turned left, I went right. I thrived on being different in youth. Therefore, it comes as no surprise to find my 'whole-body' workouts engulfed by a trend to exercise only one or two body parts per session - with one difference. This time, the contrast is not intentional.

My introduction to 'whole-body' training began at 14 when I followed "The Weider® System of Progressive Barbell Exercise" in my basement. It continued with belief in Nautilus® inventor, Arthur Jones, who viewed the physiological response to exercise as 'systemic.' The approach had become so ingrained that my reaction to a recent locker-room conversation was perplexing.

"Hey, Big John, what are you working today?"

"Chest."

John had neither time nor patience for small talk. And he was 'BIG.'

I thought long and hard. It was time for change.

Off I went to inquire among peers, trainers and 'BIG' trainees, and to read what I could. It led to confusion. In the end, the habits of youth prevailed: I developed my own plan based upon 42 years of experience.

How to divide the body was the first issue. Knowing that strengthening one limb had a positive effect on the other, I considered dividing it in half - right side one day, left side the next. Since a muscle-related split seemed more popular, however, I opted to separate my body into 365 parts, the number of training days. With over 600 skeletal muscles to choose from, the selection would include only major ones.

I then turned to Jones for other concerns. "A muscle grows when it is stimulated," he said. *Everyday training would provide plenty of that.* He also preached the need for adequate recovery time: "Muscle growth is a result of both rest and work." *To handle the 364 days of recovery between workouts, I would rely on the 'indirect effect of exercise,' whereby the stimulation of one muscle carries over to its closest neighbors. Strength maintenance between workouts would take care of itself by the sheer quantity of neighbors. To further assure success, I decided to reduce the time between sessions by rotating the workout sequence around the body's seven major quadrants: lower limbs (2), upper limbs (2), torso (both sides), and head/neck. Each quadrant would be stimulated once a week.*

"If the elements that compose recovery ability are to be available in the system," added Jones, "the body must be sufficiently rested." *To be 'ready' for the next workout, I would dedicate each night of sleep to a body section - Monday, left lower-limb; Tuesday, right upper-torso, etc. The part that slept would be trained the next day.*

Because of the importance of nutrition in strength training, I resolved to eat in parts: a high-carbohydrate breakfast for the muscle in recovery; a high-protein lunch for the one to be trained; and a fish dinner to ensure logical thinking.

To see the plan on paper is pure joy. Will it work? Time will tell. If it doesn't, I'll train everything together, rest a day or two between, eat normally and go on with life. If it does, I'll invite your shoulders to a 'power' lunch, provided my calves have had enough sleep.

And, if I can split my tongue from my cheek long enough, I'll unveil tentative plans for that troublesome leap year...

## FEBRUARY 4

---

### Lock Those Knees

Arthur Jones often distinguished fact from fiction by prefacing a response with a vocal punch. "FACT..." or "OPINION...", he'd blurt, then proceed. If it fell somewhere between, he'd call it as a "Swag," a Scientific Wild-Ass Guess or admit he didn't know the answer, then add, "Nor does anyone else."

But Arthur was certain about body mechanics and the laws of physics, and spent 22 years (and $120 million) building a tool to isolate, test and exercise the muscles of the front thigh. In the end, he had something to say about knees.

FACT: The majority of trainers instruct clients not to lock their knees during leg extensions for safety reasons. The 'danger' has wrongly become 'common knowledge.'

OPINION: Does anybody think or read?

FACT: In 1987, Jones laid out the functional dynamics of the knee (*Risks & Benefits Management*, Oct.) using what he called "third-grade math and ninth-grade physics" and concluded that the last 20-30° of extension is the least dangerous position.

The knee is mechanically inefficient. If the quadriceps muscle (front thigh) produces a force of 1,200 pounds to lift a weight (Figure 1), only 1,000 is exerted over the top of the patella (kneecap) - the remainder is lost through internal muscle friction. The 1,000 pounds is redirected around the axis of the knee (**A**) by the patella and transmitted by its ligament to the lower leg a short distance below the axis.

The effective point of attachment, however, is located a greater distance below the axis of the knee where the extended line of pull of the patellar ligament intersects the midline of the bone (**B**). There, the pull (1,000 pounds) is in the wrong direction, which means "that at least eighty percent of the force is being wasted." Furthermore, the output (now 200 pounds) is measured twice as far (as the effective point of attachment) below the knee's rotational axis, at (**C**), which cuts production in half again, to 100 pounds.

More bad news - above the patella, the quadriceps muscle does not pull in the right direction and wastes an estimated 20% of its force (not illustrated).

Therefore, an initial input of 1,200 pounds produces a functional output of 80 pounds twelve inches below the axis of the knee, which is only the prologue of a sadder tale. The enormous forces produced by the muscles of the front thigh that result in such a dismal strength output also expose the knee and upper-thigh bone (femur) to higher levels of force, depending on the position of the lower leg.

At the start of a leg extension (legs bent 120°), for example, the knee is exposed to a compression force that is 73% higher than the pulling force of the quadriceps. When legs are bent at 90°, the force is 40% higher. According to Jones, "If the legs are straightened to a point where they are only 66° short of full extension (about halfway up), the magnification of compression forces is reduced to only 9%. When fully extended, straight, the magnification of force is zero."

FACT: A man lifting 600 pounds in a leg-extension exercise (and some can) produces 7,000 pounds of pulling force with his quadriceps muscle. In the starting position, he exposes his knees to compression forces in excess of 12,110 pounds; in the contracted position, to only 7,000 pounds - **DANGER AT THE BOTTOM, LESS AT THE TOP**.

OPINION: Trainers memorize facts (for the most part) to get 'certified' but rely on opinions to get by.

FACT: Now you know the knee. Next time, get it right.

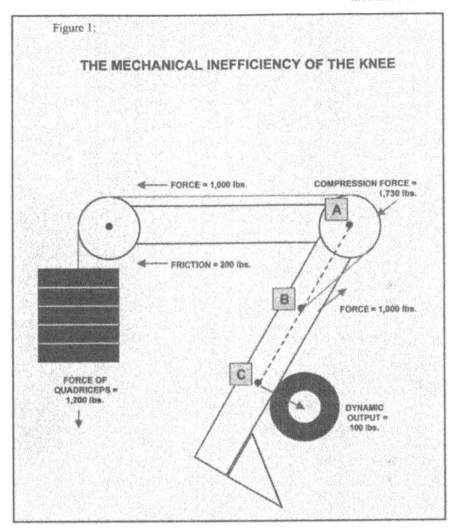

Figure 1:

THE MECHANICAL INEFFICIENCY OF THE KNEE

FORCE = 1,000 lbs.

COMPRESSION FORCE = 1,730 lbs.

A

FRICTION = 200 lbs.

B

FORCE = 1,000 lbs.

C

FORCE OF QUADRICEPS = 1,200 lbs.

DYNAMIC OUTPUT = 100 lbs.

## FEBRUARY 5

### Direct or Indirect?

Following a five-year plan, Canada declared itself 'bilingual' in 1968, forcing students like me to study seven years of French (and Latin, by choice) with nothing to show but the odd *voulez vous* and *Quis gracilus puer*. We had little conversation.

In contrast, when I went to Venezuela in 1976, without knowing a word of Spanish, I listened to street talk, watched TV and eventually recognized topics, if not content. At the same time, I headed the P. E. Department at an American high school, where only a few on the staff spoke English. I was forced to speak Spanish and became 90% fluent in 18 months - without opening a book.

Direct immersion is more effective than indirect immersion.

Arthur Jones found the same with exercise. Instead of funneling resistance through the weaker muscles of the arms, the Nautilus® inventor sought a direct route to his torso and proudly introduced his breakthrough in *Ironman* (July, 1970) - a pullover machine.

"Some new 'gimmick?' An unproven theory?" he asked. "Think what you like, but we built one test subject's lats (upper back) to a point that would normally have required at least two full years of training, in less than six weeks, on a program of three weekly workouts of exactly forty-eight minutes each...No drugs, no special diet, no marathon workouts; just a simple routine of three sets of four very basic exercises: full squats, standing presses, barbell curls, and movements on our new lat machine. No chinning movements of any kind, no rowing motions, no 'pulldowns,' absolutely nothing for the lats except our new lat machine, and only nine weekly sets on that." The subject in question gained 15 pounds of muscle and increased his arm size by two inches.

Jones spoke of 'direct' in two ways. First, the resistance had to directly oppose the direction of movement of the involved body part. If the body part moved straight up, the resistance had to move straight down. Second, direct resistance meant not being limited by the failure of weaker muscles (as with pulldowns, chin-ups or rows). Jones forced elbows against pads to lift resistance, and the results were clear.

'Direct' meant faster gains. "According to most published scientific opinion," said Jones, "maximum possible sustained gains are supposed to be limited to about 2% per week, but we have been producing sustained strength increase rates of over 30% per week, week after week after week."

'Direct' also meant less exercise and fewer workouts, but it was harder. "Most people don't make it much if any beyond two sets at first, at which point they are stretched out on the floor in a dead faint, green in the face, violently sick, unable to move."

Having the equipment was not enough. "You cannot win a horse race on a camel," said Jones, "and you cannot produce the same results that we are producing with the Nautilus equipment without using that equipment, but you can markedly improve the results you are getting from conventional training by using the same principles, where, and as, possible. Nor will you produce spectacular results even with the new equipment if you fail to use it properly." Proper use was the key, but it was slow to catch on.

In a foreword of *The Nautilus Bodybuilding Book*, 1982, Mike Mentzer (Mr. Universe and a disciple of Jones) wrote, "They (bodybuilders) don't understand or can't accept what a productive tool they have to work with. In essence, they're hitching a team of horses to an automobile and letting the animals pull the car."

Back to the books.

## FEBRUARY 6

---

### The Early Days

Dennis sat in the crude looking chair on the porch. He pressed the back of his arms to a set of pads located just above his elbows and stared at a stack of weights supported by an orange crate directly in front. His brother Walt checked the setup a final time.

"Ready?"

"Yep."

Walt kicked the crate away. The weights lowered slowly as Dennis resisted the pressure of the pads. His elbows arched forward and upward until they reached a position above his head. There he stretched for a second and reversed direction. The stack started to rise and quickly picked up an additional weight off the floor. Then another, and another. Each weight was attached by a chain of a different length, a length that was precisely measured.

By the time his arms reached their starting position again, Dennis could feel the work. He paused, squeezed his elbows against the pads and slowly returned. The guillotine-like pullover machine had taken its toll by the tenth repetition. Walt grabbed the orange crate and shoved it under the weight stack just in time.

Now it was his turn.

Dennis and Walt Anderson, at 216 and 225 pounds respectively, were college football players seeking size and strength. Although unrelated to Paul Anderson, the world's strongest man at the time, the two could hold their own. Walt set a high school 12-pound shot put record of 57'4¾" that stood for 30 years, and Dennis wasn't far behind.

Their lives changed when a friend of theirs brought soon-to-be Nautilus® inventor Arthur Jones to their home in 1968 to trade for a pair of 12½-pound barbell plates. From the start, the Andersons were intimidated by Jones' intellect and eccentric nature.

They didn't know what to make of him.

Two years later (1970) they encouraged a neighbor to train with Jones "to test the waters." When the man returned in phenomenal condition after only a month, it didn't take long for the brothers to show up on Jones' front porch in Deland, Florida.

Arthur was clear from the beginning. "I expect you to do exactly what I tell you. When you do biceps curls or any exercise, continue until the barbell falls out of your hands. Do you understand?"

They had no choice.

In 28 days, they performed 14 whole-body sessions using Jones' one-set-to-failure principle - squats in the living room, pullovers on the porch and food in the kitchen.

The first day, Dennis performed a set of squats with 250 pounds. Minutes before the final workout, Walt took his brother into the backyard to distract him while Arthur changed some 25-pound plates to 50's. Dennis performed the same exercise with 407 pounds, a weight increase of 62.8%. He returned home weighing 245 pounds; Walt, 250. They became believers in what most trainees avoid at all cost - outright hard work.

In 1971, I had the pleasure of performing a few repetitions on Jones' first commercial version of the pullover machine at McMaster University in Hamilton, Ontario. The octopus-like weight configuration had been transformed into a sleek-looking 'cam' that left nothing 'easy' about its feel. Little did I know that the machine would change the history of exercise and, more importantly, the direction of my life.

In retrospect, there was only one disappointment - it didn't come with an orange crate.

## FEBRUARY 7

---

### Chin-Ups and Dips

Chin-ups and dips work the major muscles of the torso and provide a brief, complete workout when combined with a compound leg movement (squat or leg press). Neither, however, furnishes a practical way to advance. Once you can perform 10 repetitions, there are only two paths to progress: increase the amount of exercise by attempting more repetitions or sets; or make the exercise harder by increasing the resistance with weight-belts. Most trainees opt for the first.

In 1983, a young man wearing heavy boots and a lumberjack coat (in a climate that warranted nothing but shorts) entered my gym in Caracas, Venezuela. Despite his bulky appearance, the man was quick - quick to point out that his physique was due to the performance of 300 chin-ups and dips every Sunday in a nearby park - and quick to rattle off 10 dips before a formal greeting. Bad manners and bad form, in any order, invited a dogfight.

"Let's try one chin-up, just one," I suggested.

He laughed, thinking the 'gringo' had made a numerical blunder.

"Take off your jacket and stay awhile," I urged with strained courtesy.

He left it on.

I didn't know the Spanish word for 'funeral,' so I pulled out a stopwatch.

"Sixty seconds up. Don't touch the floor. Sixty seconds down. One rep. Any questions? Adelante, caballero! Good luck."

Good thing he kept his jacket on - he didn't stay long. Forty seconds into the 'up', the mighty oak fell to the floor grasping his biceps. It was no contest.

Performed in a slow, controlled manner (as they should be), chin-ups and dips are difficult. In fact, few people ever experience the potential benefits of these exercises because they lack the arm strength to support their bodyweight.

Equipment manufacturers have long recognized this problem and offered a variety of solutions. The first device of note was called a *Gravitron*®, a computerized monster that combined your recorded bodyweight with a chosen level of difficulty to lift a hydraulic platform upon which you stood. Progress was made by reducing the amount of the 'assist' (a numerical selection) so that muscles would work harder.

Today, counter-balanced weight stacks have replaced hydraulics. If you select 100 pounds, the machine lifts 100 pounds. Your arms lift the difference.

Nautilus® inventor Arthur Jones took a different approach. He made a chin-up/dip station with steps in front to perform what he called "negative work." His premise:

If you couldn't lift your bodyweight, you could probably lower it since muscles are 40% stronger lowering than lifting.

If you couldn't lift your bodyweight with your arms, you could probably do so with your legs (that is, walk up steps to position your chin over the bar to start).

If chin-ups and dips are difficult, begin with a device that 'assists.' When you can perform 10 slow repetitions with a resistance close to your bodyweight (little help from the machine), advance to negative work if the proper equipment is available.

Regardless of ability, try the following combinations to increase your torso strength: chin-ups before or after a pullover machine, or immediately before biceps curls; and dips before or after a chest-fly movement, or immediately before a triceps extension.

You don't need to be a lumberjack to benefit...but you'd better remove your coat.

## FEBRUARY 8

### Physiological Nonsense

The well-conditioned man reached for the nearest bench and, unlike most, made it. There, head between knees, he huffed and puffed as if he had just ran his best 100 meters. Not quite - he had just finished his worst nightmare.

Ten repetitions of negative chin-ups, performed to failure, leaves trainees gasping for air and, in many cases, throwing in the towel. Yet, the instructions (when performed on a Nautilus® Multi-Exercise machine) are simple:

Set the bar at a height that places your chin over the bar when standing on the top step. Grasp the bar with a palms-up grip, place your chin over the bar and take your feet off the step. Slowly lower your body in 10 seconds. When you reach a stretched position, quickly place your feet on the steps, walk to the top (in less than three seconds) and repeat the process until you can no longer lower in control.

At first glance, performing chin-ups by lifting with legs and lowering with arms appears easier than lifting and lowering with arms only. And rightly so:

- Muscles are 40% stronger lowering than lifting.
- Strong, fresh legs can climb stairs all day.
- Chin-ups are limited by the strength of gripping muscles. Despite a biceps burn and a lesser degree of fatigue in the upper-back, at some point you will no longer be able to hold on to the bar. It's the smaller muscles that fail.

Why, then, do strong, fresh (unexercised) legs grow incapable of climbing two four-inch steps with a 10-second rest between efforts (20 total steps) despite performing no direct exercise?

Intensity. Negative work to fatigue creates a systemic impact (inroad) at least 40% greater than that encountered during normal work. If the intensity is high enough, your system can enter a state of shock that will buckle your knees.

All physical efforts - whether with legs, hips, shoulders, arms, chest or other - affect your system. When the demands of exercise exceed the system's momentary capacity, the body shuts down as a safety measure. The next time the same signal is sent, the system is better prepared, having learned in the process...which is more than can be said of its owners.

Ninety percent of today's trainees exercise 5-6 times a week on what they call a 'split' system. They divide their body into parts and work a different one (or ones) each day. In many cases, they exercise the same body part only once a week and rationalize that the routine better stimulates the selected part through more exercise while enhancing recovery between sessions. What they fail to realize is that their system takes a beating every time they train regardless of which parts are used. In time, the system cannot recover from its last session, nor prepare for its next. In essence, you train, and nothing happens. When that occurs, the intensity of training has diminished (due to sheer volume and by necessity), and lower intensity means less results.

It's called "over-training."

More exercise, the preference of those addicted to and frustrated by strength training, is a poor physiological choice. It better satisfies the social needs of performing daily exercise and conforming to the eccentricities of peers.

Think (and exercise) 'systemic.' If an arm exercise like chin-ups can buckle your legs, why can't a chest workout buckle your system?

## FEBRUARY 9

### Pecking Holes In Theory

Banging your head against a tree is probably not a great source of exercise, but you can learn from it.

As a teen, golf, running and weight training became the 'must do' activities of my life - golf, because of early success; running, because of the exhilaration it provided; and weight training, because it seemed the base of *everything* physical.

So I wasn't at all surprised and only slightly disappointed by the doctor's message concerning my low-back pain that day, "If I were you, I'd never run or lift weights again." Dr. Montenegro may have been a top physician, honest in his assessment and even a golfer, but he was no psychologist - and he certainly was not me. I thanked him and left, which was no big deal. He rang up the till and saved time.

Several years later, I had a back operation - three herniated discs. For the first time in 15 years, I stopped all activity...for a while.

At six months, I was ready to go - my way, the 'smart' way - by reducing the impact of running. The options included a softer running surface, better shoes, an improved style (which had undoubtedly deteriorated in the wait) and uphill running. I narrowed them down. A grassy surface was out. The city of Caracas was 99% concrete and I preferred the stability of something at least as hard as my head. I had the shoes, and my technique was as silent as it could be. It left one thing - running uphill.

Uphill runs provided less impact and greater demands on the cardiovascular system, but 'what goes up, must come down.' The down I would solve by walking.

A nearby highway pedestrian overpass became the site of my three-day-a-week jog-up-walk-down preparation. First 10, then 20, then 50 times; 1½ hours, three months - no pain - it was time to run on the flat.

Days later, two miles on concrete revealed that I was premature. So, I waited four more months, prepared again and ran for 10 months. After a second back operation, caused by *other* impact activities, I tried again. This time, at my wife's pace (really no pace at all) on soft grass, my back told me that my running days were through.

Nautilus® inventor Arthur Jones wrote about impact in the September issue of *Ironman* magazine, 1996. "Have you ever heard a woodpecker pecking a hole in a tree?" he asked. You haven't, according to Jones. "Nobody ever heard a woodpecker pecking wood, and they never will unless woodpeckers change their ways; what you hear is a sonic boom created by the fact that a woodpecker's head is moving at a speed of about 1,300 miles per hour when its beak hits its target, about twice the speed of sound. When the beak moving at that speed comes to an almost instantaneous stop as it hits the target, it creates an impact force of about 1,000 G's, meaning that a force of one ounce would then produce an impact force of 1,000 ounces, or more than 62 pounds."

A woodpecker has what is probably the best shock-absorption system on the planet inside its skull. It is designed to protect the bird's brain from high levels of impact. "Without it," says Jones, "the first peck would be the last."

In a similar way, runners are exposed to impact forces that amount to about six times their body weight, with shock absorbers that are far from that of a woodpecker.

High impact can be ignored, but must be absorbed by those who insist.

I once delighted in the thought of keeling over in a ditch in my running gear at some advanced age. I'm gonna miss that.

## FEBRUARY 10

### Negative Work

Negative work, the lowering of weight during exercise, is one of the most important yet misunderstood concepts in physical training.

Walk up 30 flights of stairs one day and take the elevator down. You will likely experience muscle soreness. Ride the elevator up another day and walk down, and your legs will 're-define' soreness. The adventure may lead you to believe that negative work (walking down) is of little value - it feels easy and makes you very sore. But it led Nautilus® inventor Arthur Jones to conclude the opposite. "Negative work," he claimed, "is the most important part of exercise performed for a wide variety of purposes."

Much of the confusion revolves around the difference between muscle input and functional output. To lift a 100-pound weight at a constant speed, a muscle must produce a force of exactly 100 pounds. If the input increases, the weight accelerates; if it decreases, the weight decelerates. In the same way, a contraction force of 100 pounds is required to lower a 100-pound weight at a constant speed. If the force diminishes, the weight accelerates; if it increases, the weight decelerates. When speed of movement is constant, muscle input is the same to lift as it is to lower.

Functional output - *how much* is lifted or lowered - is a different story. In one of Jones' experiments using a constant speed of movement, a muscle that was 40% stronger lowering than lifting in a 'fresh' state became 5,300% stronger (lowering than lifting) with the onset of fatigue. The difference was due to an increase in friction within the muscle itself, friction that impaired lifting but helped lowering.

It can be put to good use.

When lifting becomes impossible during exercise, it only means that the strength of the muscle has been temporarily reduced below that of the resistance (99 units of strength will not lift 100 units of weight). At that point, exercise can continue by lowering the weight. When the descent can no longer be controlled due to fatigue, a greater inroad into the muscle's reserve capacity is made, resulting in greater stimulation.

In rehabilitation, a muscle unable to lift a weight due to injury can likely lower it and eventually increase its ability to lift.

Full-range exercise - crucial to muscle size, strength, flexibility and injury prevention - is impossible without negative work. Negative work is present only when there is a force pulling in a direction opposite to that of the movement produced by muscular contraction. Without this force, a muscle cannot stimulate all of its fibers in a contracted position, nor completely stretch in extension.

Jones conducted research in the early 1970's to determine the importance of negative work and produced dramatic strength gains among athletes by lowering, not lifting, heavy weights. At the same time, the process improved flexibility and exercise form. It's tough to cheat when you're lowering something that feels like your car - which leads to the downside.

When motivated subjects lower heavy weights, it becomes dangerous for spotters to lift and transfer the weight safely (methods have since emerged that eliminate the need for help). It is also difficult to recover from negative work. For that reason, one set of negative exercise per body part per week (8-10 total sets) is recommended.

Take a good look at how you lower weights. While the reason it produces greater muscle soreness remains elusive, it is by far the most important part of exercise.

## FEBRUARY 11

### Friction in Exercise

A bicycle gliding down the street, an airplane soaring through the sky, an afternoon breeze and the blink of an eye - everything that moves creates friction, and muscles are no exception.

Muscles encounter friction from three sources during strength training: gravity, the equipment in use, and from the muscle itself.

The friction of lifting a weight against gravity is generally overlooked because gravity provides a constant force that hinders upward movement and helps downward movement, which in part is why it is more difficult to lift than lower a weight.

Gravity is constant, yet how a weight feels during exercise changes with leverage and fatigue. As leverage increases, weights feel lighter. A standing biceps curl, for example, feels heavy when forearms are parallel to the floor because leverage is poor in that position. Likewise, weights feel heavier with the onset of fatigue.

The friction inherent in exercise machines (via chains, pulleys, guide rods, levers, etc.) has a similar effect on output. Fifty pounds may feel like 100 on equipment that is poorly constructed or maintained. In the 1980's, a manufacturing firm that copied Nautilus® machines in Venezuela built a weight stack that often stuck at the top and had to be pulled down to the tune of a crash. Fortunately, friction of this magnitude is the exception, not the rule.

The least apparent source of friction is produced by the shortening and lengthening of muscle fibers. "Internal muscle friction" constantly changes during exercise because of two factors: speed of movement and muscle fatigue. The faster the speed and greater the fatigue, the higher the friction.

This time the influence is anything but subtle.

In January of 1976, Nautilus inventor Arthur Jones published an article in the *Athletic Journal* in which he speculated that internal muscle friction created the difference between lifting and lowering strength. In 1993, he designed a leg extension machine that measured the effect of friction on output during exercise. He first measured the strength of a reliable co-worker and found him 40% stronger lowering than lifting under 'fresh' conditions (a normal relationship). Jones then exercised one of the man's front thighs to exhaustion and recorded his lifting and lowering strength on each repetition.

At the start, the ability to lift and lower declined steadily. Beyond 12 repetitions, however, lifting strength dropped dramatically while lowering strength began to climb. At 25 repetitions (the end), lifting strength had been reduced by 98% (he could barely lift his leg) while lowering strength suffered a reduction of only 17% from its initial value (he could still lower plenty of weight). At this level of fatigue, the subject was 5,300% stronger lowering than lifting (compared to his fresh 40% difference) and expended more energy overcoming the increase in friction than lifting the resistance. At the same time, the increased friction greatly assisted the lowering process.

To use friction to your advantage, continue to lower a weight when you can no longer lift it - have someone else do the lifting - to take the muscle to a deeper level of fatigue. Without help, hold the last repetition as long as possible in a contracted position and then lower as slowly as you can. This keeps tension on the muscle longer than normal and increases the chance of stimulating change.

## FEBRUARY 12

---

### Designing a Workout

The purpose of strength training is to stimulate change, but you'd never know it. Most trainees straggle into the gym and wander around - a few minutes here, a few sets there. "Yeah, haven't done that yet. Ah, the abdominal machine. Nah, I'll skip that today." They treat it like a mall.

If you have the discipline to get there, plug in some quality time. Begin with a *brief* warm-up (approximately five minutes) on a cardiovascular device such as a bike, cross-trainer or treadmill. Set it in the 'Manual' or 'Quick Start' mode at a medium level of resistance and just unwind. Don't bother to select a programmed option, check your heart rate or stretch (unless you must for medical reasons). Stretching is more effective 'after' exercise (vs. 'before') because muscles are more pliable when warm. If you have walked to the gym or been physically active prior to your arrival, forego the warm-up. You're probably ready to go.

Begin your strength training with the largest muscle groups of the body – the hips and legs. Hitting those muscles early when you have the energy to put your best foot forward creates a greater impact on the system (than smaller muscles first). Perform one set of 8-15 repetitions for the rear hip, and front (quadriceps) and rear (hamstrings) thighs before you move on to the smaller leg muscles - calves, hip adductors and abductors. Select a total of 4-6 hip and leg exercises, focusing on those that suit your needs. For example, the calf plays a major role in the stability of the knee, while the hip adductors and abductors accommodate lateral movement in sports.

Next, turn to the large muscles of the torso - the shoulders, chest and upper back - and pay particular attention to the sequence. Shoulder and chest movements require help from the triceps of the upper arm, whereas back exercises generally require help from biceps. Start your upper-body sequence with either chest or shoulder movements followed by exercise for the upper-back, and then for whatever remains (of chest or shoulders). If you start with upper-back, you will likely be forced to perform consecutive triceps-related exercises without adequate rest between - and chest presses are no fun immediately after shoulder presses.

Once you have completed the torso, move to the upper-arms with, once more, caution concerning sequence. Which muscle group you start with (biceps or triceps) should be dictated by your last torso exercise. If it was a pull (biceps), start with triceps. If it was a push (triceps), start with biceps. If it was neither (such as a pullover, lateral raise or chest fly), start with the group of your choice.

Select 6-8 upper-body exercises from the torso and arm groups to bring the total number of sets in your workout to 12. If you think 12 sets is not enough, you need to work harder. Few trainees are capable of performing more than 12 HARD exercises with NO rest between. Logic suggests that more exercise only serves to reduce the intensity of the workout, and the value of the stimulation is based on intensity, not on the amount of exercise performed.

If you have any choices remaining, work the small muscles of the abdomen, neck or forearms last. Choose wisely.

At the end of your strength workout, perform 20-30 minutes of cardiovascular exercise with whatever energy you have left.

Then, shop all you want for a couple of days.

## FEBRUARY 13

### The Colorado Experiment

"Some people can and some people cannot." Nautilus® inventor Arthur Jones knew that genetics played a major role in the ability to build muscle size and strength...but believed there was more to the puzzle.

In September of 1973, he published an article in *Ironman* about a study conducted at Colorado State University in May of that year. The project was supervised by Dr. Elliott Plese, Director of the Exercise Physiology Laboratory.

Jones was looking to satisfy a few contentions, namely that:
1. Muscle growth is related to the intensity of exercise.
2. Increasing the amount of training reduces the production of results.
3. 'Negative work' is one of the most important factors in resistance training.
4. A 'special' diet beyond a balanced intake is not required.
5. The use of 'growth drugs' is not necessary or desirable.
6. Maximum size and strength "can be produced only by the use of full-range, rotary form, automatically variable, direct resistance."

Jones restricted exercise to machines only and selected Casey Viator and himself as 'subjects.' "Both," he claimed, "have demonstrated the potential for greater than average muscular mass and were rebuilding previously existing levels of muscular size."

Casey had trained on conventional equipment until he placed third in Mr. America (1970) and with barbells and Nautilus machines until he won the contest in 1971. The next year he trained primarily on Nautilus equipment, and from September to December (1972) exclusively with "negative only" Nautilus exercise, peaking at 200.5 pounds. In January of 1973, Casey lost a finger at work and almost died from a reaction to an anti-tetanus shot. For four months prior to the study, he lost "approximately 33.63 pounds" (18.75, a direct result of the accident; 14.88, a result of no exercise).

Arthur had trained sporadically for 34 years, reaching a peak muscular bodyweight of 205 pounds in 1954 (his normal weight was 145-160). He last trained for six weeks in November of 1972 with "negative only" exercise (after nothing for four previous years).

In the study, Viator trained 14 times in 28 days with steady growth. He gained a daily average of 2.06 pounds his first 14 days; 1.3, the next three days; 1.2, the next five; and 1.05 pounds, the last six. He averaged 33.6 minutes per whole-body workout and gained 4.51 pounds per workout, 8.04 pounds per training hour.

Jones trained 12 times in 22 days and gained .58 pounds per day for the first seven days, .7 pounds the next seven, and .57 the final eight. He averaged 24.8 minutes per session (1 set of 10 exercises, approximately 10 reps per set) and gained 1.28 pounds per workout, 3.06 pounds per training hour.

Strength? Viator performed 32 reps to failure with 400 pounds on a Universal® leg press one hour before the first workout and, on the same test, 45 reps with 840 pounds three days after the last workout. Leg presses were not included in the experiment.

Flexibility? According to Jones, Casey "demonstrated a range of motion far in excess of that possible by any member of the Colorado State University wrestling team."

Body fat? Viator: from 13.8% to 2.47%; and bodyweight, from 166.87lb. to 212.15lb.

Strong, massive and flexible - the result of brief, high-intensity, full-range exercise.

As Jones put it, "...the secret, if there is one, is HIGH-INTENSITY; and when you are training with high-intensity, you don't need a large amount of training."

FEBRUARY 14

---

### The Limits of Cardiovascular Endurance

There are five potential benefits of proper exercise: an increase in muscular strength, cardiovascular endurance, joint flexibility, body leanness and a reduced risk of injury. Although certain activities emphasize one over the other, all five should interest the fitness enthusiast or aspiring athlete.

Cardiovascular fitness means different things to different people, which prompted the scientific community to establish a common denominator for measurement - maximum oxygen uptake. Defined as "the body's ability to absorb, transport and utilize oxygen," it improves when we participate in activities such as running, swimming and cycling.

Our ultimate cardiovascular capacity (as our potential for strength) is determined by genetics. A review of oxygen pathways - from absorption in the lungs and transportation through the circulatory system, to consumption by the muscle - can help determine what limits that capacity.

The purpose of the lungs is to saturate blood with oxygen, a function easily met under all conditions. At rest, total saturation is accomplished in the first third of the blood's transit time through the lung's capillaries. During maximal exercise, with the heart rate and blood flow increased dramatically and transit time reduced by 50%, the reserve capacity of the lungs can easily meet the demand. At the receiving end, muscles are capable of consuming all of the oxygen in the brief period of time it takes the blood to flow through its capillaries, both at rest and during heavy exercise. Therefore, with the lungs and muscles loading and unloading oxygen at near 100% efficiency, neither appears to be a limiting factor.

The same, however, cannot be said of the circulatory system. Many physiologists believe that the heart itself is the limiting factor, reasoning that if the heart could pump more blood, the body would consume more oxygen. Accordingly, the role of cardiovascular exercise should be to increase the effectiveness of the heart's ability to pump blood. Others claim that the heart can only pump the amount of blood returning to it, and that the peripheral blood vessels restrict the blood's return by resisting every attempt the heart makes to increase blood flow.

When a muscle contracts, internal pressure rises and compresses the blood vessels within, restricting flow. Research demonstrates that such restriction begins with a voluntary contraction of as little as 20% and increases proportionately with the intensity of effort. At 50-60% (of a maximum contraction), no blood flow is present - and no oxygen delivered or consumed. The system shuts down.

There are only two ways to decrease muscle contraction intensity during activity:

- Increase the skill of the individual performing the movement, thereby diminishing the quantity of unnecessary contraction.
- Increase the strength of the muscles involved so that each contraction requires a smaller percentage of the available muscle mass.

Skill is highly specific and requires time to develop, while strength is universal and acquired more efficiently. A distance runner could become a distance swimmer by learning efficient swimming technique. He could improve at both by becoming stronger.

Therefore, in the same way genetic factors dictate our ultimate level of strength, so muscle strength limits our ultimate cardiovascular capacity. Proper strength training should be the focus of every program designed to increase physiological function.


## FEBRUARY 15

---

### Perseverance...and Thanks, Boris

Every morning was the same. The implements, the field that softened their blow, the cast of characters, the chill and the sunless sky were daily audience to a British accent that bellowed a message as if ears were far away. "M-a-g-n-i-f-i-c-e-n-t turn, Bannister. A-t-r-o-c-i-o-u-s delivery, lad. See you in the morning."

Every morning, I tested and mourned; every afternoon, I pumped homework to the nervous system. My running turn through the discus circle was balanced, rhythmic and consistent, but the delivery, adequate in distance and flight, lacked an upright left side. Learning proper technique was fun; learning enough to pass the course was not.

Two titans stood in the way: Geoff Gowan, Great Britain's Olympic distance coach, and Englishman Peter Radford, 1960 world-record holder at 220 yards. Both track-and-field professors were competent, thorough and tough.

The anxiety mounted as 20 students scrambled for a solution - Saturday was the final trial, and it came all too soon.

As expected, Gowan was on time sporting an immaculate blue Adidas® training suit. He warmed up in his usual manner, a cup of coffee and a clipboard. Traces of optimism faded as he called us one-by-one. "Magnificent turn, atrocious delivery," once more pierced the frigid air. I got back in line.

Emotion was high but morale low as we awaited the next throw. Suddenly, a voice ahead spoke through, " I don't give a (blank) any more, I'm gonna heave this one over the fence." Boris Terluk had had enough. His windup reflected a fury that Gowan thought was focus. The toss was huge. Coffee spewed. "B-e-a-u-t-y, Terluk, b-e-a-u-t-y. Fetch it quickly, lad!" Boris had stirred the throng and spread a glimmer of hope. Even my left side stood tall enough to pass the standard.

Looking back, the lesson that morning extended far beyond the throwing circle. It was about setting goals, summoning the discipline and perseverance to reach them and, from the instructor's view, creating an effective environment for learning and performance. Knowing that my grade was poor at best and that I might later require those skills as a teacher or coach, I continued to work with the discus - and improve. Gowan had fueled the fire.

In the same way, the majority of people won't do much about exercise until it becomes a need. According to health-club statistics, only a small percentage of trainees last long enough to reap the initial benefits (one month to feel more energy, 3-4 to see results). The reasons include lack of discipline, impatience, inadequate orientation, poor goal setting, exercising for aesthetic instead of health reasons, and attitude (of a less-physical, instant-result society). In many cases, the medical community must first voice a stern warning about a pending health 'risk' before more than a passing interest is taken. Yet, even at that, some are unwilling to commit.

Here are a few suggestions:

- Consider exercise a need and set aside 2-3 half-hour blocks per week.
- Select a variety of activities you like and pursue them long enough to realize a benefit. You may not want to turn back.
- Think long-term by self-injecting the small dose of fear I use with my clients, "Whether you show up or not, the weights keep going up."

See you in the morning.

## FEBRUARY 16

---

### Balanced Muscle Strength

There's a lot of talk these days about balanced strength, and rightly so. Nothing is more important than strong muscles on all sides of a joint system to maximize functional ability and prevent injury. An imbalance in strength (or flexibility) can force a structure to move in a distinct pattern and, if prolonged, create injury.

What is 'balanced' strength?

Some believe it means 'equal in strength' - that a lift of 100 pounds for 10 repetitions on a leg extension machine should be mirrored by a lift of 100 pounds for 10 repetitions on a leg curl device. Yet, judging from the resistance used by most trainees during exercise, some muscles of an opposing pair are much stronger than their counterpart. My quadriceps, for example, are 20-25% stronger than my hamstrings; my biceps 15-20% stronger than my triceps; my low back twice as strong as my abdomen; and my upper back slightly stronger than my chest.

But muscle balance determined by output alone (how much is lifted) is misleading. Output is dictated, in part, by leverage, by muscle size (larger muscles have the potential to lift heavier weights) and by the mechanical efficiency of the joint. One-hundred units of contraction by the quadriceps (front thigh) muscle, for example, results in a lift of 6-8 units of weight by the body's least efficient joint, the knee. As such, a large muscle mass is required to produce the movement. In contrast, 100 units of contraction by the muscles that extend the lumbar spine, the most efficient joint system, result in a lift of up to 400 units of weight. The lumbar spine is 50 times (5,000%) more efficient than the knee - and its muscles among the smallest in the body.

To add to the confusion, early attempts to test muscle output using isokinetic technology (motorized machines common to medical facilities) were unsafe, inaccurate and misleading. Results were biased by impact forces, non-muscular torque (produced by the weight of the involved body part and stored energy) and by friction, inevitable in dynamic testing procedures. It resulted in more than a few opinions about 'balanced' strength.

Is there an 'ideal' relationship between antagonistic muscle groups?

The advent of static testing and total muscle isolation provided by the introduction of the MedX® Knee Machine in 1994 (following 22 years and $120 million of research) reveals that there is.

According to MedX tests, the strength relationship of front and rear thigh changes at every angle throughout the range of motion (Figure 1). In the starting position of a leg extension (120°, right side of chart), the quadriceps muscle (pushing up statically) is 10-15% stronger than the hamstring (pushing down statically). At 75°, the quadriceps reaches its maximum strength and is approximately 50% stronger than the hamstring. At 30-35°, the two are equal (quadriceps strength drops dramatically while hamstring strength increases slowly). At 0° (a position of complete leg extension), the hamstring is 40-50% stronger than the quadriceps.

Balanced strength means maximum muscle strength at every angle of movement on all sides of a structure. To accomplish this, quadriceps and hamstrings (or any other pair of opposing muscles) should be trained with equipment that provides a proper change of resistance through a complete range of motion.

Full-range, balanced strength goes a long way in preventing injury.

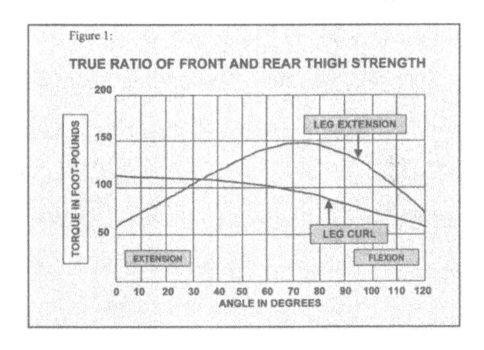

Figure 1:

TRUE RATIO OF FRONT AND REAR THIGH STRENGTH

## FEBRUARY 17

---

### Arms – Paper or Plastic?

Mike Guibilo who claimed a pumped upper-arm of 29 inches in the October 1970 issue of *Muscle Builder* magazine and Hulk Hogan who claimed a 24-inch arm in the late 1980's had something in common. They were wrong...and not alone.

"Accurately measured," concluded Joe Roark in a special issue of *Roark Report* devoted to exaggerated measurements in bodybuilding publications (1986), "a seventeen-inch arm is big. An eighteen-inch arm is very big. And anything above eighteen inches must be seen to be believed."

Nautilus® inventor Arthur Jones concurred. He measured some of the largest arms in the world - his way. He first made a measuring tape from a strip of newspaper and labeled it against a steel ruler. Cloth and plastic tapes added fractions to the actual size and tended to shrink with age. He then took the measurement on a 'cold' first flex and read the tape at right angles to the long bone in the upper-arm.

His technique resulted in accurate readings of the following bodybuilders in peak condition: Arnold Schwarzenegger - 19½" (inches); Casey Viator - 19-5/16"; Mike Mentzer - 18-5/8"; Bill Pearl - 18-5/8"; and Boyer Coe - 18-7/16".

"The largest arm I ever measured," claimed Jones, "was that of Sergio Oliva in September, 1971. It was 20-1/8 inches cold, measured at right angles to the bone with a tissue paper-thin tape, on the first flex after arising in the morning. Sergio's arm literally dwarfed the other arms I've seen since then. To obtain such a measurement, most bodybuilders would have to shrink the tape and cut off the first two inches, pump their arm for at least 30 minutes, and then add their forearm to the total."

From top to bottom, Oliva's flexed arm was larger than his head. Yet, when shown a picture of the 'status-symbol' arms of John McWilliams (a Mr. America candidate) taken in 1939, Oliva's reaction was, "They're too big!"

Jones believed that bodybuilders of the 1940-1950's incorporated less superstition and myth in their programs than do today's trainees. A massive arm back then, with nothing in the way of supplements or drugs, was quite an accomplishment.

John McWilliams visited the Nautilus complex years later. When an eager staff member asked him the 'secret' to such impressive arms, the soft-spoken champion replied, "You know, young man, that the muscles are comprised mostly of water. Therefore you must train your arms with the heaviest weight possible, then you must drink at least a gallon of water during and just after your workout, and finally you must pray that God will direct the water to your arms."

So much for the old days.

Several factors dictate how large an arm appears: head size, body height, bodyweight and overall proportion. Sergio Oliva's head was smaller than normal (22-23 inches) which made his arms look large. Lightweight champions in bodybuilding pose-downs generally appear 'puny' beside their larger peers. According to Jones, a 16-inch arm on a man of average height is very impressive; a 17-inch arm, freakish; an 18-inch arm, unbelievable; and a 19-inch arm, impossible. He was aware that a slight increase in the size (circumference) of an arm through training resulted in a disproportionate increase in its muscular bulk.

Mike Guibilo was reluctant to remove his coat for a picture, let alone a measurement of his 29-inch arms. And he never knocked on Arthur's door.

## FEBRUARY 18

### Putting It On The Line

"If race horses were trained as much as most bodybuilders, you could safely bet your money on an out-of-condition turtle - it would be unlikely that a horse trained in such a fashion could even make it around the track, and certainly not rapidly."

In the early 1970's, Nautilus® inventor Arthur Jones wanted to put to rest the idea that maximum gains from strength training required an input of "at least five days a week and several hours each workout."

He interviewed a man he thought would be 'ideal' for the experiment.

"I have been bitten by poisonous snakes more than 20 times, and have a permanently stiff thumb as a result of one such bite," said the candidate. "I was badly mauled by a lion many years ago and got a broken neck in the process, an injury that has caused me trouble ever since, involving (as it did) the nerves that lead to my arm. I have been shot through both legs and will never again have full use of either. My right arm was busted up so badly that I haven't been able to straighten it fully in more than 30 years, and my left arm had the triceps ripped out by the roots, so now I can't fully straighten either."

"Carry on."

"I have had malaria repeatedly, tick-bite fever, and 'who knows what' other tropical diseases. I have worked an average of at least 14 hours a day for more than 30 years and have probably averaged less than five hours of sleep a night during that period. Most of my teeth are gone - or ruined - from too many years in places where you didn't dare brush your teeth with the water. My ears were damaged many years ago by too many big engines and big guns, and my eyes certainly are not what they once were. The less said about my hair the better - and some people say my face looks like a map of Europe, a map made just after the last war."

"Great, when would you like to start?"

Jones hired himself for one reason, "I 'know' how I will train, and I could never be quite sure just how somebody else might train. I will train properly - very briefly, infrequently, but very hard."

To assure that he was not accused of growth drugs, overstatements or 'hanky panky,' Jones proposed the following. He would first be weighed, measured and tested by the doctors in the physiology department of a major university and then locked in a room for 28 days. The staff would "observe, monitor and carefully record literally EVERYTHING that I do." During that time, Jones planned 14 workouts: a half-hour every day for the first five days, then three times a week for the final three weeks. Each session would be less than 50 minutes with Nautilus machines only (no chin-ups, dips or squats). At the end, the same parameters would be re-measured and results published.

"If I make a fool of myself," he said, "then everyone will know it - because the results will be printed regardless of what happens, win, lose, or draw."

Jones often stuck his mauled neck out when he believed in something, and made it clear that he was dead serious.

As far as I know, the experiment never happened. Nonetheless, Jones was certain he would 'surprise' a few people and demonstrate that "almost any-body can and will make very worthwhile gains from an actually very small amount of proper training, and without the use of drugs of any kind."

It was what Nautilus was all about.


## FEBRUARY 19

---

### Free Weights vs. Machines – Part 1

Are exercise machines better than free weights? The man responsible for stirring up the controversy thinks so. When he introduced his Nautilus® machines in 1970, Arthur Jones described them as "nothing more than a thinking man's barbell" and proclaimed their superiority for reasons other than safety and convenience.

First, machines provided *direct* exercise for muscle groups that could not be isolated with free weights. Second, the machine's 'cam' varied the resistance according to the needs of the muscle as it moved through its range-of-motion. Barbells provided resistance only in the mid-range of movement, and in the starting or finishing position - but never in both. Third, machines provided resistance that rotated on a common axis with the body part moved by the muscle. It was superior to the vertical pull of gravity encountered with barbells. As Jones put it, "You can't go around a curve in the road by continuing to move in a straight line."

The attraction of bodybuilders to the new technology was short-lived. They thought the dramatic results produced by a few could be easily duplicated, but there was nothing easy about it. Coupled with Jones' belief that most trainees lacked the genetic potential for super results with any tool, it didn't take long for the word to spread - machines were for health clubs and women, not hardcore bodybuilders. That was only the beginning.

Machines were attacked from every angle. The 'cam' was wrong. They were too costly, didn't fit tall or short people, and limited movement to a pre-determined track. They eliminated the use of small joint-stabilizing muscles, restricted speed training due to friction, and destroyed the natural aspect of exercise by decreasing neurological input. Free-weight advocate Fred Hatfield even suggested that the space-age look of the machines lulled people into thinking that the tool would produce the result.

Jones remained unfazed. "Very few had sense enough," he said, "to understand the real differences between exercise machines and barbells," adding (in *Ironman* magazine, June, 1996), "(a machine) provides the capability of following any one of a great number of possible paths while lifting the weight, without the risk of dropping it. A barbell, in contrast, requires the use of a very narrow path while moving. The slightest deviation from this path results in a loss of control and potential injury." To the requirement of involving synergistic muscles to balance the barbell, Jones replied, "the most likely result is injury to the so-called 'balancing muscles.'"

Like Hatfield, Jones believed that the barbell was a miracle tool compared with anything before it and that "hard exercise - and ONLY HARD EXERCISE - produced worthwhile results in the way of muscular strength and size increases." Nautilus machines were an outward manifestation of his "harder-is-better" philosophy.

How HARD was it? Of the thousands that attempted Jones' workout in the early 1970's, no one lasted more than a few minutes. They all ended on the floor, in shock, unable to continue - due as much to the non-stop system of exercise as the equipment.

Despite the debate, the facts remain clear. A well-designed machine works a muscle more directly and more thoroughly than a barbell. In either case, muscles can't distinguish between the two; if the resistance increases, they respond.

'How' and 'how hard' you use a tool are more important than the tool itself. "If you are not willing to work hard," suggested Jones more than 30 years ago, "then forget it - there simply isn't any other way."

## FEBRUARY 20

### Free Weights vs. Machines – Part 2

Happy Birthday! The barbell is 100 years old. It arrived with the horse-and-buggy and wooden-shafted golf clubs, and has, better than all the advancements of that era, staid the course. That's the bad news.

Today, cars have become highly sophisticated and a novice can launch a golf ball out of sight. A century of technology has advanced every field but one. The field of exercise still clings to the adage that barbells are superior to anything since.

The arguments in favor are many:

- Free weights work more muscles - including those that 'stabilize' and 'balance' - which is no bargain. More energy used to 'balance' means less available for the target muscle, which leads to premature fatigue and increased risk of injury. When stabilizer muscles fatigue, the resistance might leave its ideal path. Since when does low-intensity, indirect exercise produce much in the way of a strength benefit? Aren't stabilizer muscles better strengthened with direct, full-range, isolated, high-intensity exercise on a machine? When did balancing resistance become a criterion for building strength? Muscles know only contraction and intensity of effort. They don't care about the source of intensity or the application of strength. When a muscle is called upon, free-weight strength will not prove superior to machine-based strength.

- Free-weight training simulates real-life situations and movements. Yet, the role of strength training is to strengthen muscles, not movements. Movement coordination is handled by skill training with *no* overload, and its transfer is questionable. Does performing on a Swiss ball improve a sport, or performance on a Swiss ball?
- Free weights are superior to machines for 'explosive' speed training. While it may be true that you can throw weights 'faster' with barbells than machines, throwing results in only one end - injury.

FACT: Most free-weight exercises provide effective resistance only in the mid-range of motion. Changes in resistance throughout the range rarely match the muscle's strength potential, resulting in sticking points and incomplete muscle involvement.

Overload and intensity make muscles grow, and machines provide a better overload (a higher potential level of intensity) throughout a range of motion than do free weights. As someone put it, "A set to muscle failure on a bench press is fatiguing, but a set on a (machine) will wipe you out!" As such, machines reduce work time, training volume and frequency - will get you from A to B faster with less training time.

The only people who derive a greater benefit from the use of free weights are those who require the skill of lifting weights in their sport - powerlifters. Yet, they too can benefit from machines that isolate and strengthen weak links. The combination provides the necessary variety to induce growth.

When bodybuilding legend Vince Gironda first saw a Nautilus® machine, he said, "There goes the barbell." Yet, he overestimated the ability of the average trainee to think and underestimated the ability of the powers-that-be to control.

According to Armand Hammer, politics has retarded the field of exercise. "The controlling powers of the magazines and bodybuilding contests (when Nautilus was first introduced) could not allow revolutionary thoughts such as brief, intense training... (because) it would put the truth to decades of lies promoting 'more is better'."

What's next - a gym with a hitching post, or a golf program with wooden shafts?

## FEBRUARY 21

---

### Short and Sweet

Some people love to be told exactly what to do. And bodybuilders in the early 1970's were no exception - except that they had to sift though pages of theory before they could decipher *exactly* what Arthur Jones meant by 'brief' and 'hard.' Most were stunned when they put his theory to the test. It was only the beginning.

In November of 1970, the Nautilus® inventor introduced a brief, upper-back sequence in *Ironman* magazine as follows: (1) a pullover-type lat machine; (2) a behind-neck-type lat machine; (3) a rowing-type lat machine; (4) a behind-neck chin-up; (5) a 45-degree rowing machine; and (6) a regular-grip chin-up.

The first three exercises involved no use of arm muscles other than their push against pads. The final three directly involved the biceps: the first (#4), with a weak, palms-out grip; the second (#5), with an unspecified (probably palms-out or parallel) grip; and the third (#6), with a strong, palms-up grip. The instructions were clear:

"The exercises should be performed in that order, and with no rest between sets," he said. "The entire cycle should be completed as quickly as possible, but each set should be carried to the point of total failure of the involved muscles in that position. Properly performed, one cycle will work the major torso muscles to a point of total, if momentary, failure; and not more than two such cycles should be performed in any one workout; nor should such workouts be performed more than three times weekly."

"But wait!" as the infomercial goes.

"For best possible results, each such cycle should be immediately preceded with a set of at least fifteen reps of fast, heavy squats, carried to the point of staggering under the weight, to the point of extreme breathlessness. And when I say 'immediately,' I mean just that...no slightest rest between the squats and the first set of the lat machine cycle."

There was good news. Jones recommended only one cycle of less than eight minutes (including the squats) three times a week "for maximum possible gains in the lats" (and never more than 48 minutes per week, with two cycles). His full-body workouts were equally brief. Two cycles took 80 minutes, yet, "in almost all cases, best results will be produced by a training program limited to about 48 minutes, three times weekly." It still wasn't enough for most bodybuilders. By 1972, Jones added free shipping.

"One self-confessed 'expert,'" he said, "recently remarked in one of his articles that it was a joke to even consider a brief workout as hard - but I hereby tell him very clearly that he can NOT follow one of our trainees for even as much as 10 minutes and stay on his feet; three or four minutes of actually hard training will make him vomit - 10 minutes or less will put him on the floor, 'out like a light' - and a full workout of 40 minutes or so would kill him stone dead. And if he thinks differently, let him come down here and try it - and if I am wrong, then I will pay for his trip."

Jones considered two factors:

*"No amount of exercise will produce worthwhile results if the 'intensity of effort' is too low; and if the 'amount' of exercise is too great, then no exercise will produce any worthwhile result regardless of the other factors."*

By the end of 1972, he reduced his leg circuit to 3-4 exercises (3-4 minutes) twice a week, and his total-body workout to 28 minutes. The only thing he increased was heart rate. "Thirty seconds into this routine," he explained, "the pulse rate hits a level of 160 to 190 - and will not drop below 130 until after the entire workout is completed."

Keep it short - not sweet - and don't forget to ask about free shipping.


## FEBRUARY 22

---

### Hercules From The Neck Down

As teens, we swarmed the local cinema to attempt the impossible - make a bad movie worse. Our cat-calls from all corners during such thrillers as *King Kong, Godzilla* and *The Bride of Frankenstein* wore out more than a few flashlights. On one occasion, the 'horror-horn' and 'fear-flasher' that warned of pending fright in a film whose name I can't recall took us over the top. We got the boot.

One movie of that era, *Hercules, Sampson* and *Ullyses,* featured three giants who first battled each other before joining forces (as did the ushers) to root out local evil. The film was a joke, yet one of the characters who played a minor role in that fiasco could well have been the man I met in Caracas 20 years later.

The tall, handsome Italian slipped by the reception without a word on gym policy. At the time, we did not allow multiple sets or unsupervised workouts. I briefed him as he performed a second chest press and offered to return his money.

"Do you have a station for wide-grip chin-ups?" he asked.

"Sorry," I replied. "A wide grip doesn't provide much exercise for the upper back and greatly reduces the range of motion. We won't have it here."

The 'news' triggered a discussion. He contended that a reverse grip (palms facing away from the body) during chin-ups increased the work of the upper-back by decreasing the work of the biceps. He then supported his belief by the 'look-at-me' theory, and by claiming to have participated in an early 'Hercules' movie.

I once read something about Whistler's mother. We were even.

During chin-ups, resistance is applied against the hands, which makes them a limiting factor. Failure is reached when the small, weaker muscles of the arms and hands become exhausted, long before the large, stronger muscles of the torso have been stimulated. Therefore, hands should be placed in a strong position during chin-ups and other compound movements, or the resistance should be applied directly to the torso muscles, as with a pullover machine.

Hercules was right. When you rotate your hands from a thumbs-out position to a thumbs-in position, the role of the biceps in flexing the arm is reduced. But the slack is not assumed by the upper-back. It shifts to the weaker muscles of the forearm...and failure occurs in the weak link. If stronger back muscles assumed the burden of a weaker arm position as he suggested, everyone would perform more chin-ups with a reverse grip.

They don't.

The next issue was grip width. If the value of an exercise is judged by the quality of resistance and quantity of movement, a wide-grip chin-up is a poor choice. It provides approximately 60° of motion for the upper back (a regular chin-up, 118°) and no variable resistance (rather, a random variation produced by a constant change in leverage which leaves the effective range of motion as little as 10-15°). According to Arthur Jones, 60° is less than 25% of a full-range movement. "Recently," he said, "a member of the Nautilus® staff demonstrated a range-of-movement of 270 degrees" on a pullover machine that provided a direct and variable source of resistance for the torso muscles.

I introduced Hercules to a pullover/chin-up combination that was his last.

The man who once braced the Pantheon with a lousy grip disappeared as quickly as he had arrived, and didn't learn much in the process. But I did - bodybuilders are as bad in the gym as they are on screen.

## FEBRUARY 23

---

### Ask Kermit

Five year-old Lily Miller curled up beside me on the sofa to read from a book on the human body narrated by a frog. The first line, "The body works together," mirrored Arthur Jones' first line in *Nautilus Training Principles: Bulletin No. 2* (1971), "The human body is a unit." The frog was on to something.

Jones, too, conveyed ideas in simple terms, but often less kindly. "Anybody who fails to understand this article," he once wrote, "should quit weight training immediately; because I am going to write it in such a way as to be understood by anybody."

The article in question addressed muscle function, the activation of muscle fibers and a problem with conventional exercise. He used the following analogy:

"Imagine a long line of canoes extending down a straight stretch of river; the nose of each canoe being fastened to the tail of the one in front. The first canoe is fastened to the bank by its tail, and the last canoe in the long line is attached to a large raft floating freely in the stream. In effect, we have a 'rope' made up of a line of 100 canoes. Each canoe is 10 feet long, so the rope of canoes is 1,000 feet long."

Logically, if one of the canoes located in the middle of the rope suddenly shrunk to half its length, the length of the lower half of the rope would decrease, and the raft would be pulled upstream, by five feet. If all of the canoes shrunk by half at the same time, the raft would be pulled upstream a distance of 500 feet.

"A muscle works in much the same way," he said. "Each individual fiber (canoe) works by reducing its length; and for total movement of the body part being moved by that muscle, ALL of the fibers must be working at the same time. BUT ONLY ALL OF THE FIBERS IN ONE STRAND OF MUSCLE (one rope of canoes)."

Individual muscle fibers work either all-out or not at all. If they aren't needed, they don't work. Which means the following:

- If the raft is light, then only a few strands may be required to move it.
- If it is heavy, it may require an all-out effort (despite the fact that all-out efforts only recruit a small percentage of fibers, for safety).

- If it is too heavy for one strand of canoes to move, another strand is called into play to work alongside the first. And if all canoes in both strands shrink (by half) the raft will be pulled 500 feet upstream.

Then Jones threw in a monkey wrench.

"But if, before it had moved the full 500 feet, the raft was approached from behind by a power boat and was pushed the final 200 feet of its trip upstream, then the load would be removed from the canoes before it was even possible for all of them to be involved in the work; and that is exactly what happens in all forms of conventional exercise."

"If all of the individual muscle fibers were flexed at the same time," he continued, "then the involved body part would have to be in a fully contracted position. If the load is removed or decreased, prior to the time that the moving body part has reached a position of full contraction, then no requirement for the involvement of the total number of available muscle fibers is being imposed. Yet, with one or two minor exceptions, no conventional form of exercise provides any resistance at this point in the exercise."

In other words, barbells recruit few canoes in full contraction.

If bodybuilders don't get it - and few seem to - they should rush to the nearest dollar store for a copy of *Ask Kermit*. At least the frog has his act together.


## FEBRUARY 24

---

### The Moment of Truth

The practice area of a professional golf tournament is the showcase of one glaring fact: similar results can be produced by different methods. Both a picture-perfect swing and a slash can result in similar distance, direction and ball-flight - and the reason 'why' is clear.

At the 'moment of truth' - when the club contacts the ball - there is little difference among the pros. The face of the club passes through the hitting area 'square' to its intended line of flight and produces a straight shot. To make it happen under pressure requires practice, but in the end the only thing that counts is impact.

Strength training has a similar 'moment of truth' - the final seconds of an exercise - but unlike professional golf, it is not often pretty.

"Watching a man working out properly is almost frightening - and it is frightening to some people," said Nautilus® inventor, Arthur Jones. "The intensity of effort is so great that the subject's entire body is shaking, his face will turn red - or even purple - and both breathing and heart action will be increased at least one-hundred percent, and frequently far more than that. Most people are simply not aware that such effort is even possible, and many that are aware of the possibility are totally unwilling to exert such effort; but, for maximum growth stimulation, that is exactly what is required."

Jones believed that the only repetitions capable of stimulating growth were the final few. "NEVER terminate a particular set simply because you have completed a certain number of repetitions; a set is properly finished only when additional movement is utterly impossible - curl until you can't even begin to bend your arms, squat until you can't start up from the low position, press until you cannot move the bar away from your shoulders or your chest." He didn't end there.

Once you have performed as many repetitions as you can in strict form, "cheat to make the last two or three repetitions 'possible,' not to make them 'easy.' Properly performed," he reiterated, "the cheated repetitions should be brutally hard."

Cheating involves the recruitment of other muscles to assist in the task. The extra 'help' forces a muscle to work within its existing level of reserve and generally appears in the form of movement your body 'invents' to complete a repetition. Once you can no longer lift a weight without a dangerous jerk, cheat just enough to continue movement. When movement is no longer possible, hold the weight as far toward the contracted position as you can, for as long as you can (usually 5-10 seconds), and then lower it slowly. Record only the 'good' repetitions.

One day I trained at a facility in Pompano Beach, Florida where the blasting music, busy chatter and pounding treadmills provided a background drone. Suddenly, the power went off and the room fell silent except for a single sound of human effort that echoed from the bowels of the gym - A-A-A-A-H-H-H-O-O-O-O-H-H-H-H-E-E-E-E - then silence, then again. It sounded like a truck-stop restroom. Four grunts later, the job was done and the behemoth emerged.

Research shows that a boisterous yell can help the performance of one-time maximum lifts as in weight-lifting competitions. It also shows that it should occur only once or twice toward the end of a set of exercise.

The next time you hear the cry of the wild in a gym, take it for what its worth. If it repeats too often on the same exercise, rest assured that someone is wasting energy.

## FEBRUARY 25

---

### One Set of Arm Curls

Several years ago, Ellington Darden wrote an article in *Ironman* magazine that lent credence to the challenge Nautilus® inventor Arthur Jones often issued to bodybuilders. "Have you ever vomited after doing one set of arm curls with a barbell? If not, you simply don't know what hard work really is. There is only one way to the top in bodybuilding and that one way involves *outright hard work*."

Darden, Director of Research for Nautilus Sports/Medical Industries, was present when the majority of challenges were issued. Jones essentially put his victims in an odd posture for a biceps curl - bent forward from the waist approximately 45°, knees slightly bent and elbows pinned back to the sides. From there, without torso or elbow movement, trainees slowly raised the barbell to a position of full contraction - forearms parallel to the floor. They paused and then *slowly* lowered the weight until the bar grazed their thighs - an incomplete stretch but an excellent trigger for the next repetition. Trainees continued in strict form until they were unable to move. Despite the use of only 70-80% of the resistance they could normally curl 10 times, few completed six or seven repetitions.

That was only the beginning.

When fatigue was apparent, Jones assisted the lifting phase of two more repetitions and allowed the wobbly-kneed candidates to 'cheat' minimally by rocking their torso just enough to keep the bar moving *slowly* for a few more. He then had them continue from an upright posture, pushing down on the bar as it descended in the final reps.

The majority of trainees deposited their pre-exercise meal in the back alley.

Darden also researched the effectiveness of exercise sequences and introduced a five-minute routine that he claimed would "add half an inch of muscle mass to upper arms in a week and a full inch after a month." (*The Nautilus Advanced Bodybuilding Book*, 1984) The sequence was as follows:

**Monday and Friday**:
- Multi-Biceps Curl immediately followed by 'negative-only' chin-ups on the Multi-Exercise machine. Rest 30 seconds.
- Multi-Triceps Extension immediately followed by 'negative-only' dips on the Multi-Exercise machine.

**Wednesday**:
- A one-repetition chin-up (30-60 sec. up; 30-60 sec. down) immediately followed by Multi-Biceps Curl.
- A one-repetition dip (30-60 sec. up; 30-60 sec. down) immediately followed by Multi-Triceps Extension.

Darden recommended starting the one-repetition chin-ups and dips with a 30-second lifting and lowering phase, adding five seconds each workout, if successful. He also suggested performing the routine for a maximum of one month.

In 1987, Darden produced similar results with nine men (average: 22 years, 5'9", 162 pounds) and one woman (21 years, 5'2", 129 pounds), all employees of the Gainesville Health and Fitness Center. The subjects performed two-, three- and four-exercise combinations for biceps and triceps within a full-body workout using free weights. After six weeks, the average gain in arm size was 5/8"; forearm, 3/8". From there, Darden advocated three months of regular training before returning to the special sequence.

You don't have to live in a gym to produce results, but you do have to pay the price.

## FEBRUARY 26

### How Hard is Hard?

'Hard' is a relative term. A maximum effort for one person might be a walk across the street; for another, a lift of 500 pounds. In either case, it has to be experienced to be appreciated. Nautilus® inventor Arthur Jones added another dimension - 'hard' had to be learned. Most trainees didn't have what it takes to produce best results from exercise on their own - so Jones decided to teach them.

In the late 1960's, he developed concepts and techniques that improved strength training. The concepts, for the most part, were nothing new but their application was - and the process anything but easy.

In *Nautilus Training Principles, Bulletin No. 1* (1970), Jones described his version of a 'hard' leg sequence. You be the judge:

"First you do a set of leg presses carried to the point of failure performing at least twenty full repetitions against the most resistance that you can handle, and then as many partial repetitions as you can squeeze out, stopping only when it is utterly impossible to move the weight at all in any position.

Then - IMMEDIATELY, without even two seconds of rest - you perform a set of thigh extensions; again doing at least twenty full repetitions, and again continuing with partial movements until a point of utter exhaustion is reached.

Then - again IMMEDIATELY, without even one second of rest this time start your squats with a weight that you think you can do at least ten full repetitions with, and again carry them to the point of utter failure, so that the weight must be removed from your shoulders in the low position.

Then - and yet again IMMEDIATELY - step under a much heavier squat bar and do partial range movements near the top of the squatting position - going as low as possible while still managing to come erect again, trying to make each repetition as hard as possible.

How many cycles? Are you kidding? Even one such cycle done in that fashion without careful break-in training might well kill you - and it will certainly put you on the floor for quite a while, probably in a dead faint, certainly very near a state of shock; and if you think not, just try it - exactly as outlined above."

He then went on to describe 'hard' upper-back and arm sequences and concluded, "For the benefit of any readers who feel that they are training 'hard' - or who feel that our trainees are not training a lot harder - I will make the following observation; I have been known to make wagers, for money - so come down to DeLand and run through a workout with some of our football players, and bring your money and your 'sick bag' with you. If you are foolish enough to bet, you'll need the money to pay off with - and if you try to follow our trainees through a workout, you'll need the sick bag, whether you bet or not."

Arthur and his workouts lived up to their billing. The first four years the company was in operation (1970-74), no one made it through 12 stations supervised by Jones, and few lasted more than six minutes. Most were lying on the floor in shock, clutching their wallets and a damp sick bag.

Jones knew that trainees could develop the capacity to handle the workout but warned: "DO TAKE IT EASY AT FIRST, otherwise you may literally kill yourself."

It was arguably the most productive method ever devised, but most weren't willing to work *that* 'hard' - which doesn't change the facts. Gravity is still gravity.

FEBRUARY 27

---

## Passion

When Arthur Jones introduced his strength-training concepts in the form of a machine in 1970, he had no commercial interest in the field of exercise. But the passion with which he delivered his message had such an effect on his audience that he was swamped with requests - and literally forced to commit. When he did, there was nothing 99 about Arthur Jones other than, as some suggested, his age. His commitment was 100%, and visibly so.

I first spotted him while I toured the Nautilus® facility in Lake Helen, Florida. He was having a one-way conversation with a man I later learned was Bob Hoffman, founder of York® Barbell Company. Jones' body language spelled nothing but intensity, and his tongue never stopped. I wanted to drop the tour and listen, but it would be a long time before I got around to that. In 1980, I opened a Nautilus gym with all the passion I could muster to spread Arthur's word at whatever cost.

And cost there was. I turned away potential members who wanted nothing of the regimented system, at the same time attempting to create the 'electric' atmosphere I felt at Nautilus. We pushed, prodded and delivered a service second to none. Most clients got a great workout.

One of our first members, a strong executive named Patrick, took a lot of convincing. I spewed numbers and statistics his way and relayed the message that better results were possible with 90% greater efficiency. Then, I backed it with logic and honesty - and ran into the same problems encountered by Arthur.

The hype filled Patrick's head with visions of sugarplums - a phenomenon captured in an article by Vincent Bocchicchio, "Nautilus vs. Barbells," in *Ironman* that same year:

"The appetites and expectations of the weight training devotees were whetted beyond satiability. Simply, there was no way these devices (Nautilus machines) could meet the expectations of the interested parties. As a result, the 'miracle' cure and the 'magical' machines bore the brunt of this disappointed bitterness." (May, 1980).

Part of the problem, according to the author, was the passion of the inventor, viewed by many as commercially driven. "But," he added, "which one of us would not be enthusiastic and proud of an advance (scientifically valid) in a field where virtually none had been made in all too many years?"

The major problem, however, lay with the user. Trainees failed to understand the new concepts and used the equipment the way *they* thought it should be used - when most had no idea of proper barbell use. Nautilus machines were better than barbells, but failed to produce the overnight Hercules people expected. They were a 'bust' to those seeking an easy solution, and Nautilus was anything but easy.

Passion implies energy, enthusiasm and youth - things frequently lost in the shuffle of daily life. It's contagious.

I recently worked in an environment that was, for the most part, energized by the personality of a female trainer, Jessica Parnevik of the famous golfing family. She was as dynamic and passionate about her work as Jones was about his, and brought 'energy' to the building that I hadn't felt since Nautilus. To her credit, she was more predictable than Arthur.

And Patrick? He was likely disappointed, but hung around for 10 years and sponsored a slew of new members. Perhaps he sensed *my* passion for proper training.


## FEBRUARY 28

### We've Come A Long Way, Baby

The 'featured' exercise in the September 1931 issue of **Klein's Bell**, a newsletter from Sigmund Klein's Physical Culture Studio in New York City, was a one-legged standing curl with iron shoes. The same boots were used for seated leg extensions while Klein's "Foot-Press" was performed by lying on your back, placing a barbell on the soles of your shoes, lowering knees to chest, and pressing up until your legs were straight.

Things are safer in 2003 - but not better. Professional athletes now perform the same leg curls with rubber bands, while leg-press machines have replaced far more than the "Foot Press." Sports trainers, rehab professionals and other self-proclaimed 'experts' have all but eliminated the only exercise capable of maximizing the strength of the front thigh. Leg extensions are officially evil - despite the following.

Figure 1 demonstrates that the front thigh muscles (quadriceps) cannot be entirely strengthened without the use of a leg extension exercise that provides full-range resistance. The top curve (A) represents a test of quadriceps strength *before* exercise; the bottom curve (B), the same test immediately *after* exercise continued to fatigue. The exercise was limited to the right side of the chart, the WORKED AREA. The difference between fresh and exhausted strength levels (fatigue) is pronounced where the muscle performed work, but negligible where it did not (UNWORKED AREA). If the half-range exercise were continued over time, a strength gain would appear in the worked area, but not in the unworked zone.

According to MedX® inventor Arthur Jones, approximately 80% of people react to exercise in a similar way, a pattern he called "Type S" (Specific) response. It clearly illustrates that most trainees require full-range exercise for full-range strength.

Figure 2 demonstrates a test of quadriceps strength *before* and *after* a leg press, the movement that has fashionably replaced the leg extension. As in Figure 1, fatigue from the exercise is apparent only on the right side of the chart (legs bent) despite the fact that the machine used for the exercise provided a resistance that varied threefold from flexion to extension. While 300 pounds in a bent-leg position produced fatigue, 900 pounds in a straight-leg position produced none (because of the enormous advantage in leverage provided as legs straighten). According to Jones, "In that part of the full-range movement (left side of chart) no possible amount of resistance would be high enough for your muscles to even be aware of it. A level of resistance high enough to be noticed by your muscles would crush your bones." The last part of a leg press (or squat) has no value and should be terminated approximately 15° short of a 'lockout.'

Figure 2 shows that the quadriceps muscle receives only a limited-range benefit from compound movements. An important part of the muscle that kicks in only near a position of full extension (left side of chart) is ignored. Full-range, front-thigh strength requires full-range leg extension exercise - currently being "avoided like the plague."

Rehab experts falsely believe that leg extensions expose kneecaps to high compression forces when legs are straight (forces are higher when legs are bent). Sports-performance experts ignore them because of their obsession with movement integration.

Knee stability and the ability to run fast and jump high depend on the strength of the major muscles that cross the knee joint. To maximize performance, exercise them with variable, progressive resistance; isolated, full-range movements; high levels of intensity; and proper form. Then, teach them to work together through proper *skill* training.

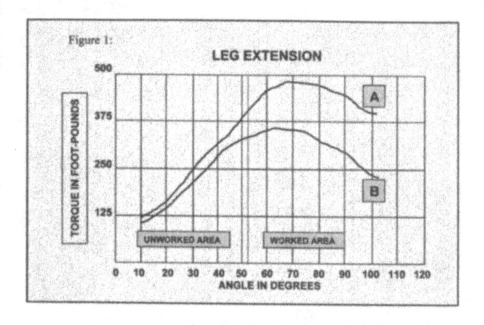

Figure 1:

LEG EXTENSION

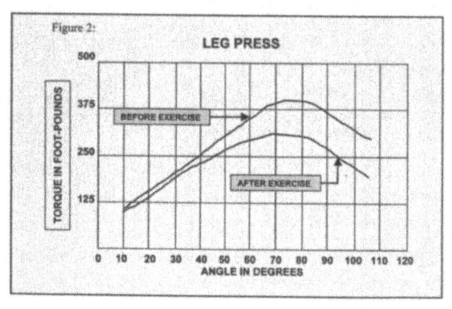

Figure 2:

LEG PRESS

FEBRUARY 29

---

## Seeing Is Not Believing

Some things are hard to take - especially when egos are involved. With 40-years of bodybuilding between them, a pair of orthopedic surgeons from Venezuela visited a gym in New York City in the mid-1970's. It was their first experience with Nautilus® machines and the 'new' system.

Both men were impressive specimens - which probably added fuel to the fire of the trainer, who flattened them in no time - and both emerged with negative opinions. First, they thought the machines put too much stress on muscle tendons, especially in positions of extension. They were accustomed to barbells, which generally do not provide adequate resistance in that position. Second, they found the instructor more interested in the kill than the workout.

He probably was.

Years later, I brought the equipment to their hometown, Caracas, with the intention of providing the same high-intensity training.

I extended an invitation to the two during a round of golf, but my attempt to prod them through a New-York-style workout was a failure. One refused to be pushed and, as I might have expected, wanted to perform additional sets following his so-called effort. The other came up with his own set of excuses - including a list of former injuries - so that he too would be spared.

Nautilus inventor Arthur Jones hosted thousands of athletes and body-builders in Lake Helen (Florida) in the early 1970's and encountered much the same. Most showed up in what they thought was a 'prepared' state.

"Less than two weeks ago," he said, "a former Florida State Powerlifting champion visited our gym for the purpose of training on the new equipment, but then left without doing so. Why? Well, I can't honestly answer that question with any real assurance of accuracy, but I do have an opinion; I think he was totally unprepared for what he saw - mentally unable to accept it. I think it 'blew his mind.' Because, while he was preparing to perform his first set of squats, one of our trainees took 15 pounds more than this recent champion's best lifetime squat weight, and then performed (12) twelve full repetitions with it very rapidly. FULL SQUATS - not half squats or parallel squats - all the way down, buttocks to heels."

The two physicians stayed for the fireworks despite their damp fuses, but they left unimpressed.

Typically, a first glance at something evokes a measure of curiosity and, at the same time, an element of rejection. The machines didn't look or feel like a barbell. Yet, they were nothing more than a thinking man's barbell - a process not often associated with the field of exercise.

Seeing the equipment was not enough. It had to be experienced. The difficulty of each exercise and the non-stop pace from one station to the next made a significant difference in workout intensity, and made believers of most. Yet, speed between exercises didn't matter (and was often not prudent) on the first workout; it only mattered over the long haul as a pre-requisite for reaching strength and size potentials.

I too was flattened on my first exposure to the training system proposed by Jones, and would have met the same fate had barbells been used. We were all unaware of what was meant by 'proper' strength training.

# MARCH

"It is a shame that bodybuilding is wasted on bodybuilders."
Arthur Jones

# MARCH 1

## Intensity vs. Insanity

By the age of "29 and many months," a man earns the right to comment on a glorious past to a trail of closed ears. Let me begin.

When "exercise was exercise" - defined, effective, efficient - it was scorned by the majority who found comfort in the old approach, and embraced only by the few open-minded enough to try something new.

The training system proposed by Nautilus® inventor Arthur Jones in 1970 was unlike anything before, and brutal to the extreme. The many facilities that opened around the country subscribed to the 'new' philosophy by whisking and prodding clients through a brief circuit of hell. It was tough.

As Jones expected, the system was attacked by the 'Master Blaster,' Joe Weider, who assembled a crew of experts to concur that:

- High intensity stressed organs and increased blood pressure to dangerous levels.
- High intensity was too much to sustain for any length of time (intensity should be cycled; high at times, low at others) and dangerous to general health.
- Machine exercise was not as effective as free-weight exercise.

The very people that should have supported any rise in interest in strength training did everything in their power to destroy it - especially if it came from Arthur Jones.

There was a lot at stake.

Jones ignored the accusations and attacks on the premise that nothing could change the facts - *a high level of intensity was required to produce best results from exercise.*

The concept was doomed. Trainees that took on its challenge were unwilling to admit that it was too difficult to do once, let alone for a lifetime. Jones warned that it took weeks, sometimes months, to build the capacity to tolerate what he called "proper strength training" without getting sick.

It was difficult to do, but even tougher to sustain. If you knew you'd be hit with a sledgehammer every time you entered the gym, you wouldn't show up. Most gyms couldn't afford to supervise workouts, and without supervision, intensity and progress came to a halt. The negative attacks, however, did not.

Jones marched on, refining his equipment and discovering parameters that further fueled his search for the truth. More facilities opened but fewer adopted the system or its offspring (super-slow; independent circuits for quick workouts; and women-only areas with downsized equipment). It was too hard for the average Joe.

I did my part by operating a gym that adhered to Nautilus principles in Caracas, Venezuela - machines only (no barbells or dumbbells; no personal training or aerobic classes), 2-3 sessions per week, 12 exercises, one set. The low cost of labor allowed 10-15 trainers on the floor during peak hours. *Every* member was supervised *every* time he or she walked in - no exceptions - for 10 years.

The only problem was the country. Venezuela fell apart in 1982 on accusations of corruption and a false economy. The banks suddenly closed for 20 days. When they reopened, it was never the same - and confirmed my belief that 14 years in Venezuela was 15 too many, a feeling that Jones must have shared from the frustrated tone of his final articles in *Ironman* magazine (1998).

*"My First Fifty Years in the Iron Game,"* as the series was titled, may have been 51 too many.

# MARCH 2

### Chemical Spills and Weapons of Mass Destruction

If 'health' is a state of not being sick, it beats the alternative, a state of non-health. But it's still miserable.

At 14, I decided to run and lift weights three times a week, and not drink alcohol or smoke (neither of which I then did) for the rest of my life. It was a good start, and one I've maintained with minor change: I exchanged running for no-impact cardiovascular exercise and lifted weights only twice a week for better results. I never missed a session the first 15 years - but I missed something.

I failed to appreciate the value of the efforts until a back operation interrupted my attendance. As I shuffled around recuperating, I realized that 'normal' health was lousy. I'd never been there before, and wanted no part of it. The same occurred after a second back operation (two years later) but recovery was quicker. Within months, I was on my way to higher ground.

On both occasions, I was left with the impression that health, to most, was nothing more than not being sick. Being fit enough to enjoy that state was where I wanted to be.

Lack of exercise is miserable, but too much may be worse (in that regard, many trainees are unhealthy). The body is capable of performing any amount of exercise, but cannot recover from the same. In essence, too much exercise can lead to losses instead of gains, and few knew more about that than the Nautilus® inventor.

Arthur Jones had both rights and wrongs in his own exercise regimen (three, 4-hour sessions a week). And while his lack of progress related more to 'amount,' he became aware of another factor - the 'indirect effect' of exercise, that "any growth somewhere produces some growth everywhere." Its magnitude was based on the mass of the muscle involved and its distance from neighbors: The larger the mass and the closer the neighbor, the greater the effect - a chemical spill.

"As a muscle works intensively," he explained, "a chemical reaction occurs that spills over and affects the entire body. Since there is a limit to your overall recovery ability, and since many of the body's chemical functions affect the entire body, it should be evident that training every day is a mistake."

It was also apparent to Jones that the effect was greatest when all major muscles were worked at the same time: "You certainly can build large arms without working your legs - but you will build them much larger, and much quicker, if you also exercise your legs."

Despite the facts, most trainees react to a lack of progress by procuring their own chemicals - supplements and weapons of mass destruction - instead of using their heads.

"Many bodybuilders are perfectly willing," he said, "to take dangerous drugs that they know little or nothing about - simply in an effort to improve their 'recovery ability,' which is the purpose of such drugs; and it never seems to occur to such people that their normal recovery ability would be more than adequate for any amount of possible growth if they didn't waste it performing unnecessary sets and exercises."

The training method Jones introduced provided its own anti-overtraining ingredient - hard work. "Up to this point," he assured, "nobody using this system has actually kidded himself by attempting to overtrain." The intensity was high, as it should be; and workouts, brief. No one wanted to return for days.

Elevate your fitness without living in a gym and begin to enjoy the state of not being sick. You may never go back.

# MARCH 3

## The Triple Whammy

Ellington Darden rushed toward a silent mass of flesh lying face-up on the floor. He touched it - the body was cold, clammy and unresponsive. "He looks dead to me." Suddenly the corpse opened its left eye and smiled. "Arthur wouldn't let me die - at least not until I've finished the workout."

Sergio Oliva, then the largest man in the history of bodybuilding, had just completed a brief cycle of leg exercise - according to Darden, "the most demanding pre-exhaustion routine ever devised by Arthur Jones."

Jones recognized the full squat as the most productive lower-body exercise because of the large-muscle involvement of the thighs, buttocks and lower back. He was also aware that the lower back fatigued long before the thighs had been worked thoroughly. His solution: fatigue the thighs *before* the squat so that the lower back would be temporarily stronger and that failure would more likely occur in the thighs.

First up was a leg press with 480 pounds. Jones demanded 20 reps but Sergio was forced to catch his breath at 17. He slowly squeezed out the remainder. Jones nodded to the spotters (two football players) to rush him to a leg extension loaded with 200 pounds. The goal again was 20 reps but Sergio was ready to pack it in at 10. "Somehow," said Darden, "with Jones hurling insults about his manhood, Oliva managed another seven or eight repetitions." Jones nodded. They rushed Sergio off to a squat rack on thighs that couldn't have made it alone. He barely completed the second and third reps with 420 pounds (he could not perform one rep with 400 pounds three weeks earlier). The goal was 12. Eleven was slow; twelve, even slower; and thirteen, a dead stop. Jones nodded. The spotters removed a few plates and rushed him back in.

"Okay, Sergio, any champion bodybuilder ought to be able to squat with 300 pounds."

He had no choice. Six repetitions, perfect form and then, boom, he hit the floor. Jones allowed a clammy 20-minute rest before starting the upper-body sequence.

Sergio Oliva was famous for the size of his upper body. Two friends of mine, both bodybuilders and physicians, spotted him in 1973 walking the streets of Sabana Grande, a suburb of Caracas, where he was starring in a film called "Black Power" with Venezuelan actress, Lila Morillo. They couldn't believe his size. I later saw the film and his mass was 'beyond belief.' Yet, because of the size of his torso - and the beauty of the actress - few noticed the development of his legs.

The same occurred with three-time Canadian gymnastics champion, Digby Sale (McMaster University, Hamilton, Ontario). No one noticed his legs until the day he entered the weight room with a loose shirt that hid his massive upper body and left his lower extremities exposed from the top of the thigh. They were impressive.

Darden watched Jones put many candidates through the same leg cycle that, properly performed, took less than five minutes, and came up with the following suggestions:

- The routine, at first, will make you nauseous. Take two or three sessions to 'break in.' After four or five, the nausea should disappear.
- Take a five-minute rest after the cycle, before performing upper-body exercise.
- Perform the cycle, at most, twice a week for three consecutive weeks. From there, use it no more than once a week, or once every two weeks.

"Done properly," said Jones, "it is simply too demanding on your overall recovery ability."

## MARCH 4

### On Rest and Recovery

Emil Zatopek didn't fool around when he went out to run. In the late 1940's and early 1950's, the Czech distance runner's daily regimen consisted of sixty 440-yard intervals framed by five 220-yard intervals of warm-up and cool-down. He timed each phase and never missed a day, including the day before an important meet. Called the "Iron Man" by his peers, his work ethic was the exception, not the rule.

But even the best go down.

Two weeks before the 1950 European Championship, Zatopek was hospitalized with a serious stomach ailment. For 14 days, he lay bedridden and untrained. His doctors grew annoyed with his impatience and determination to run. Within an hour of his discharge, he was on a plane to Brussels. The rest is history.

Zatopek almost lapped the second place finisher in the 10,000 meters and won the 5,000 meters by an astonishing 23 seconds. Distance historian Peter Lovesey called the performance "the most decisive double long-distance victory in any major international championship."

Was Zatopek that much better than his competitors, or did they simply have a bad day? Was it a fluke, or was the prolonged bed rest a blessing?

Many coaches and runners believe that everyday training is a 'must' for optimal performance, that continuous hard work is the only way to achievement. The same sentiment is embraced in the world of strength training and bodybuilding where most trainees perform far too much exercise and don't allow sufficient recovery time between sessions. As such, their rate of improvement suffers.

According to Dan Riley, strength coach of the NFL Washington Redskins, "Exercise is performed to stimulate an increase in fitness. If an athlete overloads the muscles properly and allows adequate time to recover, he should stimulate such an increase (regardless of how small) each and every workout. If an increase is not recorded, the athlete is performing too much exercise, not allowing adequate time to recover, or not properly overloading the muscles involved."

Riley was highly influenced by the Nautilus® inventor, who advocated the same in the early 1970's. Arthur Jones typically reviewed the exercise regimen of a bodybuilder and, without regard for its content, drove him to a hotel on a remote beach where the only "iron" was in the tap water. Days later, he brought the victim in to train.

One candidate, Chuck Amato (Mr. Oregon), regularly performed 60 sets of biceps curls during each of his workouts with "no results in several years." Using Jones' system, he increased the girth of his upper arm 13/16ths of an inch after five workouts in 10 days. The arm portion of each session lasted seven minutes, 20 seconds and included biceps, triceps and forearms (front and back). The spectacular result was due to intensity of work and adequate recovery between sessions.

Jones used similar tactics for those who prolonged their stay. When training reached a plateau, he always trimmed the *amount* of exercise performed and increased the intensity of what was left. In doing so, he produced results that were superior to that of anything that had gone before.

Research at the University of Florida recently confirmed the same - that less exercise produced more results. The formula is simple: **Hard Work + Rest = Success.**

Be forewarned - less exercise is *not* the "easy" way out.

## MARCH 5

---

### What Next?

It was one of those 'female' things in 1901 - the selection of attire for an outing - and a long skirt seemed a poor choice as Annie Taylor climbed into the metal-framed wood barrel. Two friends sealed the lid, forced air in with a bicycle pump to 30 psi., rowed it out to a swift current and cut the rope. The plunge over the falls was only minutes away. Below, in the roaring surge of Niagara, a crew waited to rescue the remains.

"There it is," hollered a man pointing to an object bobbing like a cork in the foam. The crew scrambled to fetch it and popped the lid as quickly as they could. Annie stumbled out, roughed up but alive. It was little more than a bad hair day.

Daredevils and inventors are alike - their wheels constantly turn. One involves a risk to the very life the other is trying to improve. Such was the case with Arthur Jones.

In his youth, the Nautilus® inventor "designed, built and tested damned near anything possible just short of a nuclear submarine" and tinkered with his major interests - filmmaking, flying and exercise - without risk to life, almost. "I've spent a good deal of my life avoiding danger," he said. "Any time you've looked out the plane window and seen an engine burning off the wing, you've had all the adventure you want."

In the late 1940's, Jones befriended Percy Cunningham, an American Airlines® pilot, while training at a YMCA gym in Tulsa, Oklahoma. "With the money for the required materials being supplied by Percy (a total cost of $9)," he said, "I then built the first serious attempt in the direction of what eventually lead to Nautilus machines; a machine that was suppose to provide direct, full-range exercise for the large muscles of the back. During the next 20 years, I designed and built later versions in Oklahoma, Louisiana, Texas, Florida, New York, Mississippi, Mexico, Colombia, Singapore, Africa and several other places. Everywhere I went I built one or more new versions. And none of them satisfied me. All had problems that I did not then understand and thus could not solve."

Jones eventually solved those problems and moved on to a greater challenge - the construction of a strength-testing tool, starting with the knee. His efforts soon exposed seven problems "related to the introduction of errors into positional measurements."

In his first prototype (1972), the double chain he used (rated for continuous high-speed use with a load of 7,200 pounds) wasn't sturdy enough to resist the torque of a strong man. It stretched under load, changing the position of measurement by as much as 30 degrees. In later prototypes (1973 and 1975), Jones had such little confidence in his measurements that he refused to publish the otherwise excellent results.

"Some of the things I tried actually did produce at least some of the results I was seeking, but most of them failed, sometimes miserably, often painfully."

Twenty years later, he solved the final problem related to the knee machine.

"Primarily, that is how you learn," he said, "from your mistakes. When something fails, it should get your attention, and that should lead to a careful examination of the situation, which sometimes leads to a solution; but when something appears to work, then you believe you already know the answer and quit looking; which is usually a mistake, because even when something appears to work, we usually give the credit to the wrong factor, seldom really understand the actual cause and effect relationship."

Jones once build a non-nuclear submarine (fortunately, Annie was long gone) which he described as "a bit short of a success, it went down like a rock but did not come up worth a damn. Fortunately, the guy who tested it was good at holding his breath."

## MARCH 6

### Anybody Out There?

Education is one of the greatest gifts anyone can pass on to the next generation. Unfortunately, the relay requires someone at the other end.

Years ago, I was invited to address five 'fitness' classes at a new high school in Royal Palm, Florida. The physical education teacher who invited me wanted her students to hear the basics of proper strength training from someone with the same philosophy.

The setting was spacious, airy and new - that's where it ended.

When the bell rang, a group of 10th graders trudged in looking as if they might not make it to their desks. Most dropped their gear, plunked arms on a desktop and cradled their weary heads. There was little interest in the 'special guest.'

I narrated a series of slides selected from the presentation I made to gym members. When the lights went out, so did eyes. I strengthened my resolve and upped the volume to no avail. Stimulating a discussion was like milking a bull.

At the bell, a second group entered with the same energy. I jazzed up my delivery and added stories about athletes and Arnold Schwarzenneger - again, to no avail.

By the end of five classes, I could have won the National Speech Contest. Yet, the most I could squeeze from my audience was two questions: "Where do you work?" and, "How much can you bench press?"

Formal education is not the ticket to success for everyone, but education is. Nautilus® inventor Arthur Jones didn't have much of the former - he was busy running away from home. His first escape occurred at the age of eight and he was "rather successful at it by the age of eleven...(and) gone most of the time from eleven (through) fourteen." It didn't mean that he was uneducated.

At the age of five, he could read the newspaper in English and German (and became "reasonably fluent in eight languages.") By 10, he had read his father's entire medical library. By 12, he built a working machine gun, and by 14, "had visited every state in this country, parts of Mexico, Canada and British Honduras, hitch-hiking, riding freight trains and tramp steamers; working where and when (he) could find work of any kind."

"I am driven," he said, "always have been - by curiosity. Yes, I hated school but I loved to learn. Asking 'WHY' has been central to my constitution. And I don't quit until I discover what I seek to discover."

According to Jay Block, Jones did four things that all inventors do to become successful: (1) He envisioned the end before he began; (2) He had the insight and courage to scrap all previous assumptions and 'go back to scratch;' (3) He made key adjustments along the way (by changing his approach); and (4) He studied and learned more and more - self-education - and used that knowledge to create his breakthrough. "Success," suggested Block, "is largely a matter of hanging on long after others have let go," or as Jones put it, "There are no such things as unrealistic goals, just unrealistic timetables."

When Vince Gironda first saw an early prototype of Jones' work in 1970, the 'Iron Guru' saw more than a machine - but he may have been alone. "After listening to 10 or 12 conversations between Art Jones and bodybuilders who were asking questions about his equipment," he said, "I discovered that the two major questions in all of their minds were the same, because they obviously did not understand the basic principles behind this equipment. They asked, 'Does it work?' and 'Who have you turned out?'"

Sounds like, "Where do you work?" My return to formal education is on hold.


## MARCH 7

---

### Squats – Part 1

A pair of two-pronged, hole-infested steel columns supported by a cross-frame crept upward from the floor. Fortunately, the demand for use was low. When the squat rack was loaded, the pins that supported the weight somehow held.

The workout room at college was so small that few could find it. Fewer cared. Nobody lifted weights back then, which was both good and bad.

With everything set, I dislodged the bar from its pins and shifted back until it clanged the frame behind. Head up, chest out, feet forward, down I went to the sound of scraping metal. Slowly I touched my butt to a chair, thighs parallel to the floor. Then up, and down and up - 10 times with 240 pounds.

I added 20 pounds at a time and repeated the same until I reached 320. The process was difficult and dangerous, but my legs were the strongest they would get. As Nautilus® inventor Arthur Jones said, "You cannot hunt elephants without running at least some risk of getting stomped by an elephant."

Squats are, by far, the most productive exercise for the lower body. Because of the muscle mass involved, they also provide great 'overall' stimulation. But they are not without concerns, and one relates to depth.

"The danger in a full squat, a low squat," says Jones, "is not a result of the position of your legs in relation to your torso. The danger is a result of the direction from which the force is imposed." The force is trying to bend the bones of your lower leg and pull your knee apart - the same as a leg extension. Although the direction of force is worse in a leg extension, the amount of force is greater in a squat. Results are about the same.

Nevertheless, Jones had trainees and bodybuilders perform squats to a level where their thighs, in photographs, were below parallel to the floor. According to Ellington Darden, who worked for Jones, "Squats should be carried to a point where the thighs first start to contact the backs of the calves. At that point, the squat should be stopped by muscular action instead of by bouncing the thighs off the calves. Performed in the correct manner, there is no danger to the knees. On the contrary, squats can do more to prevent knee injuries than any other barbell exercise."

A slow, controlled speed is more important than depth. Why then, you might ask, are parallel squats (rather than full squats) included as one of three basic lifts in competition? Easy. Heavy power-lifters have trouble getting their thighs parallel to the floor because of leg thickness, and speed of movement is difficult to control with heavy weights.

If you have 'concerns' about squats, try the following:

- Use a device (such as a Smith Machine) that allows you to bail out when needed.
- Pre-exhaust your thighs, then squat with approximately 50% of your normal weight. "Your muscles don't know how much weight you are using," said Jones. "If the weight is enough to require a maximum output on the part of your muscles, that is all that is required - whether this is two ounces or two tons is of no slightest importance insofar as building muscular size and/or strength is concerned."
- Increase your repetition guideline to 15-20, using less weight.
- Move at a slow speed. Joints are not damaged by normal movements or by speed of movement alone, but by sudden changes in speed of movement.
- Pause briefly at the bottom of the squat; don't lock your knees or linger at the top.
- Perform squats early in the routine to maximize control and overall stimulation.

## MARCH 8

---

### Squats – Part 2

Arthur Jones was rarely satisfied with his accomplishments in the field of exercise.

In November of 1970 he wrote an article in *Ironman*, "The Final Breakthrough," that signaled the end of a quest to build a machine more productive than squats. In May of 1971, he wrote a sequel in which he claimed the new machine "will certainly become one of the most important contributions to physical training within this century, and perhaps literally for all time. And if you think otherwise - then attack it with all due vigor; but I clearly warn you in advance, any such efforts would be better directed towards an attempt to tear down the pyramids with your bare hands."

As sure as he sounded, Jones wasn't satisfied. He failed to market the machine along with its advanced versions used in the 'The Colorado Experiment' (1973) and 'Project Total Conditioning' (US Military Academy, West Point, 1975). By 1982, it was ready.

"Solving the problems involved in designing a proper squat machine," he said, "has a great deal in common with flying a helicopter...it looks easy until you try it, but...it is just damn near impossible. If the passengers in a helicopter could read the mind of a pilot then there would be very few passengers, and no sane ones at all."

Some of the issues he faced included the following:

- The large amount of weight required for the quantity of major muscles involved.
- The magnitude and direction of force on the knee and spine.
- The unique pattern (variation) of resistance required. "In a squat, the proper resistance must start fairly high, go down as you approach the so-called sticking point, and then increase rapidly when the sticking point is passed."
- The design of the movement-arm. The movement of the weight during a squat formed an approximate straight line, although the 'straight' movement was a result of rotational movement around three joints: the ankle, knee and hip.
- The proper transmission of the torque of the movement-arm to the weight stack
- Getting the weight to the top of the lift at the start and finish (an entry/exit issue). As he put it, "Blood does not make a satisfactory lubricant, particularly your own. Which point you may learn very quickly if you ever find yourself stuck in the low position of a deep squat with a 500 pound barbell on your shoulders."

Jones varied the resistance on his new device by using a 'negative' cam. Instead of altering the torque by changing the radius as in a normal cam (larger radius = greater resistance), the negative cam maintained a constant level of torque while changing the force in inverse proportion to the radius (smaller radius = greater resistance). In plain English, it converted a 510-pound weight stack to a 1,174-pound force toward the end of the squat, which, in turn, meant work for the muscles that stabilize the knee.

He then solved the problems (inherent in a squat) of stretching the knee and bending the leg bones by imposing the forces in line with the lower leg, which allowed a safe, unlimited range of motion. The exercise was performed one leg at a time (two-leg and akinetic exercise were options), which allowed safe entry and exit in the mid-range of motion and reduced spinal compression...and I emphasize reduced.

I purchased a Duo-Squat Machine when it first came out - it didn't take long to appreciate Jones' input. The exercise was brutal with a challenging weight, but tough on the spine. An upright seat on a later version better deflected the compression force.

If you ever get the opportunity, try one for the ride of your life.

## MARCH 9

### Bu...Bu...Bu...Benny and the Jets

Eighteen was never enough. With a few beers down the hatch and loose lips flying, the entourage stormed from the clubhouse to prepare the carts for battle. Bets were on.

First up, a PGA Tour player with a red nose and cheeks followed by 10-15 opponents led by a man named 'Benny.' Off they drove, down the hill to the fairway that led to the first hole - one group, a dozen carts. When Bobby Mitchell came home, the Glen Oak Country Club in Danville, Virginia was lawless.

Bobby was home only a few times a year - a time to celebrate and a chance to make a buck. He played the 'best-ball' of a group of low-handicap cronies and spotted 'The Jets' one shot per nine. At that, Bobby still had the upper hand.

Too much of anything can lead to problems. Too many rules can create insurrection. Too much golf can erode skill. Too many beers can increase bravado. Too much exercise can lead to atrophy, which is only half the issue in that arena.

With exercise, it's either feast or famine. Most people are turned off by the gym scene, afraid of the 'look' it creates (a false impression), or just lazy. Those lured in are buoyed by their heroes - the biggest guys in the gym - to do stupid things in excess.

It doesn't have to be that way.

In 1970, Nautilus® inventor Arthur Jones introduced logic into training by seeking middle ground. Intensity had to be high - "Work of normal intensity is incapable of producing high levels of muscular ability regardless of the 'amount' of such work" - but amount had to be low. "A pilot should understand," he said, "that increasing his cruising speed by as little as five percent may require increasing his power output (and fuel consumption) by as much as 100 percent -

and that doing so will obviously reduce his range (flight distance); and a weight-trainee is faced with much the same situation, but with a difference - inducing growth-stimulation requires maximum-possible power production (intensity), which will unavoidably 'reduce the range,' make long workouts literally impossible."

Sessions had to be infrequent. "Muscles are capable of recovering from work carried to the point of exhaustion in a very short period of time - but in order to make such rapid recovery, muscles must make demands upon the system as a whole, and THE SYSTEM CAN NOT RECOVER QUICKLY." Jones advocated a 48-hour rest between workouts and added, "It really doesn't matter 'why' high-intensity exertion is required to induce muscular growth or exactly 'how' this is brought about. It is equally unimportant for us to understand the actual reasons for the limitations in our recovery ability. But it is necessary to know that hard work is required, and that recovery ability is limited."

He also came up with a practical method of determining a state of 'overtraining.' "Once properly conditioned, an athlete should be able to complete a hard workout," he said, "and then, after not more than thirty minutes rest, go through the entire workout again at the same pace without reducing his number of sets, number of repetitions, or number of exercises, and without reducing the amount of resistance by more than five percent. If he cannot do so, then he is overtraining; overtraining insofar as the 'amount' of exercise is concerned - not insofar as the 'intensity of effort' is concerned."

The golf bet that day was a way to attain middle ground. To make it fair, right-handed Bobby Mitchell played left-handed. As Jones often said, "Some can, and some cannot."

Seek middle ground with the 'amount' you train and re-discover your potential.


## MARCH 10

---

### When Bigger is Better

I once volunteered to dismantle a Nautilus® multi-station exercise machine, which resulted in a 10-hour day, a near-broken window and a bruised finger. The machine had a lot in common with the football player that helped. The larger it was, the longer it took to go around. The heavier it was, the tougher it was to move - which helps rationalize the protruding guts on some of our so-called athletic heroes.

Look at a football player's arms. A 300-pound lineman has large, smooth arms with no definition, while a 220-pound receiver has smaller, more defined arms. Then listen to the crap about their speed. Simply put, fat men don't run fast, as fast as they could. Nor, according to Arthur Jones, do they perform to their potential.

"Paul Anderson (weightlifter) is certainly strong," he said, "but he is just as certainly too fat - he would perform better with less fat, whether he is aware of it or not. Your car may run well with the trunk full of sand - but it will run better without the sand."

Jones found similar misconceptions in the field of bodybuilding, beginning with the common practice of 'bulking up' (eating as much as possible and performing a reduced amount of heavy exercise for large muscle groups). He agreed with a reduction in training for most and with heavier exercise in general, but not with increasing the amount of food. Extra calories are always stored in the form of fatty tissue.

"In spite of great evidence to the contrary," he said, "there are still those, including well-known top bodybuilders, who believe that the maximum in muscular size cannot be reached without a resulting loss in definition, which, of course, is utter nonsense."

He proved his point with a subject named Casey Viator.

In 1969, Viator trained under the tutelage of former Mr. America, Red Lerille, for the Mr. USA contest, in which he placed respectably. When he won the 1970 title in spectacular fashion, Lerille, a contest judge, commented on Viator's improved definition, thinking he was "smaller" than in the Mr. America competition two months prior. But he was wrong. Viator was 12 pounds heavier, with arms larger by a half inch. According to Jones, who was then training Casey, Lerille "would not have believed that Casey could improve that much in a year if he hadn't seen it personally."

A competitor asked Jones how much more weight he thought Casey could gain without losing his definition. He replied 20-30 pounds with an increase in definition, at which the man implied Jones was a fool. "So long as additional weight (bulk) is added in the form of an increase in muscular tissue, rather than intramuscular or subcutaneous fatty tissue," said Jones, "then such an increase in size will actually increase the existing degree of definition, literally must make the individual more defined."

Viator won the 1971 Mr. America contest in record fashion, weighing 218 pounds, but Jones wasn't satisfied. "I wanted him to weigh-in at the Mr. America at a bodyweight close to 240 pounds...and I think he could have done so, if I had actually trained him during the entire period while he was in Florida."

Then, as now, most trainees lacked the genetics and the concepts of proper training to gain 30 pounds without becoming 'over fat.' So, why do football coaches ask players to put on 30 pounds? And why should athletes be forced to add body fat when it only hinders their speed and ability to circumvent an overweight coaching staff in order to reach the field in time to avoid a 'delay of game' penalty?

It's time to control intake and be an example, rather than part of the problem.

## MARCH 11

### What Started It All

The growing use of fast speeds of movement during progressive resistance training is not substantiated by research. Nonetheless, the trend has brought to light 'the grandfather of research studies' published by Moffroid and Whipple in the *Journal of the American Physical Therapy Association* in 1970 - the one that started it all.

In that study, one group of subjects trained on an isokinetic knee-extension machine at a high intensity and slow speed (36° per second). A second group trained at what was called a fast speed of movement, 108° per second (limbs are capable of speeds in excess of 1,000° per second). A third group tested before and after the training period but did not exercise. At six weeks, all subjects were tested for strength gains in a static fashion, and at six different speeds ranging from 18°-108° per second.

The authors concluded that training at a fast speed produced strength gains at all tested speeds, whereas training at a slow speed produced strength gains only at slow tested speeds. The results have been cited thousands of times as evidence that strength training should occur at fast speeds and with low intensity.

Not so fast.

The data from the study was examined using 'analysis of variance' instead of 'analysis of covariance' (which statistically equates the groups on pre-test data so that post-test data can be accurately compared) and does not support the conclusion. In review, proper analysis demonstrates that the slow group produced the only statistically significant strength gains of the study - nearly twice that of the fast group - at two lower speeds. Where the fast group out-gained the slow, the difference was not statistically significant, and could not be attributed to the training method.

Since 1970, exercise literature has been flooded with hundreds of isokinetic studies suggesting the same - that fast movements are superior to slow for the production of force. The flood caught the attention of coaches and athletes searching for ways to recruit the powerful fast-twitch muscle fibers during athletic performance. Years later, the work of Nautilus® inventor Arthur Jones, backed by research at the University of Florida, clearly demonstrated that isokinetic technology, the only thing available then, was dangerous, inaccurate and misleading.

According to Michael Wolf, Ph.D., "It is the intensity that determines which and how many muscle fibers will be used. There is no evidence that the speed of contraction determines fiber recruitment. In other words, the brain recruits muscle based on how much force the muscle must create, and not on how fast it must contract."

Despite the facts, ignorance and poor research have led to an epidemic that has already become 'tradition' in many sports applications.

Our gym recently introduced a program designed to teach athletes to run faster, the "Frappier Acceleration Program." The staff - all graduates in exercise science - is 'certified,' but I can't bear to look. Most of what they do ignores physiology, common sense, laws of physics and, while not life-threatening, poses a threat to athletic careers.

*No valid research* shows that fast repetitions in the gym produce speed on the field. On the contrary, the slower you move during exercise (the best way to gain strength), the faster you'll be on the field. Fast repetitions produce nothing but injury.

As Jones once commented on the 'closed' nature of the medical community in regard to muscle testing, "An open mind is not the same as an empty head."

## MARCH 12

### Power Production

The practice of developing 'explosive power' by moving quickly against resistance has become the gold standard in sports performance programs. Is it valid, or safe?

Arthur Jones stressed the importance of "power production" in his early Nautilus® bulletins when he said, "Demands for work inside the existing levels of reserve ability can only be produced by forcing a muscle to produce more power - by lifting more weight the same distance in the same length of time, or by lifting the same amount of weight a greater distance in the same length of time, or by lifting the same weight the same distance in less time."

Although no one knew much about speed of movement during exercise at the time, physics dictated that more speed was more power. It was different at ground level.

"In general, speed of movement should always be as great as possible," said Jones. "But in practice, this does not mean that the actual movement will be very fast - because if resistance is as high as it should be, then maximum possible speed of movement may in fact be quite slow."

Speed created problems with form and safety. Its application had to be 'timed.'

"Maximum-possible strength-size," he said, "absolutely can be produced without ever producing maximum power - even though maximum power production is a requirement for maximum growth-stimulation, and there is no paradox involved; for maximum growth-stimulation, it is only necessary to produce the momentarily maximum-possible amount of power - and this can be done (and should be done) only after the momentary ability has been reduced by the performance of at least three immediately-preceding repetitions that did not involve maximum power production."

Accordingly, any attempt at maximum speed should occur at the end of a set when fatigue is too great to produce much of any speed. Its application is dangerous at the start because muscles have the potential to produce high forces when fresh, and any such increase results in geometrical increases in the strain imposed on connective tissues, whose ability to resist is less than a muscle's ability to increase strength. Fortunately, the connective tissue's resistance to strain remains constant during exercise.

Jones believed that "mass - the actual size - of a muscle clearly indicates (and limits) its ability to produce power." And since size is related to strength, the key to producing power lies in strengthening the muscles involved.

Yet, what do we see in sports performance programs? Explosive movements from the first rep, speed at the expense of form and resistance, momentum that limits the potential for full-range strength and, last but not least, the alleged measurement of such nonsense.

An article in the Summer 2002 issue of *Frappier Acceleration* unveiled an equipment breakthrough that quantified power during the performance of plyometric leg presses. It measured peak torque and fatigue rates over a 30-second interval but failed to identify which muscles made what contribution to the outcome. It also ignored factors that greatly affect the output of dynamic tests such as muscle friction, gravity and impact forces.

To improve power, isolate and strengthen each muscle involved using a repetition scheme suited to its fiber type. Then plug the new values into simultaneous, but separate, skill training. You can't strengthen movement patterns, but you can strengthen the muscles that produce them - and measure their progress by static, isolated testing.

Anything else is a step in the wrong direction.


## MARCH 13

---------------

### Recovery From Exercise

Rather than pound shoes on the pulpit, he rolled up his sleeves. Nautilus® inventor Arthur Jones believed that failure to progress in exercise was related to one of two things - or both: lack of stimulus, or lack of full recovery. In the first case, the solution was 'harder' exercise, taking muscles beyond fatigue; in the second, less exercise per workout and fewer sessions. Sometimes it wasn't enough.

'Muscle' and 'system' recovery are not necessarily related. That is, a fully recovered muscle may have little or no bearing on the status of the system, and a recovered system does not ensure the recovery of muscles. With nothing more than a training log and subjective feelings to gauge systemic recovery, Jones set out to discover the nature of muscle response to exercise.

Figure 1 demonstrates the results of three strength tests of the isolated muscles that extend the lumbar spine. The highest curve (#1) shows a subject's fresh strength; the lowest curve (#2), his strength following an exercise that was considered light (200 foot-pounds for 6 repetitions) and not continued to failure. The other top curve (#3) features his strength four hours after the first test - in essence, his recovery.

Based on the difference between curve #1 and #3, the subject recovered 99.79% of his fresh strength, with the greatest deviation in flexion (right side of chart) at 4.9%.

Figure 2 shows the addition of a recovery test taken two days later, the lowest of the top curves (#4). The subject's fresh strength had declined by 3% throughout the range of motion, a fact that Jones (who tested the subject more than 100 times) knew was unrelated to error or daily variation. It was this subject's individual recovery pattern.

"Tested at a fresh level of 100, then exercised lightly and re-tested for remaining strength," said Jones, "he will show a remaining level of about 45. Tested for recovery five hours later he will show a level of 100. Tested two days later he will show a level between 96 and 97. A week following the initial tests he will again show a level of 100; and two weeks after the first tests he will show a level of 110."

The muscle would then be ready for further stimulation.

Figure 3 shows a three-part recovery test taken one hour and 26 minutes after the initial test (same subject, weeks earlier). This time, the exercise was heavy (800 foot-pounds for 8 repetitions) and continued to a point of failure. Recovery (#3) was incomplete. At 24°, fresh strength was within 1% of its original value (#1), but not close in extension and flexion. This was a universal phenomenon, not an individual pattern. "Recovery from exhaustion is selective in nature," said Jones, "the midrange of motion regains its level of fresh strength faster than the flexed and extended positions."

The graphs demonstrate several additional points. The exhausting exercise in Figure 3 produced a strength loss of 67.3%. Yet, the easier task in Figures 1 and 2 produced a loss of approximately 55%. The greater-than-average 'effect' of both exercises indicates a high percentage of fast-twitch fibers in the muscles. The subject cannot tolerate much exercise, even if it is light. And the fact that he appears to recover completely in five hours is not the entire story.

The data provided by recovery tests should help therapists and trainers determine an appropriate protocol for exercise, with one caution. Chronic pain subjects may not tolerate a recovery test that soon after exercise.

One question remains. What happens to recovery when you add 10 other exercises?

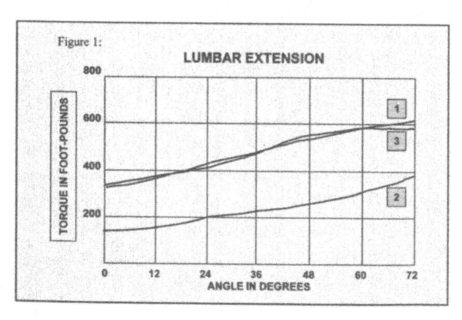

Figure 1:

LUMBAR EXTENSION

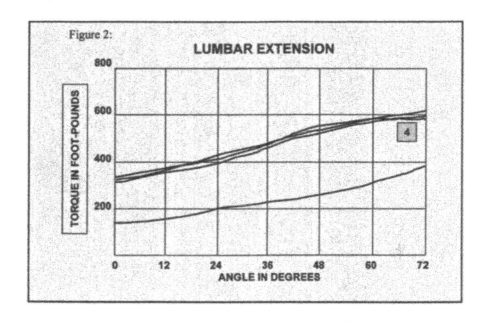

Figure 2:

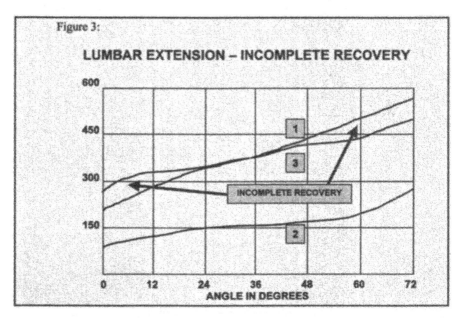

Figure 3:

## MARCH 14

---

### Blisters and Calluses

"I'm the only man on the planet that can hit a golf ball straight every time I swing at it," declared the man on the practice tee. "That's not my opinion. It's the opinion of the people that have seen me. I'm going to hit 400 balls this afternoon. If you see a crooked one, tell me," he said as he scanned the crowd, "...because you won't."

From pitching wedge to driver, shots pumped off the face of his clubs faster than sweat from his pores. Every shot was a carbon copy of the one before - long and straight, mostly straight. Ironically, the introverted Canadian was at his best on stage - and today would be no exception.

"How did you get so good," hollered a spectator.

"I hit 800 balls a day for 40 years. That helps."

According to his book, *The Feeling of Greatness*, Moe Norman practiced until his hands were covered in blood. He then doused them in cold water or wrapped them in damp towels that he later discarded to the ire of the pro-shop staff. Moe learned early that hitting too many balls produced a negative effect - including in a way he never imagined. It built his grip strength to a level that discouraged anyone from shaking his hand. As PGA pro Ted Kroll described, "It would take about a week to recover (from Moe's handshake)." His calluses were so thick he had to shave them with a razor.

Physiologists call the development of a callus 'overcompensation.' If you repeatedly expose a body part to an abrasive object, the thickness of the skin may not be sufficient to protect it. With overcompensation, the body replaces the normal thickness of the skin that was reduced by the pressure of the object, and then overcompensates by adding extra tissue in the form of a callus.

The body develops a callus in the exposed area *only as long as the conditions are right*. For that, the work must conform to the following:

- Be *hard* enough to stimulate the growth of a callus, but...
- Not reach an *amount* that will prevent growth or create a blister.

In essence, no amount of gentle rubbing will stimulate growth. But if you rub your hand once, hard, with a file and repeat it every 48 hours, a callus will begin to form immediately and grow quickly to great thickness. If you rub your palm too many times or too often, no callus will result because the rubbing removes the overcompensation tissue at a rate faster than it can be supplied.

Muscle growth takes place in the same way. While part of such growth is normal, growth beyond that point must be stimulated. Extra growth *will not occur* unless it is signaled by heavy demands on the existing levels of muscular size resulting from natural growth. And it *cannot occur* unless the recovery ability of the system is able to compensate at the same time. If the system's recovery ability has been depleted in efforts to compensate, no energy is available for the overcompensation that can produce greater-than-normal growth.

Most bodybuilders exhaust the majority, if not all, of their recovery ability due to the amount of training they perform, making growth impossible. Besides that, they seldom train hard enough to stimulate overcompensation, so that little or no growth can occur (even if their system is capable of overcompensation).

Repetition may be required in a high-skill sport like golf, but it doesn't work with the physical demands of strength training.

## MARCH 15

### Beyond Failure

I never thought I would encourage athletes to fail - especially as a former coach - but I did. According to 'experts,' it was an absolute requirement for success. One of those advocates was Arthur Jones.

"If you do 10 repetitions of an exercise when you could have done 12," said the Nautilus® inventor, "you may as well stay in the parking lot. You'll get *nothing* from strength training." Jones knew the value of intensity and was driven to make exercise harder, to take exertion to failure...and beyond.

One method he used to take muscles beyond the point of no longer being able to *lift* a weight was to fatigue them until they could no longer *lower* a weight. His quest was paralleled by the work of Scandinavian physiologist, Paavo Komi who claimed the "superiority of eccentric conditioning (lowering weight) over concentric (lifting) or isometric (static) conditioning to improve muscle strength" (*Ergonomus*, 1972).

Both Jones and Komi believed that lowering weights to fatigue provided an increased loading tension, and sent a stronger signal to the body.

Jones put his belief into action with pure "negative only" exercise (no lifting). Several assistants raised the weight and passed it to a trainee who then lowered it from a contracted position in 10 seconds. They lifted, he lowered, until the descent occurred in less than three seconds - the definition of muscle failure when lowering. The technique was effective but not without problems: The resistance became so heavy that spotters could not get close enough to the weight to lift and transfer it safely.

Jones introduced an alternative called "negative emphasis" training. In this method, a trainer helped lift the resistance only when fatigue was evident (in the final repetitions) and then pushed against the movement arm as it lowered. It was difficult to measure progress because the *amount* of push could not be gauged.

Jones eventually came up with a third approach - "negative accentuated" exercise - that required no assistance. Using approximately 70-80% of the normal weight, a trainee lifted with two limbs, paused in the contracted position, transferred the weight to one limb and lowered in 10 seconds. He then lifted the weight with both and lowered with the opposite limb, until the weight could no longer be lifted.

Besides techniques, Jones introduced equipment that allowed the performance of negative-only work *without* help. His Omni-Biceps and Omni-Triceps machines (1972) had foot pedals that lifted the movement arm to a contracted position from where it could be lowered with the arms. His Multi-Exercise machine featured three steps in front of an adjustable chin-up/dip station. Trainees walked to the top, placed their chin over the bar, removed their feet, lowered in 10 seconds and then walked up quickly for the next descent. Negative chin ups, when performed to failure, were so difficult that Nautilus orthopedic representative, Dr. Michael Fulton once commented, "If I read a trainee's heart monitor from my office, I'd know exactly when he was performing negative chin-ups. His heart rate would be at its maximum."

Negative work was effective, but demanding. After several negative-only studies with bodybuilders and football players in the early 1970's, Jones concluded that best results were achieved by the *infrequent* use of negative exercise. His suggestion: one set of 8-12 repetitions per body part per week.

Muscles worked beyond normal fatigue require more time for recovery.


## MARCH 16

---

### Early Problems...and Solutions

It doesn't really matter that exercise machines - as poor as some are - work muscles harder than barbells. Most trainees aren't willing to work hard. Hand them one or the other and they look for the easy way out.

When the Nautilus® inventor opened his doors in DeLand, Florida (1970), hundreds of bodybuilders left an impression: "Almost without exception," said Arthur Jones, "the bodybuilders of today simply don't know what hard work is - most are convinced that 'more' work equals 'harder' work, and that belief, of course, is ridiculous. Secondly, a very high percentage of them are downright fat; and thirdly, very few are anywhere near as strong as they should be."

Jones directed his efforts toward searching for ways to make exercise harder and trainees stronger. He built machines that enhanced the 'miracle' of the barbell and introduced brief, intense cycles of exercise that, combined, covered the major muscle groups in the same session. It was nothing new.

The so-called 'PHA' system of training (briefly in vogue years before) involved a circuit of non-stop exercise that greatly improved the cardiovascular system. But most bodybuilders saw little value in anything unrelated to building maximum muscle size. "The appearance of great strength," stated Jones, "seems to be of far greater importance than actual strength."

Jones' system had much in common with the 'old' but the cardiovascular result was a mere bi-product. "Maximum-possible increases in muscular size and strength," he said, "literally CANNOT be produced without such cycle training."

'Circuit' or cycle training was the only way to involve a higher percentage of the total number of available muscle fibers without depleting recovery ability. "Performing endless sets is not the answer," he reasoned, "because you are simply working the same few muscle fibers over and over."

In 1971, Jones proposed the following arm cycle: one set (8-10 reps) of standing arm curls "until the bar literally drops out of your exhausted hands;" immediately followed by one set of equally hard pulldowns to the chest on a lat machine (palms-up, close grip); one minute rest; one set of triceps curls (on the lat machine) immediately followed by one set of parallel dips "carried to the point of utter failure;" one minute rest; one set of palms-up wrist curls immediately followed by one set of reverse (palms-down) wrist curls. Rest two or three minutes and repeat the entire cycle.

The combination of arm exercises forced exhausted muscles to work beyond fatigue by calling on fresh muscles to assist in a second effort and "should be performed last - because, if you do it right, you literally won't be able to do anything else afterwards; and if you can do anything else afterwards, then you didn't do it right."

How effective was it? Mr. Oregon pumped his upper arms 1.125" (in 7 min., 20 sec.) during his first workout; 1.5" (in less than 8 min.) during his second; and gained a full half inch to his 'cold' arm measurement only 48 hours after he had arrived.

It leant credence to the question often posed by Jones - "Have you ever passed out cold after three or four exercises for your arms?" - but contributed little to its acceptance.

Circuit training is, by far, the most productive way to train for muscle size, strength and overall condition. Yet, as Jones suggests, "Most people are not really interested in the truth, especially when it leads to unavoidably 'hard' solutions to their problems."

## MARCH 17

---

### There's Push and then There's PUSH

"Sounds like they're trying to kill somebody," I said as the grunts of a scuffle echoed through the building. Three adults vs. one teen did not seem fair, but it was effective. In the end, the kid lay in a heap on the floor in the corner of the room, victim of a high-school football workout at the Nautilus® complex.

It was my first view of what Arthur Jones called "outright hard work" - a routine of 17 minutes and 20 seconds, that, according to one instructor, "would be *less* effective if we added five minutes to it's duration."

Jones was a master motivator. In 1970, he trained bodybuilding hopeful, Casey Viator for five months in preparation for the Mr. America competition. On November 1, he left Viator in the hands of others for the next five months. According to Arthur (and confirmed by pictures), "his muscular size, strength, and degree of muscularity steadily declined." Jones immediately reduced Viator's weekly workouts from six to three, removed half of his exercises, cut the number of sets to one and two, assigned a football player to push him, and then, pushed them both.

In less than a month, Viator's high-repetition leg presses soared from 400 to 750 pounds; his pre-exhaustion squats from less than 400 to over 500 pounds. Said Jones, "He was almost back into the shape that he had attained earlier." Two days before the competition (June 10, 1971), Viator performed the following leg sequence in 3-4 minutes: one set of presses (750 pounds, 20 reps); one set of extensions (225 pounds, 20 reps); and one set of full squats (502 pounds, 13 reps). Every set was carried to "absolute failure" with no rest between movements.

Viator was the youngest in history (at 19) to win the event, and first to win everything - Best Arms, Best Back, Best Chest, Best Legs and Most-Muscular.

Ellington Darden, Ph.D., witnessed the final workout with Dr. Elliott Plese of Colorado State University and remarked, "It would be interesting to know just how much of the results are produced by the machines and how much by Jones' pushing."

"You can't push with a rope," replied Jones, "you must have a pole - regardless of how much I push, the machine must still be able to do the job, otherwise the results would not be produced."

It was only the beginning.

Jones ran the two top professional bodybuilders of the day, Sergio Oliva and Arnold Schwartzenegger through the same circuit. On his first workout, Oliva performed one set of three exercises to exhaustion in less than five minutes - leg press (460 pounds, 17 reps), leg extensions (200 pounds, 16 reps), and squats. On the latter, he collapsed twice with 400 pounds, performed seven repetitions with 300 pounds and then hit the floor for good. When he recovered enough to continue, he completed a 12-minute torso and 7½-minute arm circuit.

"I've often experienced times during a workout where I had difficulty walking," commented Arnold after his ordeal. "But this is the first time that I've ever had difficulty lying down." His normal leg workout was 90 minutes; his torso, two hours.

Personal training could stand a lesson from the past - intensity improves results. Yet, the chance of pushing as many people out of the program as in has led trainers to take a conservative, if not passive approach.

Everyone has to be coaxed, but intensity can't be ignored.


## MARCH 18

---

### Push and Pull

They didn't know what hit them, but they knew it wasn't light. The exercise routine I used for advanced trainees who disregarded what I had to say was 'do-able,' but rather inconvenient. A large carcass can take up a lot of floor space.

It started with a leg press followed by a leg extension on a Nautilus® Compound Leg Machine. The 'animal' instinct of the press allowed the release of the conflictive energy I inspired at the door. It also left trainees dead for the next task - a leg extension after a press is nearly impossible with even 50% of the normal weight. It revealed what I called "character."

The non-stop sequence continued with a prone leg curl immediately followed by a Nautilus Hip and Back machine, a difficult rear hip and thigh exercise. In less than five minutes, the routine had their attention - if they were still around.

From there - and few got beyond *there* - the upper-body sequence was 'push and pull.' One exercise pushed weights from the body; the next pulled weights toward it. It started with an overhead press and proceeded as follows: regular grip chin-ups, chest press, pullover (which is neither push nor pull), behind-the-neck pulldown, dips (positive or negative, depending on the trainee), biceps curls and triceps extensions.

The 'push and pull' workout was tough because it used compound movements and larger numbers of muscle groups. It was also based on sound physiology.

Following an exhaustive exercise, the transport system within a muscle is clogged with waste products. There are three options to assist in the disposal: rest, light exercise for the same muscle, or immediate exercise for an antagonistic (functionally opposite) muscle group.

A muscle begins to rid of waste products if it is allowed complete rest after heavy exercise, but recovers more quickly when it performs 'light' exercise instead. This is why a cool-down is recommended after a workout - movement aids recovery. Performing a light set of triceps exercise between two heavy sets of triceps exercise is effective, but *adds* exercise to the workout. Performing a heavy set of biceps curls between two heavy sets of triceps exercise provides the same low order of triceps work, without adding exercise to the workout. It should be obvious that working biceps and triceps on separate days is a poor style of training - yet a style common among bodybuilders.

To design a 'push and pull' routine, first classify your exercises as *push, pull or neither.* The words 'press' and 'extension' are push movements; 'curl' is a pull. Lifting resistance *from* your center is a push; lifting *toward* it, a pull. The following may help:

- **Push:** Leg Extension, Leg Press, Squat, Hip Extension, Abduction, Calf Raise, Shoulder or Overhead Press, Chest or Bench Press, Dip, Triceps Extension.
- **Pull:** Leg Curl, Hip Flexion, Adduction, Pulldown or Torso Arm, Rowing, Chin-Up, Abdominal Curl or Crunch.
- **Neither:** Pullover, Lateral Raise, Shrug, Chest Fly or Arm Cross, Rotary Torso.

Next, sequence your exercises so that a push is followed by a pull, and vice versa. Exercises that are neither can be sprinkled in to allow arm muscles an occasional 'break.'

Perform one set of 4-6 leg exercises and 6-8 upper-body exercises. The 'rush' factor between movements is not critical in 'push and pull' routines. Therefore, reduce your total training time *gradually* to increase the overall intensity of the workout.

Remember - there's not much floor space left.

## MARCH 19

### For Your Viewing Pleasure

Nautilus® inventor Arthur Jones spent a lifetime searching for ways to make exercise harder and more productive. On many occasions, a single solution would produce more questions than he bargained for, but his response was always the same, "Let's find out." For a man who often gave the impression that he knew something others didn't, Arthur was not afraid to admit that he did not know the answer.

He just didn't *like* to.

His commitment to "what works and what doesn't" resulted in changes that revolutionized the field of exercise...but not everyone saw it that way.

Many detractors and a few supporters tried to match egos with him. Those who refused to acknowledge his efforts reacted as most to innovation: ignore, ridicule, attack, copy, and steal. Others modified things to suit their needs. After all, "What did Jones know that they hadn't already discovered?"

My first Nautilus purchase was shipped to Venezuela where the curiosity of "Where did they come from?" and "How are they used?" soon turned to "How can we make them here?" and "How can we block their import?" Attempts at both were bold, but disastrous. What started out as an *exact* copy of the machines took a turn for the worse when decorative touches and functional modifications were added.

The import issue was handled under the table.

I lacked the arrogance to modify function, but my penchant for 'fiddling' led me to believe that I, too, could make exercise harder.

I started by watching weights go up and down. Every repetition produced a movement of the resistance to a height that varied with the weight itself and with the lifter's anatomy. Heavier weights traveled less distance - less again with shorter limbs, smaller people and certain joint structures. In time, I established a high and low range-of-motion for every exercise that featured a view of the weight stack, and then:

- Placed a series of different-colored, plastic rectangles (approximately ¼ x ½ inch) on one of the tubes that framed the weight stack, and
- Fastened a yellow electrical wire to the top of the weight stack so that it would align with the edge of the rectangles during movement.

The creation provided a height (and color) target per repetition and, more importantly, motivation during final efforts. It also assured an accurate count and served as a speed trap. If movement was too fast, the wire 'bounced' at the top of the lift, and a pause in the contracted position was now beyond dispute. I was adamant about 'slow' - they were lucky I didn't attach it to the fire alarm.

My next project was to time repetitions during negative work on the Nautilus Multi-Exercise machine, where the brutality of chins-ups and dips often resulted in a reduction of the recommended lowering time of 8-10 seconds. To prevent cheating, I attached a large digital timer to the adjustable front bar of the machine. The timer remained the same distance from the trainee during exercise and allowed a normal head and neck alignment throughout. It also provided motivation and assured an accurate speed and repetition count.

Most clients hated the gadgets because they removed the 'fun' from something that was not much fun in the first place. I agreed with them on one thing - it was tough to distinguish colors when your eyeballs were about to explode.


## MARCH 20

------------

### Bannister Rules

Two foursomes milled around the first tee. Sunday morning was a time to get away, to share the camaraderie of golf, to sort the chaff from the bran, bad backs from knees and sleep-deprivation from hangover. It was also a time to set the format for the match, to reinforce the old maxim that "figures lie and liars figure."

It was 'fun' time at the Lagunita Country Club in El Hatillo, Venezuela.

"Caballeros," proclaimed a Doctor who stepped to the fore once things had settled. "Today, we play Bannister rules. Hit from the back tees, no 'mulligans,' no touching the ball ('winter rules' never made much sense down there) and no 'gimmies' - putt everything out."

The gang agreed to what seemed a subtle honor.

The first foursome teed off. I played in the second.

Minutes later, we watched a player putt from 25 feet as we stood in the third fairway waiting for the group ahead to clear the green. The ball remained 'above the sod.' He walked over, bent down, picked it up and put it in his pocket.

"H-h-e-e-y-y," hollered one of my playing partners with a shoulder shrug and two-arm gesture that suggested, 'What are you doing?'

The accused indicated the length of the ball from the hole with his hands - one foot.

My partner threw his arms in the air again, this time using a less distinguished North American gesture that was echoed by the culprit.

It was the end of the 'Bannister' rules.

The Bannister rules of strength training, almost as short-lived, are the same as those introduced by Arthur Jones more than 30 years ago. Without beating a dead horse:

- Limit weekly workouts to three sessions for the entire body.
- Select 12 exercises (4-6 lower body; 6-8 upper body) that involve large muscle groups and full-range motion. Select the toughest ones and perform them in the hardest manner possible.
- Work the large muscles first, the small muscles last.
- Perform one set of each exercise, terminating only when additional movement is impossible. Move quickly from one exercise to another.
- Perform 8-15 repetitions and increase the weight by 5% when 15 is reached.
- Limit the length of each workout to 20-30 minutes. Perform cardiovascular exercise, if you must, *after* strength training.
- Pay attention to style or form. Don't just go through the motions.
- Try to improve in every set of every exercise. Chart progress by comparing weight and repetitions to prior efforts, but don't compare yourself with others.
- Eat a reasonable, balanced diet. The 'amount' is more important than the content.
- And, as Jones suggested, "Avoid so-called 'growth drugs' like the plague."

An upcoming project with a business associate from Venezuela looks interesting. The establishment of medical/exercise centers in Europe and the United States might once again provide trainees the opportunity to exercise the old way with the finest equipment, training methods and proper supervision. Bannister rules.

If Jones had tried to establish guidelines for golf as he did exercise - where myth, fraud and deception ruled - he probably would have played with a machine gun.

## MARCH 21

---

### The Other Gym - Part 1

We are great creatures of habit, but not creatures of great habits.

For as long as I can remember, I have bitten my fingernails and if someone gave me 10 reasons why I shouldn't, I would probably ignore the advice. Habits are hard to break. So, I'm not at all surprised by what I face each day on the exercise floor. Whether through evaluation, observation or in suggesting an alternative, I hear the same thing time and time again, "Oh, that's what they told me in the other gym."

The best I can do is throw in my 50 cents, support it with fact and hope for the best. Some of the common ideas from the 'other' gym include:

- Perform only cardiovascular exercise (for those who are overweight or dislike strength training). Body fat represents stored calories and when calories are burned at a rate that exceeds consumption, weight loss occurs. *Cardiovascular training promotes indiscriminate weight loss (from muscle tissue, organ tissue and fat tissue). It is also three times slower than strength training (at losing body fat), burns fewer residual calories when the body is inactive, results in a loss of strength and flexibility, and increases the chance of injury.*
- Perform strength training and cardiovascular training on separate days (for those who don't want to spend hours at a time in the gym or who choose to workout on a daily basis). *Recovery is a problem with daily training. Every workout stimulates corporal change, a change the body makes the next day - if it can. When the intensity and/or duration of each workout exceeds the body's recovery ability, however, the system cannot respond. Each daily session, whether cardiovascular- or strength-related, interferes with the last. Best results are produced by training both entities on the same day and doing nothing the next.*
- Perform a cardiovascular workout before strength training (suggested as a matter of little importance or to those more interested

in cardiovascular exercise). *Strength training has more potential benefits than cardiovascular conditioning. Warm up for five minutes, train for strength first (while you are fresh) and then perform cardiovascular exercise with whatever energy you have left. And remember, proper strength training includes a cardiovascular benefit.*

- Perform only cardiovascular exercise as a first step toward weight loss. Essentially, burn the extra calories first and then tone up what's left. *Backwards. Exercise is a slow weight-loss solution. Ten sessions on a bike, for example, at 350 calories per session consumes one pound of body fat (chewing a fingernail after will put you about even). Ellington Darden, Ph.D. allows no cardiovascular training during his fat-loss programs (a reduced caloric intake combined with strength training only) because it burns off some of the muscle the program is designed to create. Only when the body reaches its goal does he add cardiovascular exercise.*
- Never straighten or lock your knees during strength training. *Hogwash. Locking the knee ensures full muscle contraction during leg extensions and standing calf raises and a better stretch during leg curls and calf exercise. Knees should remain unlocked during squats, lunges and leg presses because locking allows the muscle to rest (not because of any inherent danger).*

With the dissemination of that kind of information, you'd think the other gym would be empty. Just the opposite - it's full.

## MARCH 22

### The Other Gym - Part 2

At the 'other' gym, they tell trainees what they expect to hear based on trends. Most of the ideas, however, counter both logic and physiology, like the following:

- Train the body in parts for emphasis. *When asked the best way to divide the body into parts for training, my response is standard. "I divide mine in half. Today, I worked my left half; tomorrow, my right." When the laughter subsides, I add, "It's the same dumb thing you're doing." Anything that adds exercise to a training routine is generally a step in the wrong direction. It leads to less inten-*

*sity (just observe those who train every day on a 'split' routine), a state of over-training and turns exercise into a social event. Muscle groups can recover with a few days rest, but the system never gets that opportunity (and the system is what feeds the muscles). Brief, infrequent (2-3 times per week), high-intensity, whole-body workouts are still, by far, the most effective means of providing systemic stimulation and recovery.*

- Spot train for fat loss or perform extra exercise for your problem area(s). *The body cannot lose fat in one area without losing it in all areas. By the time your hips and thighs are up to par, your face may be too thin. Performing extra inner-thigh exercise (for women) or abdominal exercise (for men) is about as effective as performing wrist curls to lose 20 pounds. Small muscle groups do not burn as many calories as large ones during and after exercise. Therefore, strength workouts should include intense exercise for the muscles that send the strongest signal for change - gluteus, front and rear thigh, upper back, chest, shoulders and upper arms. Your stomach will take care of itself without exercise.*

- Performing sets. *If you shot someone between the eyes, would you fill the rest of his body with bullets? Do you continue to crank the key once you've turned on the ignition of your car? Muscle stimulation is much the same. The body's mechanism for change is initiated when the intensity of effort reaches a muscle's threshold of stimulation (a percentage of its momentary ability). Once 'turned on', the muscle needs **no further stimulation**. Recent research at the University of Florida demonstrated that one set of exercise was as effective as three sets for building strength. Twenty years before, Nautilus® inventor Arthur Jones said, "If you are capable of performing a second set, you didn't do the first one right." The intensity of effort triggers the result, and intensity is what most trainees try to avoid. One hard set taken to a point of muscle failure is more difficult than three easier sets. Another reason behind performing multiple sets is to reduce the chance of injury through warm-up. Hogwash. The first few repetitions of an exercise (using a weight you can lift only 10 times), properly performed (slow and smooth), provide a sufficient warm-up for a muscle that has emerged from the deep freeze.*

- Rest between sets. *The issue is not if, but how long. Why rest between efforts when it interrupts workout intensity and frustrates those waiting? If you insist:*

1. *Perform other exercises between sets. Russian research on 'active rest' showed improved recovery when antagonistic muscle groups were worked between sets.*
2. *Time your rest and reduce it to a minimum (muscle recovery is initially rapid).*
3. *Although not as effective because it adds exercise, perform a drop set by lowering the weight at failure and immediately continuing as if it was the same set.*

You came to the gym to work. Rest at home.


## MARCH 23

---

### The Other Gym - Part 3

More sound advice from the 'other' gym:

- Stretch after every exercise. *This is a poor way to rationalize a benefit. Stretching a muscle immediately after a resistance exercise is based on the idea that it is easier and safer to stretch a warm (vs. cold) muscle. But stretching a muscle while it's hot is not more effective or efficient. First, you interrupt the intensity of the workout and negate potential cardiovascular gains by resting after each exercise. Performing 12 exercises in 20 minutes is harder than the same effort in 30 minutes. Second, stretching between exercises adds time to your workout. Recent research demonstrated better strength and flexibility increases when stretching followed the workout. Don't make your gym a second home.*
- Use lighter weights and more repetitions to tone. *The word 'tone' (from tonus, which the Greeks should have changed to a feminine noun) leads to the belief that, through fear or laziness, a large benefit can be derived from a small effort. Toning is as much a waste of time to expose as it is to do. First, most trainees don't have the genetics to make the changes they fear, regardless of what they do. Second, why settle for a little health when you can have a lot - by a slight increase of input? The root of the problem lies in the word 'effort,' something that disappeared with the Greeks.*
- Speed of movement. *Nautilus® inventor Arthur Jones said, "It's impossible to lift weights too slowly." That's all that needs to be said. Yet, it's hard to convince someone in a sport like karate, foot-*

*ball or wrestling that the slower he moves in the gym, the quicker he'll be on the field. The reason? SLOWER IS HARDER, and harder improves strength, cardiovascular response and the body's muscle-to-weight ratio. A loss of body fat reduces friction during movement. More muscle, less friction and only a slight increase in body weight creates speed. When hospitals fill with fast-repetition advocates, someone will finally realize that 1 + 1 = 2.*

- Sport-specific training. *The same quadriceps strength that improves tennis will help soccer, basketball and golf. But, because athletes demand something specific to improve performance in their sport, gyms respond as expected, with something commercial. 'Specificity' is exactly what it implies, specific - the same movement, with the same implement, under the same conditions. Subjecting a muscle to added resistance through a skill movement is more likely to throw the train off the track than add a positive. Because it feels different, the nervous system becomes confused about the path it's supposed to take. The solution - strengthen the muscles involved without regard for how they are to be used, and then apply the 'new' level of conditioning to practice of the skill itself.*

- Core training. *Suddenly, the abdomen and low back have become areas of focus, with Pilates and sports training leading the parade. At least half of it is false. The muscles that extend the lumbar spine cannot be strengthened in a meaningful way through traditional exercise (U of Fl. research, 1986). And the abdomen? It may help stabilize things while the body is in flight, but it is rarely the prime mover. Follow your stomach during a golf swing and think "Core training for golf?" Spend your time strengthening and sequencing the larger, more productive entities.*

Don't get sidetracked. Brief, infrequent, high-intensity exercise is still the best way to get from A to B, regardless of what B may be.

## MARCH 24

---

### Black Coffee and Burnt Toast

Beginning in 1986, an entourage of employees traveled the country attending trade shows and exhibitions to showcase the new line of MedX® rehabilitative testing and exercise tools. The chairman and founder of the corporation, and inventor of the computerized equipment, Arthur Jones, made an occasional appearance, but the bulk of the responsibility fell on the shoulders of General Manager, Jim Flanagan. At six feet, four inches and a solid 240 pounds, Jim could handle anything - except predicting the actions of his boss.

The morning of one such exposition, the crew met in the hotel restaurant for an early start. The menu was nothing fancy, but the orders reflected the busy day ahead - until it was Arthur's turn.

"A cup of black coffee and two pieces of burnt toast," he growled in a tone that declared meals an intrusion.

Minutes later, the waitress delivered the toast as ordered - black and burnt.

"These aren't burnt enough. Run 'em through another time."

Despite the request, Jones was aware that the opposite was required for best results from progressive resistance exercise. He found "absolutely nothing progressive about the training of most bodybuilders."

"Once having learned to spell your own name," he said, "you cannot then improve your spelling - nor your vocabulary - by writing your name over and over again; your writing, perhaps, in effect, your form or style, but not your spelling."

He understood that mere repetition of things already easy was not the way to go. "Yet most weight trainees - bodybuilders, power lifters, and Olympic lifters alike," he said, "seldom continue an exercise to a point anywhere near the required intensity of effort; while usually attempting to justify their easier styles of training on the grounds that they compensate by performing more exercises or more sets of each exercise."

"Given enough time," he added, "an ant could move the pyramids from Cairo to Capetown - and in the process he would perform an enormous amount of work; while the intensity of work would never be high enough to measure in meaningful terms."

Jones backed his stance by looking at the past:

"More than a century ago, by a study of the bones of men who spent their lives at manual labor, it was determined that the intensity of work is a factor of great importance; even the chemical composition of the bones is changed by hard work. How much you work - the actual amount of work - is a factor of only secondary importance. Men who spend years working at a job that requires constant repetition of fairly light movements seldom if ever develop much if any more than average levels of size-strength; while men who work much less - but harder - usually develop above average muscular mass."

Despite the obvious, things never change.

Trainees continue to spend hours in the gym when minutes would do - and do more. Most are slaves to habit, ignorant of alternatives or unwilling to pay the price (of high intensity). Yet, they are eager to share their 'knowledge' with a new generation - which burns more than a few slices of bread.

Repetition may improve toast for some, but does not improve physical ability - especially size and strength in any timely fashion.

As Jones put it, "It is a shame that bodybuilding is wasted on bodybuilders."

## MARCH 25

### Three Sets of Ten

If advice from trainers is the sole arbiter, three sets of 10 repetitions is one of the few *Commandments of Strength Training* upon which there is agreement. Yet, if fitness publications are the guide, three sets of 10 lies somewhere between the single set advocated by Nautilus® inventor Arthur Jones in 1970 and the 60 sets of biceps curls performed by bodybuilder Chuck Amato.

How much strength training is enough to produce best results?

Dr. Michael Pollock (School of Medicine, University of Florida) launched a project to find out in January of 1996. He carefully considered the results of several research studies conducted by his staff and reviewed "everything ever published on the subject (one set vs. multiple sets) in any scientific journal" dating back to 1962.

In that year, a man named Berger compared the results of one set vs. two vs. three on a chest press exercise with 177 untrained subjects for 12 weeks. One set increased the strength of the group by 23.6%; two sets by 24%; and three sets by 26.3%. The slight differences fell within the range of random variation.

In a 1975 study at West Point Academy, a group of trained cadets increased their strength an average of 59.8% in six weeks using only one set of 13 different exercises.

In 1982, a man named Sylvester, using 48 subjects, compared one set of barbell curls to three over an eight-week period. One set of exercise increased strength by 24.6%; three sets by 26.2%. The difference was not statistically significant.

In 1983, a man named Stowers used 28 subjects in a seven-week study that compared one set to three in both the bench press and squat. His result was the same as Sylvester's.

In 1986, Wayne Westcott compared one set to two with 79 subjects for four weeks. Although better results were produced with one set (11.2%) than with two (10.8%), the difference was not significant.

In a 1989 10-week study involving 127 subjects (men and women), Westcott found no difference between one, two and three sets using chin-ups and dips as exercises.

In 1993, Dr. Pollock's group found no meaningful difference when they compared one set to two on a cervical extension exercise for 12 weeks with 140 subjects.

In 1995, Dr. Jay Graves recorded a significant result in favor of one set over two using a MedX® Lumbar Extension machine with 141 subjects for a period of 12 weeks.

In 1995, a man named Starkey used 88 subjects for 14 weeks and compared one set to three on leg extensions and leg curls. One set proved superior on both exercises.

Dr. Pollock concluded that the difference between one set and multiple sets was time.

Because only slight and often insignificant variance is found between one set and multiple sets in research, the American Council of Sports Medicine recently adopted an official protocol of "one set to failure, not more than three times weekly."

Hardcore trainees scoffed at the thought, but Arthur Jones believed the amount was "too much for most people and required by nobody. While some exercise is good," he added, "it does not follow that more exercise is better; in fact, more is usually worse. Exercise does not 'produce' results; instead, if properly performed, it stimulates results."

Perhaps we should reconsider what was written 80 years ago when lengthy workouts were in vogue among those who exercised at all. "Instead of trying to determine how much exercise we can tolerate, perhaps we should try to determine how little we actually require."


MARCH 26

---

## Of Weak and Strong Links

When I began coaching in college, I didn't know a basket from a backboard, so I sought information that would make it look otherwise, starting with an old book from my college days. The players weren't dumb. When I introduced the two-handed jump shot, a dinosaur of 30 years, I might as well have sung "Oh, Canada!" I was the weak link in the chain, the effect of which I understood from years of hockey.

- You didn't dare pass the puck to certain players for fear they'd lose it.
- You couldn't rely on the third line for more than holding the opponent scoreless for two minutes (the league had rules that dictated equal play for everybody, which further emphasized that weak links held you back).

Fortunately, I knew something about conditioning and vowed never to lose a game on that account. There was more to it. Recruiting was out - the school could barely afford uniforms - which forced us to work on strengths and weaknesses related to individual and team skills. The basketball team was only as strong as its weakest link - whether an individual, a skill or a team deficiency. Success involved the full preparation of every player and their integration into a functional unit.

In that regard, it was much the same as physical preparation for a sport. Each muscle must be fully prepared and then integrated by the nervous system into a team to perform a task - which is where the problem begins.

Strength training used to stand on its own merits. Now, it has fallen prey to the whims of those who believe that it's not enough. Self-proclaimed experts continue to add things to the point that the original has all but disappeared. "Strength" has slowly become "strength for..." and must now connect to function.

As a result, almost all strength exercises are compound movements that involve several muscle groups and joint systems. The purported advantages are greater muscle-mass involvement; better stimulation of the weak link in the chain; and better coordination (that is, muscles learn to work together under load). The disadvantages are an output limited by the weak link; a poor, if any, stimulation of larger, stronger muscles and a questionable transfer to the skill itself.

The current trends in exercise - functional and sports-specific training - are steps in the wrong direction. Their focus on compound movements and small muscle groups - even when performed in conjunction with proper strength training - adds a burden that can lead to over-training. What was once accomplished in 20 minutes has been extended to hours - like bodybuilders who train in excess because of a perceived need.

The formula proposed by Arthur Jones in 1970 was simple and sound: isolate and strengthen each muscle involved; then coordinate them through skill training. If the bomb he dropped then wasn't enough, there's little hope in today's environment, which shouldn't sound so negative. I'm not dead yet, and there are still many of his disciples injecting common sense into the stream.

Arthur Jones underestimated the influence he had on people. Perhaps I, too, have had some influence on the next generation.

In 1972, the Averett College men's golf team consisted of anyone I could find in the parking lot before the van left for the match. In 2003, they won the NCAA Division-III National Championship.

## MARCH 27

---

### Feast or Famine

In the May, 1974 issue of *Ironman*, Nautilus® inventor Arthur Jones detailed the size and strength gains he expected from a program he designed for 36 players of the DeLand High School football team. Other than limited exposure the year before, most had no experience with resistance training; and only one had trained with weights, for eight months prior to Jones' arrival. It showed. At 17 years old and 5'8", the young man had gained 41.5 pounds (from 132.5 to 174) and added three inches to his arm.

"During initial strength tests," said Jones, "he was able to perform 21 repetitions with 260 pounds in the full squat - and the second strongest (on the team) was able to do only one repetition with 255 pounds, with the average performance being far below that."

Besides superiority in *all* strength performances, he was extremely flexible - touched a point 10 inches below his feet with his knees locked and had 240° of elbow range-of-motion (average was 150°). He was also among the fastest in the 100-yard *and* 660-yard runs, despite not running for two years. The kid was a rare bird.

The bird, however, didn't live up to expectations. "Being almost totally lacking in incentive," said Jones, "he simply refused to push himself in training - and avoided training entirely if at all possible."

Coaches face the same dilemma in every sport. Some kids are loaded with talent, but have poor work habits; others have little talent, but work like animals to make the roster. Knowing that they need 'talent' on the field, coaches typically funnel their efforts to motivate the lazy and improve the skills of those who work.

On the other hand, the talented individual recognizes his superiority and tries less. He can stand on the sidelines, smoke a cigarette and still save the day. Why give 100% when 80% can beat most?

I coached several high school and college athletes in that category and left them the thought: "One day, you'll meet your match." When you stand at the bottom of the scale, you are forced to try harder, as in the case of many novice bodybuilders who have taken things too far.

In an article entitled "The Frequency and Extent of Exercise" (*Ironman*, Sept 1974), Jones referred to one such case. "A recent article described the training routine that one young man has followed for a period of seven years, four hours a day, seven days a week - twenty-eight hours of weekly training; and his results, in the end, have been fairly good - if not spectacular. But it is the author's contention that far better results would have resulted in far less time from the practice of a training routine that required only about fifteen percent of the weekly training time that this individual spent training - and if even the same degree of results could have been produced in one third of the elapsed time, then it is obvious that only five percent of this subject's training was actually required...I think that this individual has merely developed a tolerance to this amount of exercise - and I cannot believe that it is an actual requirement...There have been literally hundreds of examples of individuals who have shown far better results...while practicing a total of less than three percent of the number of exercise movements that have been employed by that subject within a period of seven years."

Too much or too little leads to the same end. Hard, brief and infrequent workouts are the key to reaching your strength potential. If you can motivate your 'best' athletes to "go for it," you will have contributed to the making of a 'super' athlete.

## MARCH 28

### Steroids

The old man grabbed the bodybuilder by the scruff of the neck, hauled him out to the parking lot and repeatedly banged his head into the rear bumper of a car. It was time to make a statement about the drugs the youth had mistakenly offered his son.

Nautilus® inventor Arthur Jones had seen enough of the drug scene at Muscle Beach in California - where the city was forced to shut it down - to know the potential risks of offering an 'open' invitation to train using his revolutionary system of exercise. He made it clear from the start: "It won't happen here and I think that some people, at least, know it won't happen, now. 'That which is necessary' will be done to stop it from happening - WHATEVER that may prove to be."

"If you are using drugs of any kind," he warned, "don't bother to come to DeLand, Florida, hoping to train...we 'don't shoot sick children and we don't pet mad dogs,' but we can do rather nicely without either."

That same year (1970), Jones introduced the inaugural "Mr. Nautilus" competition, offering $25,000 to the winner and $50,000 in total prize money (at the time, first-place money was generally $1,000). He also promised widespread publicity (when contests were known only to the few in the sport) through a made-for-TV movie on physical training, with the contest as the highlight of the film. And more. Participants would receive free housing for the duration of the event.

In return, Jones demanded that all entrants "present themselves a week in advance of the contest, and submit to a wide variety of physical tests, any reasonable tests." Testing was to be conducted by Dr. Elliott Plese (Colorado State University) and a staff of exercise physiologists from a number of universities and research foundations around the country. "Of particular importance," he noted, "a number of tests to determine drug usage - and the results of such usage - will be conducted, and the results of these tests will be published." The contest suddenly suffered from a lack of interest.

Arthur's stance on drugs was marred only once. He made an exception for Sergio Oliva who trained in DeLand two months before the Mr. Universe contest in London (Sept., 1971). "He (Oliva) will continue to use them (growth drugs) during his period of training here," Jones clarified, "because he is now at least temporarily 'hooked' on them. If he stopped using them now he would undoubtedly lose muscular size for at least six months...we don't approve of his use of such drugs but we will at least permit it under the circumstances. However, there will be no other such exceptions."

Jones remained true to his word. In 1983, he terminated a contract with Boyer Coe (Mr. Universe, 1975) until the detected use of steroids had ceased.

In the early 1980's, a New York physician examined more than 300 athletes taking 'significant' amounts of steroid drugs. Clinical damage was detected in 100% of users up to six months *after* they had discontinued. Twenty-five percent were left with permanent damage including testicular atrophy, enlarged prostate, high blood pressure and pituitary, kidney and liver malfunctions.

The facts are clear. Steroids kill, but they are not likely to kill sports if the powers-that-be have their say. In their minds, harsh legislation and threats of permanent disqualification only empower the belief that some advantage can be gained by using drugs - which has led to the current absurdity of wrist slaps and fourth chances.

When all else fails, take 'em out to the parking lot.

## MARCH 29

### Left and Right Discrepancies

The difference in strength between my left and right arm was apparent the first time I used a Nautilus® Multi Curl machine (an independent-arm biceps tool). My left failed after nine repetitions while my right could have continued for at least four or five more. My initial reaction was the same as that of most - perform another set with the left so that it can catch up.

I refused.

The machine's inventor, Arthur Jones was an advocate of harder exercise - not more - in the case of strength deficiencies. He believed that my left had to work *harder* than my right to get to nine repetitions and - because of the intensity - would eventually catch up without performing additional exercise. He was right.

After six months of no supplementary exercise, the left equaled the right in performance, outgrew it, and to this day, is superior in strength.

Ellington Darden disclosed the same in *The Nautilus Bodybuilding Book* (1986) - that most right-handed bodybuilders have larger left arms. Like Jones, he believed that the non-dominant arm "must work harder to perform its share of an equally divided work load. The left arm does not work more, nor differently - it works harder, with a greater intensity of effort. And it responds by growing larger than the right arm."

The non-dominant arm may lack the coordination and balance control of the dominant arm, but it is generally stronger in tests that do not involve muscular coordination or balance. When bodybuilders become aware of that fact (whether perceived or demonstrated), most perform *another* set of exercise with the weaker limb - always *more*, when it was really *harder* exercise that produced the better outcome in the first place.

The result of their actions is evident.

Once they have graduated from Strength Training 101, the majority of trainees take a 'more is better' approach. When they reach a plateau, they increase the *amount* of exercise - more repetitions, more sets, more time per session, more sessions or more days (by using a split system) - in an effort to produce more results. They rationalize their actions by the fact that everyone else is sharing the same information. And while some may find what best works for them by attrition, most remain mired in a sea of low-intensity work or quit because they are unable to produce the result they once thought was possible. Frustrated, many turn to steroids and growth hormones - something everyone else seems to be doing as well.

The fact of the matter is few people have the genetic potential to reach the muscular development illustrated in today's bodybuilding magazines, and few 'stars' have the potential to reach that level without steroids. Even fewer care about long-term health or the future of their sport.

The body has a reserve of energy to help it recover from exercise. The reserve can be increased with exercise as the body adapts, but its ultimate capacity is limited. When the capacity is exceeded, the body requires time to recover. If time is not forthcoming in duration or amount, the body will not take kindly to further stimulation.

Plateaus are a function of *too much* exercise and can be surpassed by reducing the *amount* of exercise, by re-focusing on form and intensity, and by allowing more time between workouts.

Questions? Call your left arm.

## MARCH 30

### In the Land of Giants

The packet arrived several months before pre-season training. The ninth-round draft pick from Lehigh University and the youngest (at 20) to play in the league grasped the letter within. "Welcome to the New York Giants' six-week training camp at Fairfield University (Fairfield, Connecticut) on July 15, 1963...Enclosed you will find an 'isometric' rope with complete instructions to help you report in top condition."

In the early 1960's, pro football had no strength training - no barbells or machines - just calisthenics and stretching. Tackle Reed Bohovich, the only rookie to make the Giants' offensive starting lineup that year, had to rely on a rope to prepare for the NFL.

Things weren't much better by the end of the decade when teams flirted with pre-season resistance training only to abandon it when the games began. The result was a loss in strength and an increased risk of injury as the season progressed.

In the early 1970's, Arthur Jones introduced his Nautilus® machines and high-intensity training system to Miami coach, Don Shula, whose success stirred the league. Within a year, most teams had the new equipment; but few used it properly. Washington Redskins conditioning coach, Dan Riley was one of the few to carry the torch for Jones.

In *Strength Training by the Experts* (1977), Riley reiterated that physical efficiency depended upon cardio-respiratory fitness and muscle strength. "Most athletes are conditioned so that their cardiovascular system is capable of meeting the demands of competition at the desired level of intensity. However, too few possess a level of strength commensurate with their skill level. Therefore, successful athletes could become more successful by increasing the strength of the musculature involved in their sport."

Jones concurred: "Most athletes finish their careers with absolutely nothing in the way of strength training," he said, "...and very few, if any, are producing even 50% of the potential benefit of a properly conducted program of exercise."

It was his introduction to business associate, Dick Butkus. "Dick was probably the best in the world at his particular specialty (middle linebacker)," said Arthur, "but not as a result of great strength; instead, he was a naturally strong man who also happened to have every possible advantage for a particular activity...great skill, ideal bodily proportions for a specific function, at least adequate cardiovascular ability for the same function, and outstanding neurological efficiency. He was the best in the world with absolutely nothing in the way of strength training. Like most outstanding athletes, he was a natural... and the great athletes are the ones who have the most to gain from strength training, and are the most unlikely to use it. He (Butkus) now realizes this after the fact, too late to be of any help."

Former Redskins offensive tackle, Guy Earle entered our facility the other day. At the mention of Dan Riley, he remembered "going down a line of machines with Coach Riley making us count slowly as we lifted and lowered each weight."

I thought I was in for a treat until his lightning-quick repetitions on a seated leg curl led me to believe that Riley's work was wasted. Jones said it best when he described the experience of training Casey Viator (Mr. America, 1971), "...from all appearances, I can only say that he displayed very few signs of any real learning." (*Nautilus Training Principles: Bulletin No. 2*)

At least Casey, Guy and Reed passed their respective exams. The way most trainees perform exercise, they'd be better off with a P.O. Box and a rope.

## MARCH 31

### Pre-Exhaustion

According to Nautilus® inventor Arthur Jones, "If you work a muscle to a point of momentary failure, it can recover more than 50% of its strength in less than three seconds." He also realized that a greater degree of fatigue (and stimulation) was possible if a muscle was forced *beyond* the point of failure with the help of a fresh, secondary muscle group. To that end, he created a series of 'double' exercise machines that satisfied the physiological principles of what came to be known as *pre-exhaustion*.

Double machines - one machine with two exercises - offered a direct, isolated exercise for the major muscle group and a secondary compound exercise involving the same muscle and a helping group. Jones unleashed his torture in five versions:

- Double Shoulder (a lateral raise as the major exercise followed by an overhead press as the secondary)
- Double Chest (an arm cross followed by a decline press)
- Behind Neck/Torso Arm (an upper-back exercise followed by a behind-neck pulldown)
- Pullover/Torso Arm (a pullover followed by a front pulldown)
- Compound Leg (a leg extension followed by a leg press)

The handles and pads used for both exercises were easily accessible from the same seat, making it possible to begin the second exercise in less than three seconds from the completion of the first. It was necessary, however, to use less weight (than normal) on the second exercise because it involved one exhausted and one fresh muscle. With practice, both exercises flowed into one...but felt like four.

Double machines were so demanding that advanced trainees were warned not to include more than two in any 12-exercise workout because of recovery demands. Both exercises, taken to a point of momentary failure and performed with an interval of less than three seconds between, confirmed what Jones often reiterated about the stupidity of performing what has become the national pastime - multiple sets.

Proper performance of the basic combinations produced a degree of stimulation (and soreness) that was impossible to attain using traditional methods. Ellington Darden, Ph.D. (who wrote the Nautilus books throughout the 1970's and 80's) took pre-exhaustion a step further by devising combinations of double machines with other exercises. One of the most popular was the use of a double machine in reverse order (secondary exercise first, then the primary movement reduced by 20%) immediately followed by a compound movement that involved *both* muscle groups.

Jones often treated bodybuilders to a leg press followed by a leg extension and barbell squat. Other effective combinations were front pulldown, pullover and negative chin-ups; and decline chest press, arm cross and negative dips.

Properly performed, they left trainees looking for a spot to hide.

Despite the success of the machines in working a muscle directly and with pre-exhaustion, their popularity waned. They were brutally hard and from a time perspective kept trainees at one station too long. In the end, their demise had nothing to do with physiology, psychology or time. It related to concern over the bottom line. The sale of two machines created more profit than one.

Double machines are history. Rapid, productive exercise sequences in gyms have now been replaced by other physiological combinations - mainly a snooze with a nap.

# APRIL

---

"Twenty years ago, I finally learned that an actually-proper workout with barbells had to be brief in the extreme – so brief that I was always tempted to increase the number of exercises or sets, since the workouts never seemed to contain 'enough:' but when I did increase anything in the workouts, the production of results was always reduced, ALWAYS."

Arthur Jones

## APRIL 1

---

### First Things First

The 'pep' talk we probably didn't need was followed by a knock on the dressing-room door that we did. It was championship night and excitement ran high as our team shuffled down the rubber-floored corridor toward the thick, hinged door. From there, it was a long step to the ice for a five-year old.

Dad slipped behind the bench with pride, having coached his boys to the big game. As he scanned the slick surface, he noticed a player standing in front with a disgruntled look on his face. Danny McLean was pumping his arms and hockey stick in vain. Dad bent over the boards, spotted the problem and pointed down. Danny had forgotten to remove the plastic runners that protected his skate blades. When he hit the ice, he went nowhere.

It was my first lesson in strength training.

You can't advance in physical endeavors as quickly as you'd like if you don't first grasp the basics; and you can't progress from there if you don't return to the basics every once in a while. Both errors are all too common in strength training where the basics are simple, but often ignored.

Adopt the following as part of your approach:

**Form**: Good form begins with proper set-up, good posture and a slow speed of movement. As Ellington Darden suggested in reference to the momentum initiated by most trainees during the first 10-15° of movement (*High Intensity Bodybuilding*, 1990), "Barely start (to move the resistance), then slow down." When in doubt about speed, always perform repetitions at a slower pace.

**Intensity**: The higher the intensity during exercise, the greater the chance of stimulating change. "It should be obvious," said Nautilus® inventor Arthur Jones, "that an intensity of effort anything less than an outright 100 percent is probably a mistake, and that much less is a major mistake - with no 'probably' about it. Since it is impossible to measure any degree of effort less than 100 percent, the only way to be sure that you are working hard enough is to go all the way."

When the intensity is high, the workout won't last long. "Twenty years ago," he said in 1971, "I finally learned that an actually-proper workout with barbells had to be brief in the extreme - so brief that I was always tempted to increase the number of exercises or sets, since the workouts never seemed to contain 'enough;' but when I did increase anything in the workouts, the production of results was always reduced, ALWAYS." He recognized that "increasing the 'intensity of effort' requires a disproportionate reduction in the 'amount' of exercise."

**Progression**: Steady progress requires increasing the resistance and number of repetitions performed, and having adequate recovery ability. In that regard, allow 48-72 hours of rest between workouts. As training advances, pay attention to recovery ability (harder exercise takes a greater toll on the system). If it is inadequate, perform less exercise (less frequency, fewer total exercises, or both). If it is adequate, review your form (strict, slow, isolated muscle training) and intensity. Are you working as HARD as you can, or merely going through the motions? Is each exercise continued to a point of muscle failure?

Whether playing hockey or lifting weights, use what Jones called "the classic example of a clear explanation..."

"'...how to make a rabbit stew; first, you catch a rabbit...'"

## APRIL 2

### Worth The Price?

In the 1970's, I reached the pinnacle of my golf career and "packed it in" without regret, although I still entertain thoughts of "What if...?"

I focused efforts on playing famous courses with an eye on the Mother, St. Andrews. Twenty years later, I saved enough pennies, called in advance, flew northeast to arrive on a brisk Scottish morning and waited four hours in the blustery cold before they called my name. When all was said and done, I was disappointed. St. Andrews was not as charming as Turnberry, Prestwick or Troon. In fact, it was flat and ugly - if I had been trodden upon for more than 500 years, I might look and feel the same - a reaction as common as the adage, "The more you play her, the more you appreciate her." But it was still St. Andrews, stately and reverent. There was 'something' at the top.

The same, unfortunately, cannot be said of other sports.

Throughout history, strong men such as Sampson, Hercules and Milo were looked upon with reverence; yet, it might have been different if they were much larger or stronger. "If an advanced bodybuilder had suddenly appeared on the scene 400 years ago," said Nautilus® inventor Arthur Jones, "he would probably have been burned at the stake. If you have the potential for unusual muscular size, and if you actually build such size to a maximum possible degree, you will undoubtedly be looked upon as an outright freak. In my opinion, a realistic goal is far better."

Most bodybuilders do everything they can to attract attention both in the gym and out, and are surprised by the reactions they produce. In that sense, they are much like Mark Twain's "two-headed stranger." When one boy saw him, he commented that he wouldn't want to be like that. When another saw him, he took a more practical stance, saying, "Oh, that would be dandy - eat for two but only stump toes for one."

According to Jones, the invention of the barbell in 1902 may have provided a catalyst.

"In a very real sense, the barbell was literally too productive for its own good: For the first time in history, at least a few men appeared on the scene who were so muscular that they seemed to most people to be freaks. Rather than being admired, such men were usually ridiculed, looked upon with scorn."

Things haven't changed.

Friends of mine recently attended their first bodybuilding show in West Palm Beach and were appalled at both the freaks on stage and those in the audience. It confirmed Jones' belief that the few who make it to the top "are surprised to find that there is nothing there, no rewards, no applause, literally NOTHING. Average people look upon them as freaks, most girls avoid or ridicule them, nobody outside a very narrow circle of close associates has any respect for them - so, was it worth the price?" To add insult to injury, the powers-that-be 'fix' the winners.

Shortly after Casey Viator won the Mr. America contest in 1971, Jones encouraged him to go back to school and get out of bodybuilding despite the fact that it's difficult to tell someone at 19 how to live his life or that few actually 'make' it. But when making it requires the use of dangerous drugs and exotic diets, it's time to consider more 'realistic' goals.

Wouldn't you settle for great health, Hercules?

A nearby, public golf course my brother calls "a five-star dump" charges $185 during the winter months. I'd rather, cross the pond again for $90.

## APRIL 3

---

### Strength Training and Flexibility

Around 1940, one of the bulkiest muscular men in history, John Grimek, remarked, "You can lift weights and be called 'muscle-bound', or not lift weights and actually be muscle-bound."

Nautilus® inventor Arthur Jones agreed.

"Grimek," he said, "was capable of touching both elbows to the floor from a standing position without bending his knees, performing full splits and many other movements far outside the ranges of possible movement displayed by the average man."

In the 1970's, Jones trained bodybuilder Casey Viator and took the notion - the same exercises used to increase strength can vastly improve flexibility - a step beyond. "Heavy exercise," he said, "is not only capable of increasing flexibility but is actually required for that purpose."

Despite his efforts, the myth that great size is incompatible with flexibility lives on.

When a body-part is pulled into a position that cannot be reached by the muscular contraction of an antagonistic muscle, stretching occurs. Hold your elbow over the edge of a table (palm-up) so that your upper arm is flush with its surface, and contract your triceps muscle (to straighten your arm). The weight of your lower arm will begin to stretch the ligaments of your biceps. If you hold an additional weight in your hand, the stretch will occur at a faster rate, and to a greater degree, if the limits of the joint structure have not been reached. And if you hold a heavier weight, and everything else remains constant, the stretch will be *more* effective and efficient.

The secret of gaining flexibility *during* exercise is to reach a fully extended position with a resistance heavy enough to create a stretch.

But that's not all: the speed at which you approach full-extension is equally important. If the weight is lowered into a stretch position with too much speed, the muscle contracts instead of lengthens - a phenomenon known as a "stretch reflex;" or functionally, a "pre-stretch."

"Pre-stretching," according to Ellington Darden, "occurs when a relaxed muscle is pulled into a position of increased tension prior to the start of contraction." Sensors in the muscle warn of pending danger and trigger a contraction. This 'safety' contraction, when added to that of lifting the weight, results in a higher level of intensity.

Pre-stretching involves the muscle and nervous system, and is important for strength. Stretching involves joints, muscles and connective tissues and is important for flexibility. Speed of movement approaching full-extension dictates the outcome.

It is possible to increase strength without increasing flexibility, if full-range exercise is not practiced; and possible to increase strength while losing flexibility, if antagonistic muscles are not strengthened to the same degree.

Besides form and speed, choice of equipment is a factor.

With few exceptions, exercises using free weights, Universal® machines and pulley stations offer only one of three choices in regard to resistance: resistance at the start, in the mid-range or at the end of the movement. Most traditional exercises provide mid-range resistance only, which does *nothing* to stretch the involved muscles.

To gain flexibility *during* exercise, relax and move slowly when approaching full-extension, and pause briefly in that position. "Pre-stretch" only during the last few repetitions, when the potential for injury has been reduced by fatigue.

## APRIL 4

---

### Wanna Bet?

A high-school buddy with an MBA in hand quit a four-year teaching stint at college to pursue his love, music. He started by picking up where he left off - strumming guitar and singing in bars as a student. But Charlie was no dummy - he found a way to make extra cash on the side.

Charlie kept himself in shape and found a practical way to strengthen his legs on the road. He assumed a seated squat position against a wall (thighs parallel to the floor) and timed how long he could stay there. Initially, he felt a burn at one minute and the urge to scream at three, but practiced until he could last a grueling 15. Then he'd bet a few drunkards and win (fortunately, he was seated for the music).

Charlie knew exactly what to expect.

Nautilus® inventor Arthur Jones loved a challenge in the same way. While conducting research at the United States Military Academy in West Point (May, 1975), he met a young man on the staff who later became the strength coach of the Washington Redskins. Dan Riley was Arthur's size and weight, but had larger arms by an inch and a half. Jones bet he could build his arms larger than Riley's in one month.

"He accepted the bet," said Jones, "and immediately started a literally frantic training program for his arms. The agreed-upon time passed and we re-measured our arms, 'cold' and accurately; and I won the bet...by a larger margin than I expected because Dan lost some arm size during that period as a result of overtraining."

Jones kept records of his irregular training for 37 years. He knew what to expect.

Whenever he ceased training, his weight dropped to 160 pounds and arms to 14 inches, where both remained without exercise. Within weeks of resumption, however, he rose to 172 pounds and his arms to 15-3/8 inches - Jones was a fast gainer. He would not bet beyond that, however, because he usually got 'stuck' there and had no patience for lack of progress - the reason he frequently quit.

When progress came to a halt, Jones was performing four sets each of 12 exercises to muscle failure. One day, he scaled back to two sets, 12 exercises, and quickly progressed to levels that were previously impossible. He later reduced his program to two sets of eight exercises and reached a bodyweight of 205 pounds with 17-1/8-inch arms, his best. By then, he understood why.

"After I cut my training from 48 sets to only 16 sets, a reduction of 66 2/3%," he said, "I was no longer overtraining and thus additional growth became possible for the first time."

In retrospect, he believed that training only twice a week using one set of exercise - a reduction of 90% - would have been better: "Such an additional reduction in the amount of training might not have produced any better final results, but would have, I believe, reduced the time required to reach that same level."

If you suggested a reduction of 90% to a current bodybuilder, you would be shot on the spot before you could take a bet. A 10% reduction would be suicide - though a good start for most.

Note: Arthur Jones worked HARDER than most. If the average trainee cut his program by 90% and performed it with today's intensity, the miracle would not occur.

Most people remain unaware of what they can do because they focus only on what they are willing to do. Progress would be music to their ears.

## APRIL 5

---

### Inroad

The brief, high-intensity training philosophy advocated by Nautilus® inventor Arthur Jones in the early 1970's proved a success with most, but not with some - which led him to believe that failure to produce results was genetic. By 1986, his measuring tools proved that he was right and revealed a surprise in the process - the range of genetic differences was greater than expected.

"The purpose of exercise intended to increase strength," he claimed, "is to fatigue a muscle through its full range of possible movement; to fatigue it to a certain level but not much if any beyond that level...because exercise that does not produce enough fatigue will not stimulate growth, and exercise that produces too much fatigue will not permit growth, or may even produce losses in both muscular size and strength. Thus exercise must be maintained between certain limits, neither too much nor too little, neither too easy nor too hard, neither too seldom nor too frequent." (*The Lumbar Spine*, 1986).

Jones believed there was an 'ideal' level of stimulation (what he called "inroad") that produced best results from strength training. To measure the immediate effect of exercise on starting strength, he tested strength immediately before and after exercise. Most subjects lost approximately 2% of their strength per repetition when exercised to exhaustion.

The ideal inroad, according to Jones, was 20-25%. That is, if an exercise failed to decrease starting strength by at least 20%, it was not hard enough (or the number of repetitions too few to stimulate change). If it decreased starting strength by more than 25%, it was too strenuous (or the number of repetitions too many to allow growth).

Besides high intensity, the number of repetitions and time spent performing them ("time under load") became crucial. If 17 repetitions produced an inroad of only 10%, more reps with a lighter weight would produce a greater effect. On the other hand, if six repetitions produced an inroad of 53%, fewer reps with more weight would produce less effect. A 'deep' inroad affected workout frequency and the ability to recover from exercise, necessitating (in some cases) the use of as little as 30-60 seconds of exercise once every two weeks. The trick was to determine the amount of exercise that produced the 'ideal' inroad.

Jones found that 70-80% of 10,000 test subjects produced best results using a repetition scheme of 8-15 (a 2-second lift, 1-second pause and 4-second descent per repetition) and an ideal time under load of 56-105 seconds. Recent research at the University of Florida used a 90-second limit per exercise and disregarded the number of repetitions (one study allowed only two repetitions per exercise). If subjects lasted more than 90 seconds under load, they were greeted with a higher resistance.

To calculate the number of repetitions required to produce the ideal inroad of 20-25%, perform as many repetitions as you can with 75-80% of your one-rep-maximum weight (1RM, determined by testing). If you perform 15 repetitions, use 14-16 as a guide for that muscle group; if you perform six, use 5-7. And keep in mind, the fatigue characteristics of muscle groups in the same individual may vary greatly. Some muscles quiver at the sight of a weight stack; others thrive.

If you care to avoid the dangers of a one-rep-maximum strength test, use a time limit. When exhaustion occurs *after* 90 seconds of exercise, increase the resistance by 5%.

It puts a refreshing twist on slavery to numbers.

# APRIL 6

## Intensity and the Work-Rest Ratio

It's hard to perform when sick, dizzy and flat on your back - but it's a great way to improve 'performance.' A 30-mile run at age 21 and heavy sets of negative chin-ups at 32 left me in that state, but what happened between *really* caught my attention.

In the summer of 1972, I set a goal to run a five-minute mile by interval training - six 75-second quarter miles to start and a 3-minute rest between (a work-rest ratio of 1:2.4). From there, I gradually decreased the 'rest' until the increased heat, humidity and intensity forced me to abandon the plan at a work-rest ratio of 1:2.

Arthur Jones toyed with the same in strength training. "If you double the intensity," he said, "you must reduce the amount of training by more than 80% to compensate for the increase. If not, you will produce losses instead of gains." His message was lost in time.

A recent issue of *Personal Fitness Professional* (July, 2003) featured an article on high-speed 'performance' training by Juan Carlos Santana. "Extreme Training" was, in essence, interval training: 1-6 sets of a leg routine performed at a fast pace (84 reps in 105 seconds); 3-4 sets of a chest routine

(90 reps in 80 seconds); and 3-4 sets of a pulling routine (70 reps in 60 seconds). Each routine was characterized by four exercises, rubber bands for resistance and a 2-3 minute recovery between sets.

'Gut-check' day included six sets of legs (8-10 minute total), three sets of chest (10 min.) and three of pulling (9 min.), with a 3-minute rest between sets. "When most clients finish this protocol (50-55 minutes)," reported Santana, "they believe nothing they do in life or sport is this tough; thus they are ready for just about anything."

Including a hospital - there are more efficient and effective ways to reach exhaustion.

One, the author advocates too much exercise. The entire body can be worked in less than 20 minutes by increasing the intensity. Plus, it's better to perform one leg, one chest and one pulling set in succession and repeat the process three times with *no* rest between than water down something already bad. Better yet, don't do it at all.

Two, it can't be hard if it lasts 50 minutes. And sets? "If you are 'pushed' to an all-out effort in each of 12 exercises," says Ellington Darden, "you will not want to do more than one set. In fact, your body will literally 'not be able to stand' more than one."

Three, what (other than mental toughness) is gained in the suggested program?

- Strength - less than you think. Most exercises fail to isolate or provide full-range strength for large muscles due to poor resistance (bands) and excess speed.
- Flexibility - none. Mid-range movements offer little resistance in stretched positions.
- Cardiovascular - excellent, if rest is minimized.
- Protection from injury - poor. Full-range strength is compromised by speed, limited range of motion, and poor resistance. Survival is no proof of benefit.
- Loss of body fat - some. Greater strength gains would accelerate fat-loss.

Compare Santana's workout with that of Miami legend, Mercury Morris in the 1970's.

| | # of Exercises (sets) | Training Time (min) | Exercise/ Rest Time (min) | Work-Rest Ratio | Total Reps |
|---|---|---|---|---|---|
| Extreme | 12 (48) | 50-55 | 30-33/ 17-25 | 1.25:1 to 2:1 (50-65%) | 984 |
| Nautilus | 12 (12) | 13:06 | 10:45/ 2:21 | 4.557:1 (82% work) | 142 |

Morris averaged 54 seconds per exercise at a slow speed and 13 seconds of rest between. If I recall correctly, Mercury was training for 'performance,' speed on the football field (a product of strength and reduced body fat, *not* of speed *during* training).

The 'old' system is more efficient, effective and safe.


APRIL 7

————

**Modestine and The Exercise Puzzle**

I stood at the top of the hill pondering survival. I'd been there before with a golf club in hand, but this was winter and I had skis strapped to my feet, and no clue how to use them. Off I went - slow to fast to faster, with no means of deceleration - and soon bailed out in a puff of white. By the end of the day, with two arms, two legs, a torso and a head - small at that - still in tact, I quit while I was ahead.

It was unlike the 'Donkey Baseball' game I played that summer where there were enough stubborn animals, besides yours truly, to slow anything down and only one tool to speed things up - a carrot on a stick. The pace was comically slow by design.

Which is where "comically slow by design" should end, in a baseball field full of donkeys. But it doesn't. It extends to the heart of fitness centers.

Good results from exercise relate to issues of work and rest, issues that most trainees have reversed. Where they should go fast, they go slow; and where they should go slow, they go fast. The performance of a repetition should be painfully slow, both up and down, while movement between exercises should be carrot-stick quick. Yet, most people race through each movement and rest in excess between. Other than an occasional burst of energy on a treadmill or stepper, the pace of most workouts resembles that of Modestine, the mule of Robert Louis Stevenson in *Travels with a Donkey*. "What that pace was," he uttered, "there is no word mean enough to describe; it was something as much slower than a walk as a walk is slower than a run."

Granted, there are obstacles and distractions along the way, like mirrors, whose use was best described (without intention) by William James: "What our human emotions seem to require is the sight of the struggle going on...Sweat and human effort, human nature strained to its uttermost and on the rack, yet getting through alive, then turning its back on its success to pursue another more rare and arduous still - this is the sort of thing the presence of which inspires us." (*What Makes a Life Significant*)

Inspiration, perhaps, but from a practical perspective, mirrors slow the pace of a workout. People look and look again, seeking the same post-exertion reward provided by a water fountain, a chat with a member of the opposite sex, the sharing of an exercise station (your turn, my turn) or the sharing of the burden at hand with peers who embrace the same posture - rest. Small escapes from physiology can ruin the potential benefits of exercise.

No one likes to rush to a funeral, especially his own, but come on. I once saw a sloth cross a fairway in Venezuela at a pace that was faster than that of most trainees to their next station in gyms. And pace only scratches the surface.

I have seen great form, lengthy pauses in contracted positions, super-slow repetitions, excellent posture and high levels of intensity in gyms, but rarely have I seen *all* parts of the puzzle. As the Nautilus® inventor put it, "You can have an elephant's body, an elephant's head, four elephant's feet, and all the other required parts, but you still won't have an elephant if all of the required parts are not fitted together properly."

Without compromising good form during exercise, pick up the pace between efforts to reap maximum benefits. Glance at the clock the moment you start and record your *total* workout time. Then, gradually reduce it to 15-20 minutes.

The way things are going, gyms may soon be forced to use organic carrots for something more than smoothies.

## APRIL 8

---

### The Commercialization of Anatomy

The most confusing (and traumatic) part of an anatomy course is the study of muscles and their functions. Origins, insertions and function quickly merge in the complexity of human movement. To this day, do we really know exactly what muscles are involved, the extent of their involvement, or in what sequence they are called upon?

The study of anatomy has led to many positives in the field of physical training but, just as certain, fueled a lot of controversy.

Nautilus® inventor Arthur Jones spent a lifetime trying to isolate muscle function. When he finally said something about a muscle, it would be 100% of that muscle; and his findings, beyond dispute. The task of isolation, however, was anything but easy.

"Anatomical charts of the human muscular structure," he said in the early stages, "unavoidably give a somewhat distorted impression of the major muscles - it is thus a common misconception that the muscles are entirely separate, that each muscle is an entity unto itself; but in fact, the actual interweaving of muscles is such that it is sometimes almost literally impossible to separate and accurately identify them - and secondly, recent work on neurological patterns makes it obvious that many of the previous assumptions regarding the actual contributions of particular muscle structures to specific movements were invalid. Careful tracing of nerve patterns has indicated that nerves frequently pass entirely through one muscle and terminate elsewhere. In the past, it was generally assumed that these nerves served the first muscle, but it is now obvious that in fact they are involved in the functions of the second muscle in such situations."

The implications were clear.

"Human muscular structures," he continued, "are capable of an almost infinite number of individual movements if we consider all of the possibilities and combinations, and attempting to provide a separate exercise for each of these possible movements would certainly be impractical at the very least - but if we consider only major movements, then the number of possibilities is reduced to manageable proportions, and since the interrelationships of muscular functions are such that 'almost all muscles are involved in almost all movements' (at least in gross terms and in a general sense), it becomes obvious that an actually very limited number of exercises can provide the required work for all of the muscle structures."

According to Jones, only a few basic exercises were required to produce significant gains in size and strength. He judged the value of exercise by the quality of resistance throughout the range of motion (especially in contraction), the number of major muscles (and total muscle mass) involved, and the vertical distance the resistance moved.

Since walking stairs and curling dumbbells elicited the same systemic response - an elevated heart rate, increased body temperature, and local and general fatigue - he emphasized whole-body workouts as the most effective and efficient way to stimulate growth. He also determined (through fact and logic) that a swimmer's program should not differ much from that of a football player or a golfer - not a popular stance.

Things have changed. We now split bodies into parts for targeted training, conduct special classes for special areas (abdomen, hips and buttocks), and provide athletes with specific training suited to their sport. Then, we cross fingers and toes hoping that the stimulus has a positive, rather than negative effect.

The field of exercise has sold out to money, and there's no end in sight.

## APRIL 9

---

### The Big Leagues

If you knew nothing about baseball, you might be led to believe that the requirements of a fan are a red hat and a large stomach; and of a fanatic - a red hat and a larger stomach.

Throughout the month of March, thousands of eager spectators flock to the grounds of Roger Dean Stadium in Jupiter, Florida - spring-training home of the St. Louis Cardinals and Florida Marlins - to witness the spectacle of professional baseball.

The sight isn't pretty.

Gut after gut after gut, men and women alike, parade by our windows (across the street) every day - a reminder that obesity has become the national pastime.

According to statistics, more than half of Americans are over-fat, that is, their body fat percentage is higher than standards recommended for good health. Obesity, by definition, refers to a level of body fat that is 5% or more above those standards.

Genetics plays a major role. If both parents are obese, the chance that offspring will be obese is 80%. If one parent is obese, children have a 40% chance of obesity. If both parents are lean, the odds are reduced to 6%. A new generation of obese youth slowly penetrates the gene pool as physical education curriculums disappear, computers occupy free time and fewer students participate in demanding sports. Some children (and their children) will eventually be dealt a poor hand.

Age contributes to the problem - but is often used as an excuse. The average female peaks at 14 in regard to body fat (16.7%); the average male at 20. From there through 50, both lose approximately a half-pound of muscle and gain one and a half pounds of body fat *per year*. At age 50, the average female has 47% body fat - nothing to cheer about. The average female who enters our facility has 25-35% body fat (ideal: 16-18%); the average male, 18-25% (ideal: 10-12%). The results are what we see during 'Fantasy Camp' where baseballs rarely escape an infield of over-stretched jerseys - over, maybe, but never through.

The solution?

Amid the hype of fast-fix remedies lies the ignored recommendation of the American Medical Association, diet and exercise. Yet, as factual as it may be, diet has become a 'dirty' word, and exercise is too much to ask of anyone. It's not what people want to hear.

The best way to lose body fat, according to Ellington Darden (*Living Longer Stonger,* 1995), is to combine proper strength training with a gradual decrease in caloric intake. In his research, men lose an average of 21 pounds of fat and gain 4-5 pounds of muscle, while women lose 12 pounds of fat and add three pounds of muscle in six-weeks. The approach is sane, logical and effective - but is *not* the 'easy' way out.

The players are not far behind. The other day, a friend and I watched a platoon of red-shirts execute what was once called 'wind sprints.' From a stationary jog, the group sauntered into a moving jog of approximately 20 yards, then walked back.

"Maybe they were warming up," I thought.

"Maybe they were the guys making only $2 million per year," he thought.

When they repeated the drill 10 times at the same speed, I was sure my grandmother could have made the squad. On second thought, she was too slim.

With proper conditioning, baseball may one day become something more than millionaires perfecting jumping jacks.

APRIL 10

---

## The Day I Quit Golf

University of Houston golf sensation, Wright Garrett nestled into a leather-backed chair at the Glen Oak Country Club in his hometown of Danville, Virginia. "I remember the conversation as if it was yesterday," he said. "Teammate, Fred Marti headed straight for the phone after his final round."

"I don't know what happened, Dad. I was three shots up, went out and shot a 65 and lost by seven."

That day Marti was struck by a Texas hurricane named Homero Blancas who fired an all-time 18-hole-record 55, 15-under par at the Premier Invitational at Longview, Texas, on "a reasonably demanding course with a par of 70."

I got a taste of the same in the 1969 Brooke Invitational at the Lookout Point Golf Club in Fonthill, Ontario. The event boasted "the largest amateur trophy in Ontario" and attracted the likes of Nick Westlock, Bill Bevan, George Stokes and a host of local hot shots. Normally, a score of 70 or 71 was good enough to win.

A one-over-par 37 looked solid as I approached the tee to the 'easier' nine, where I heard a roar from the club bar. Suddenly, the double doors flung open and out crashed former club-champion, Bob "Moose Jaw" Mason, with a beer in hand. He had just fired a six-under-par 30 on the front nine. Two beers later, he birdied the tough par-3 11th and stumbled home with a 67. My 71 was a distant second.

Some days your best is *not* good enough.

Four years later, I ran into a hurricane of greater magnitude in the Porter Cup at the Niagara Falls C.C. The 'invitation-only' fixture on the US Amateur circuit drew the best players in the country with 20 spots open for local qualifiers. I threw my hat in the ring with 180 low-handicappers and qualified with "the highest score in a decade," 74-72.

It paid. The next day, I was paired with Bill Rogers from Texarkana, Texas, who later became rookie-of-the-year on the PGA Tour and 1983 British Open champion. Behind us, were Craig Stadler and Gary Koch; behind them, defending champion, Ben Crenshaw. I was on the outside looking in.

Rogers strutted around as if he owned the place. On the par-3 6th hole, he sunk a shot from the bunker fronting the green and showed no emotion. The next hole, he rifled his approach shot at a pin located in the back of the green and found another bunker - a shallow, downhill-to-the-pin, no-green-to-work-with bunker. "OK, Mr. Rogers," I thought, "let's see what you do with this." He looked it over briefly, chopped it onto the putting surface and watched it trickled in - this time with a minor fist-pump. It was a wonderful day in the neighborhood.

The 15th hole was a short, dogleg par-4 with high trees and a cement canal blocking attempts to cross the corner. After conversing with his caddie, Rogers held nothing back and finished in a bunker 30 yards from the elevated green. He blasted out 20 feet from the pin, climbed out of the bunker and slammed his club to the ground. "That's the worst bunker shot I've hit in three years," he pouted. For someone who had never seen the course, his 66 was serious.

If I had to play the likes of Bill Rogers every day, I thought, I'd probably eat peanut-butter sandwiches the rest of my life. After the tournament, without hesitation or shame, I put away my competitive golf hat.

One day you'll meet your match. React well.


APRIL 11

---

### The Detroit Experiment

In 1972, Canada's legendary coach and trainer, Lloyd Percival sat in the back of a taxi headed for the Olympia (hockey arena). He had been asked to establish a developmental conditioning program for the Detroit Red Wings based on ideas from his 1958 classic, *The Hockey Handbook* - the 'Bible' the Soviets used to establish their dynasty. The Wings were in dire need.

The taxi driver was more a fan of golf than hockey, however, and eventually brought up the name George Knudson, Canada's finest professional.

"Knudson," he said, "had a chance to become a great golfer until some idiot gave him a lot of weight-lifting exercises and ruined him."

It was a bad start to the day for Knudson's friend and exercise consultant.

Months before, the Red Wings' management, coaching staff, scouts, trainers and players held a meeting and agreed to implement a three-stage physical training and skill development program for the entire organization. During the summer, players were evaluated at Percival's The Fitness Institute in Toronto and given a program to follow. Some worked out there while others trained in a new state-of-the-art facility installed within the Olympia. Approximately 40% of the organization got involved.

When they re-tested at the beginning of pre-season training camp in Port Huron, Michigan, those who complied showed excellent gains in strength, endurance, flexibility and total fitness. Phase II, the pre-season program, was initiated amid great enthusiasm. Only a few players, like Alex Delvecchio, rejected what they perceived as a drastic change in procedure. Gordie Howe supported the project.

The organization got off to their best start ever - the Red Wings won their first six games and led the league - but all was not well. The radical program received a lot of publicity and Detroit coach, John Wilson felt threatened. He modified and de-emphasized the plan despite agreeing that all changes would go through Percival. The team began to slide. Wilson looked for an out.

He first blamed the losing streak on managerial interference (not the case) and later claimed that he, too, was a trainer, and that the system needed tweaking. Percival withdrew his support, and added, "There was nothing 'way out' or extreme in the program; just a few established, scientific principles of conditioning and skill development applied to hockey."

Percival was fighting more than the Red Wings organization. Like Nautilus® inventor Arthur Jones, whose revolutionary ideas about training were attacked and ridiculed, he was up against the establishment.

Both men were ahead of their time - both were eventually copied.

In the late 1960's, I visited The Fitness Institute as an exercise physiology student and listened as a balding Percival outlined the fitness programs of two of Canada's leading golfers, George Knudson and Al Balding. I absorbed tips and golf drills that formed the basis of my approach to training for the next decade. Anyone who could persuade Knudson to exchange cigarettes for barbells was worth listening to.

Percival was intense and passionate. His enthusiasm turned heads, and he shared something else with the Nautilus inventor. Arthur Jones refused to go to restaurants where he would have to leave a tip.

That day in Detroit, Percival got a little revenge - he forgot to tip the taxi driver.

APRIL 12

---

### "In-Season" Training

My brother, Al and I crawled through a mound of trees to get to the cigarettes. Once there, like Indians in a tee-pee, we let a trail of smoke drift skyward through branches and leaves. Our home-away-from-home wouldn't last.

The orchards behind our house would soon be replaced by a subdivision, which meant new neighbors, one of whom would provide a better 'example.'

Ed Learn, a nine-year veteran of the CFL's Montreal Alouettes (1958-66), moved in near the site of our pow-wows, his lot adjacent to the cemetery we crossed on the way to high school. If we took the back way, we often saw him lifting weights in a basement gym, training in the off-season. We never saw him in-season.

Ed wasn't big, but he was strong and talented, and had a great work ethic. His tool of choice was a barbell - there wasn't much else. What a set of Nautilus® machines could have done for Mr. Learn!

In the November 1971 issue of *Ironman*, Arthur Jones placed an ad for "Nautilus Progressive Weight Training Equipment for Football Players' 'In Season' Training." The ad was unique. It advocated training with weights *during* football season, something most teams couldn't find the time or interest to do, having just adopted it in pre-season. It also advocated a workout (two or three times a week) that took less time than tightening a pair of cleats - 10 minutes. It was anything but nonsense.

Jones claimed that strength could be maintained in the major muscles of the body by using one set each of six machines: Pullover-Type Torso, Torso-Arm, Double Chest, Leg Press, Thigh-Extension and Squat Machine (at a total cost of $4,335). "The Kansas City Chiefs Professional Football Team," he said, "is training in this fashion NOW - under the direction of Alvin Roy."

Jones didn't stop there. In a later issue of the same, he addressed the need for year-round training and outlined a 28-minute 'total body' workout he was using for other athletes. "The above-mentioned routine," he said, "is the exact training program that we will use with the Cincinnati Bengals Professional Football Team starting in May of this year (1972) - it is the exact program that almost anybody should use, regardless of 'why' they are training, no matter what their goals may be. It is the program (or, at the very least, very close to the exact program) that almost everybody will eventually use."

The impact of Nautilus on professional football was great, but the commercial bias on the part of its trainers gave way to the avalanche of nonsense that now prevails - ballet, Pilates, yoga, power-lifting and anything but efficiency. Dan Riley, strength coach of the Washington Redskins, is one of the few who still hangs his hat on Arthur's door.

Year-round training is crucial to success in any sport. Training like a madman for a few months only to 'let things go' during the season makes as much sense as bulking-up in hope of a 'size' carryover for a bodybuilding contest.

I once trained a group of LPGA players who, for the most part, took too long a break after their season. With only two months before the next season's start, they took their sweet time to arrive. By the time some did, it was too late. Fitness can't handle a break of more than 7-10 days.

The 'when to workout' of each sport is different, but the fact remains: two weekly sessions, one hard and one easy, can maintain strength in-season. As Jones suggests, if 10 minutes is enough for football - and it is - why spend more?

## APRIL 13

---

## Project Total Conditioning

There must have been something about football huddles that annoyed Nautilus® inventor, Arthur Jones. A team whose athletes had optimized their strength, flexibility and cardiovascular capacities should have no need to huddle; simply, line up and play, line up and play until the defense was strewn out on the field. The method he advocated to attain such a condition was called "proper strength training," a 20-25 minute circuit of non-stop, high-intensity exercise.

At first, coaches and athletes ridiculed him. It was "not enough exercise" to produce the claimed results. Yet in 1972, Don Shula adopted the system and led the Miami Dolphins to the game's only perfect season. Within a year, most teams in the NFL had the equipment. Jones, however, was more interested in proving theories than selling machines and, in 1975, conducted a research study called "Project Total Conditioning" with the football team at the United States Military Academy in West Point, New York.

The team was "ready to play." They had practiced football twice a day, performed an unsupervised circuit of strength training and ran two miles three times a week for several months. Jones took half the team at random and changed one thing - the strength training was supervised on his machines. The other half continued to train the traditional way.

For the first two weeks, Jones' group familiarized themselves with the equipment to minimize the learning effect (initial strength gains are generally attributed to nervous system changes). At the start of the third week, the West Point staff initiated testing and training, and re-tested six weeks (18 sessions) later. Each workout consisted of 10 exercises and averaged less than 30 minutes.

The results were conclusive. The supervised group increased their strength 58.54% - a significant amount for athletes who were considered 'strong' before the project began. They also increased their flexibility an average of 11%

on trunk flexion, trunk extension and shoulder flexion by performing exercise through a complete range-of-motion. The control group improved less than 1%.

In concurrent studies, the vertical jumping height of the supervised group improved 6.49% compared to 1.42% for the control group. In the 40-yard dash, a measure of speed in football, the circuit-trained cadets improved twice as much as their teammates.

Cardiovascular results were equally impressive. The supervised group decreased their time to run two miles by 88 seconds while the control group improved by 20 seconds. On 60 different measures of cardiovascular fitness including at-rest, sub-maximal and maximal-work conditions, there was such a dramatic improvement that Dr. Kenneth Cooper, Director of the Aerobic Institute in Dallas, Texas called the results "impossible" and trashed them. At the time, the leading authority on aerobic exercise refused to acknowledge that strength training had any cardiovascular benefit.

The good news - the results were impossible to produce using the training methods advocated by Cooper and others: They could have only been produced by proper strength training. The bad news - Cooper's staff measured the results.

"Project Total Conditioning" should have revolutionized the thinking of coaches and trainers involved in the preparation of athletes for sports such as football, but the world was asleep and remains so. Today, football teams continue to huddle, yet produce their best results when they can't - in the final minutes of a game.

Insist on becoming your best by using proper strength training.


## APRIL 14

---

### Between Exercises

The 26 year-old cross-country runner huffed and puffed through an exercise circuit, his speed between machines hindered by a pulse monitor attached to his body. Rick had volunteered for a study to determine the heart's response to proper strength training and to changing levels of activity between exercises.

During his first workout, Rick was 'pushed' to fatigue on each of 12 machines as he moved quickly from one to another. His heart rate was recorded every minute. By the time he finished the third machine, a leg curl, his heart rate had entered the "training zone" (an age parameter that defines cardiovascular benefits). It reached its peak during torso exercises (back, chest and shoulders), dropped slightly during the arm segment and remained in the zone for 18 of 21 minutes.

Rick performed the same circuit a week later, with one change - he rode an upright bike for one minute between exercises at a rate that kept his pulse at 150 beats per minute. This prolonged the workout by 11 minutes, but elevated his heart rate by only a few beats throughout (compared to the machine-only workout).

The next week, Rick pedaled at a "maximum" rate for one minute between machines. Midway through the ninth exercise, with his pulse and system nearing their limits, he headed for the alley behind the gym.

Two ingredients are necessary to produce best results from strength training - good form and high levels of intensity. Intensity is a function of two factors: input during exercise, and time spent between efforts.

After a few weeks of break-in, I encourage trainees to work as hard as they can during each exercise even if they have to lie on the floor between efforts. As their condition improves, I advocate a reduction in time between exercises to increase the overall intensity.

The following are 'between-exercise' suggestions based on research and logic.

- Systematically reduce rest time by using a watch with a second hand. Muscle and aerobic systems respond to the *degree* of stimulation, as demonstrated by "Project Total Conditioning" (USMA, 1975) and Boyer Coe's (former Mr. Universe) non-stop Nautilus® workouts in 1983. An exercise routine completed in 20 minutes creates more 'shock' than the same routine in 30.
- Perform 1-2 minutes of cardiovascular activity between exercises. Make sure the activity is vigorous enough to sustain the heart rate within your "training zone."
- Stretch between machines. A recent study by Wayne Westcott revealed that stretching a muscle immediately after exercise produces greater increases in strength (19.6%) than not stretching (16.4%). Stretching at the end of the workout produced the best gains in strength (19.8%). With this choice, expect a reduction in cardiovascular benefits.
- Exercise an antagonistic (opposite) muscle group. Russian research on "active rest" demonstrates faster muscle recovery when an antagonistic muscle group is exercised between sets. In other words, a

biceps-triceps-biceps sequence with *no* rest between is more productive than a biceps-rest-biceps sequence.

Don't just sit there between exercises, do something. It's the same price.

## APRIL 15

---

### An Introduction to High Intensity

For a man who rarely showed emotion or moved his mouth when he talked, exercise physiology professor, Digby Sale was in tenth gear as he led me to his office. There, he opened an envelope that displayed glossy prints of a body-builder and a bikini-clad model posing beside an odd-looking device. Claims about the effectiveness of the device made even Digby's lips move. It was my first glimpse of a Nautilus® machine.

Months later, he rushed me to the basement of the physical education complex where I performed a number of repetitions on McMaster University's (Hamilton, Ontario) latest acquisition, a plate-loaded Nautilus Pullover machine.

Two years later (1973), I received an invitation to the 'grand opening' of a Nautilus gym in Danville, Virginia where I was teaching. It was a no-brainer. Surely, a decade of running and lifting weights was preparation enough.

The new center had 10 machines, as ominous as they were sturdy. I told the owner that I was in excellent condition. It really didn't matter.

The first device was the size of my room, a Compound Leg machine that featured a leg extension and press. Although I normally squatted 320 pounds in a safety rack for 10 repetitions, I wasn't used to being 'pushed,' and less, having my face bury in a carpet when I finished. I scrambled to the next machine, a Leg Curl, more determined to show that I was equal to the task.

The fourth exercise, a Super Pullover, was the version I'd seen in the photos. By now, I was puffing like a train. After four repetitions, I felt light-headed and wobbled to the bathroom, sick.

It was a rude awakening, unacceptable. Less than seven minutes of exercise rendered the remainder of my day useless. Apparently, I'd done better than some.

In 1970, Nautilus inventor Arthur Jones invited anyone in the world to train with his novel system. Despite the fact that there were only four machines built at the time (Universal® equipment and free-weights were used), no one completed a 12-exercise circuit the first four years the company was open. After a few minutes with Jones, most ended up, as I had, on the floor - in shock, sick, unable to continue.

The scenario repeated when I opened my own Nautilus facility in Caracas, Venezuela in 1980. Approximately 30 bodybuilders came by the first year to try out the new system. Only one made it to the fifth exercise. The others finished in a horizontal state of dysfunction, having learned an age-old lesson - it's better to give than to receive.

It wasn't the equipment that made the difference (I could have done the same in their gym using free weights); it was the all-out, non-stop barrage of exercise.

Brief, high-intensity workouts were not easy. By combining the elements of strength and cardiovascular training, Jones uncovered a third level of physical fitness he called "metabolic condition" - the ability to work at a high level of intensity for a prolonged length of time. The state of shock encountered was a result of the body's inability to make chemical changes quickly enough to meet the demands of the sustained effort. Metabolic condition improved with training, which provided a challenge for some but left the majority seeking other venues of pleasure.

In 1994, I returned to the physical education building at McMaster. Smack in the middle of a new gym, high on a pedestal, sat the old plate-loaded pullover, still in use.

It was a fitting tribute to a tool that changed much more than the face of its users.

## APRIL 16

---

### The Negative-Only Years

In the early 1970's, several exercise equipment manufacturers began bashing negative work, the lowering of resistance. Their new machines featured "positive-only" exercise that allowed trainees to lift weights, but not lower them. The claims came hard and fast, and sparked the curiosity of Nautilus® inventor, Arthur Jones, who hadn't given it much thought until then. It was time to investigate.

Jones introduced "negative-only" exercise to a staff that included 1971 Mr. America, Casey Viator, to find out how 'bad' lowering weights could be. When initial results were anything but bad, he took the plunge himself.

On November 21, 1972, Jones started a six-week training program of negative-only exercise after not having trained for three and a half years. Toward the end of the second week, he submitted an article about his results to *Ironman* ("The Facts Are...," March, 1973). After six workouts in 11 days and 48 total sets (45 negative-only and 3 normal sets as progress checks), the self-proclaimed "old man" boasted a gain of one full inch on his cold upper-arm measurement.

His sixth workout (one set each of approximately 10 reps) was as follows: Nautilus Pullover machine, Torso-Arm (pulldown to chest), Behind-Neck Machine, Torso-Arm to neck, Bench Press with parallel grip, normal barbell curls (STRICT), Triceps Machine, Biceps Machine, parallel dips, and barbell wrist curls.

He then sought to make it official by conducting a "negative-only" research study in the exercise-physiology lab at Colorado State University in May of 1973, a project he called "The Colorado Experiment." The subjects were Casey Viator and himself.

Jones, who hadn't trained since January 1973, performed 12 workouts in 22 days and averaged 10 sets of exercise in 24.8 minutes per workout (total training time of 4 hours and 58 minutes). He performed 54 negative-only sets, 14 negative-accentuated sets (two limbs up, one down) and 54 normal sets, for a total of 122.

He increased his bodyweight by 13.62 pounds, lost 1.82 pounds of body fat and added 15.44 pounds of lean muscle mass (arms increased by 1.625 inches). He was hospitalized with flu toward the end and was disappointed he didn't gain the 30 pounds he expected.

Casey Viator, who had not trained for months due to a work accident, performed 14 workouts in 28 days (33.6 minutes per workout; total time, 7 hours, 50.5 minutes). He increased his bodyweight by 45.28 pounds, lost 17.93 pounds of body fat and added 63.21 pounds of lean muscle mass. His strength increased accordingly: Leg press from 400lb. x 32 reps to 840lb. x 45 reps (110% increase); Chin-ups from 217lb. x 10 reps to 287lb. x 11 reps (32%); Standing press from 160lb. x 8 reps to 200lb. x 11 reps (25%); and Parallel Dips from 217lb. x 12 reps to 312lb. x 16 reps (43%).

Meanwhile, back behind the DeLand High School in Florida, a number of professional football-players were producing similar results with "negative-only" training. In two months, a Canadian player went from 275 pounds on a pullover to over 675 pounds. Lou Ross (Buffalo Bills) gained 20 pounds, cut his already fast 40-yard dash time by 2/10 of a second, added 5.5 inches to his vertical leap and doubled his strength on many machines. Mercury Morris (Miami Dolphins) gained seven pounds of body weight and ran the fastest 40-

yard dash of his life. Dick Butkus (Chicago Bears) trained with negative work the month before signing a five-year contract on a knee that was barely there.

All the while, negative work was somehow 'bad.'

## APRIL 17

### Good vs. Evil

Throughout his writings, Nautilus® inventor Arthur Jones portrayed *intensity* as the good guy and *amount* as the bad guy. Any increase in intensity represented a step in the right direction; any increase in amount, a step in the wrong direction, which is why he spent a lifetime seeking ways to make exercise harder.

His logic was clear.

If you walked 10 miles at a normal pace on level ground, you would not be out of breath, tired or sore when you finished. If you repeated it every day for a week, 10 weeks or 100 weeks, you would get the same result - no soreness, no muscle growth.

But if, instead, you ran "like a mad grizzly was after you" for 1/10 of a mile (1% of the walk), you would likely not be standing when you finished, become sore and grow. The reason, according to Jones, was simple, "You worked HARDER."

He found the relationship between intensity and amount of exercise one of mutual exclusivity (if you had one, you couldn't have the other) and geometric (doubling the intensity required a reduction of more than half - about 80% - of the amount). He also realized that muscles had three levels of strength: lifting (positive); holding (static); and lowering (negative). They could hold more than they could lift, and lower more than they could hold - all of which raced through his head.

"Negative-only resistance," he claimed, "gives you the highest possible intensity, higher than you could even begin to attain with either positive-only or normal positive and negative exercises...When performing normal exercises you are always limited to performances within your weakest strength level, the positive strength level - because, obviously, you can NOT lift more than you can lift. But with negative exercises you are working with your strongest level, the negative level - a level so high that it is impossible for you to move the weight in a positive direction, or even impossible to 'hold' it."

But it was not dangerous - intensity had nothing to do with the amount of weight used. "Instead," said Jones, "It is determined by the 'percentage of momentarily-possible effort.'" Nonetheless, the weight used for negative exercise was 40% higher than normal and could be lifted for at least a few repetitions, but it was not. It was lowered to the point where control was lost - and the results were stunning. Yet, the immediate effect of negative exercise had the greatest impact on Jones.

"Even though negative-only resistance is capable of giving you an intensity that is utterly impossible to produce in normal exercise," he claimed, "it does so without causing a racing pulse, and without making you gasp for air, and without even causing you to sweat very much. Why? Because your breathing increases from exercise in proportion to the amount of exercise - and your circulation does precisely the same thing - and since the amount of work also determines the heat-rise involved, and thus the requirement for cooling by sweating - it thus logically follows that negative-only exercises do not make much in the way of a demand for increased circulation, or breathing, or sweating. It is, I think about as close as you can get to a 'no work' workout."

The hardest and most productive form of exercise seemed as if it wasn't. "Now all that apparently remains to be done," he said, "is to determine just what balance is best for producing the greatest degree of results in the shortest period of time."

He started with three negative sets per muscle group per week but later settled on one.

As expected, more good meant less evil.

APRIL 18

---

### The Coaching Dilemma

Fresh out of graduate school, I was hired to coach the men's basketball team at Averett College in Danville, Virginia. At the time, I understood the value of conditioning but didn't know much about basketball or coaching, so I turned to books.

It wasn't enough.

In one of our initial encounters, Rockingham Community College - whose students mistook our longhaired players for the homecoming 'rock' band - ran us out of the building with their fast-break offense, despite a patchwork solution. I returned to the books for preventive medicine.

The second lesson came at the hands of Southern Wesleyan University in Central, South Carolina. Their two-building campus, a dorm and a gym, lulled us into thinking we could easily prevail, but their towering, scholarship athletes hammered us to the floor. I apologized to the players for the scheduling error at halftime and, despite a valiant effort on their part, prayed for an early buzzer.

Consolation for our 2-13 record that year came from Nautilus® General Manager, Ed Farnham who wrote, "A novice coach usually formulates a game plan or methodology based on the opinions and philosophies of his coaches or peers. His initial success is largely dependent upon luck; luck in what kind of genetic 'pool' he falls into in his first job. If he produces a winning season (because of, perhaps in spite of, his efforts) he gains credibility. Credibility gives him recruiting power. Recruiting power gives him more genetically superior athletes. More superior athletes give him another winning season. Another winning season gives him more credibility and so on."

He continued: "Most coaches base decisions on the say-so of their peers who happened to produce a winning season last year." This eventually leads to coaching and training practices in most sports that can best be described as 'traditional.' Yet, tradition doesn't always dictate success.

That same year (1972), Bill Bradford was relieved of his duties as football coach of Deland High School. He hooked up with Nautilus inventor Arthur Jones who had built a training facility behind the school. Bradford was impressed by the results Jones produced with 'negative-only' exercise and decided to start a weight-lifting team.

"At the time," said Jones, "I doubt that he really knew the difference between a barbell and a palm tree, but he was not stupid." Bradford trained his team using negative-only exercise (lowering weights) as Jones suggested: "two weekly workouts, only one set of each exercise, from six to eight repetitions in each set."

His teams went undefeated and untied for seven consecutive seasons.

Arthur was right: Bradford *was* smart and quit while he was ahead. The new coach started losing because, as Jones said, "he went back to using conventional training methods," adding, "And having been regularly trounced by Bradford's team for seven years, how many other coaches adopted his training method? None. Why not? Damned if I know; but I do know that it is impossible to explain insanity."

According to Jones, nothing succeeds like failure. Success reinforces what you already believe to be true, whether right or wrong. Failure forces you to stand back, analyze and make appropriate adjustments...unless it goes against 'tradition.'

The four-year basketball experience was a struggle; and if you truly learn *only* from your mistakes as Jones suggests, Averett College fired a walking encyclopedia.


## APRIL 19

---

### Golf, Then and Now

"Back in my day..." has long been recognized, but often ignored, as a great way to lose an audience. Times change, but history repeats. And what one sees as progress may be anything but in the eyes of others.

I attended the 2001 Masters tournament in Augusta, Georgia and was shocked by two things: the topography of the land, and the changing nature of the game.

One was positive. The Augusta National Golf Club sat on a stretch of undulating terrain to which television can do no justice. Everything but the tees pitched - up, down and sideways. Yet, with 60,000 spectators trampling its surface, the landscape remained as impeccable as it was stunning - in greens, browns, pinks and whites.

The other was negative. The par-five holes and many of the fours had fallen victim to the distance players hit the ball. On the eighteenth hole, Tiger Woods stood 78 yards from a green that, 20 years before, required a mid-iron to its surface. Advancements in the game have rendered courses obsolete. And it's not a first.

When wooden shafts crawled to extinction in 1934, golf writer Bernard Darwin commented on the reduction of golf to a putting contest in his book, *Playing The Like*. "Any of us can remember many a hole," he said, "that called for three good shots to the green... (now) every hole is for long hitters a two-shot hole." He recalled the extinct Leith course in Edinburg whose five holes measured 414, 461, 426, 495 and 465 yards respectively (then, feather-filled balls traveled 150 yards). "As they (golfers) set out on each of those holes, they must have felt that they were only at the beginning of a very big adventure, and that fortune might many times incline this way and that before they got to the end." He advocated reducing the number of holes from 18 to 12 to put what he called "adventure" back into the game.

The reasons for the current crisis are twofold. Today's athletes are in better physical condition, which allows them to generate and tolerate greater clubhead speeds. This contrast (of generations) was never more vivid than in the Masters practice area where 70 year-old, Gay Brewer, a cigarette dangling from his mouth, pitched balls beside a trim and fit David Duval. To his credit, Brewer was hitting shots that others could only envy.

Second, equipment manufacturers continue to fuel excitement with club and ball innovations. Today's metal woods have a thin-faced hitting surface that acts like a trampoline to "spring" the ball forward on contact (an idea first introduced by Spalding® in 1902). Solid, two- and three-piece balls that defy gravity are on the verge of replacing wound balls, a technology that created its own stir in 1898.

Publisher, Robert Macdonald recently reviewed the difference between 'then' and 'now.' "What is just as bad (as the current crisis)," he said, "few people seem willing to stand up for the traditional game."

Last month, I purchased a "BAKSPIN" mashie (a collector's item) that was 'banned' in 1922 because of the depth of its clubface grooves. Back then, a banned club spelled death; people refused to buy it. Nowadays, manufacturers (most recently, Ping® and Callaway®) market products in defiance of bans. And the demand is high.

In the end, let's hope that the governing bodies of golf have the wisdom to uphold the integrity of the game. If not, Tiger's tee shots will appear puny 50 years from now and a Wednesday Par-Three Tournament at the Masters may not be necessary. The four-day event will provide plenty of one-shot holes.

## APRIL 20

---

### The Best Nautilus® Machine

The discarded prototypes that filled a prefabricated building at Nautilus headquarters in DeLand (Florida) provided proof that Arthur Jones was probably not satisfied with any machine he made. The few that made the grade were all about function.

"Please don't tell me how big the tail fins are on your car," he said, "tell me how far it will go on a gallon of gas, and how long it will remain in one piece. And don't tell me how many exercises you can perform on a particular exercise machine (which was then a trend) - instead, show me something in the way of worthwhile results."

Worthwhile results for Arthur started with hard exercise for major muscles. "The most productive barbell exercises," he said, "are the basic movements - squats, standing presses, deadlifts, pullovers, etc. But these are also the HARD-

EST exercises - and for that very reason, many trainees avoid them like the plague. Substituting endless sets of lighter, easier exercises - and then wondering why their progress is slow or non-existent."

He delighted in the prospect of providing hard work for major muscles that had never been exposed to direct exercise.

"If you double the size of a rabbit," he said (*Ironman*, Jan. 1972), "you have increased its mass by 700%, because he will then be 'twice as long,' and also 'twice as wide,' and also 'twice as high' so he will weigh eight times as much as he did before you 'doubled him;' but he still won't be very large. And if you double the size of an elephant, then your 'rate of increase' will be exactly the same as it was in the case of the rabbit; but with a great and obvious 'difference' - in the case of an elephant you will add as much as 160,000 pounds to his weight. Whereas, in the case of the rabbit, you might add only 40 pounds. Thus, while the 'degree' of increase was the same in both cases - the 'actual' increase was very different."

He went on.

"Doubling the size of the major torso muscles - or increasing their mass to any degree - will thus produce a far greater increase in muscular size and strength than would be produced by an equal degree of improvement in the arm muscles; simply because the torso muscles are (at least potentially) much larger that the arm muscles."

There were added benefits. "Growth of a 'big' muscle," he clarified, "will cause more secondary growth as a result of indirect effect than would have been produced by the growth of a 'small' muscle. If the arms grow in response to exercise, the lats (upper back) will also grow 'some,' even if they receive no direct exercise - but if the lats grow in response to exercise, then the arms will grow to a greater degree and to a greater 'amount' than would have been produced by the opposite situation."

Jones first developed a pullover machine for the large muscles of the upper back that was near perfect, but not practical. It weighed more than 2,000 pounds, was 11 feet long, seven feet tall, cost $15,000 to build and took two people to help a trainee enter and exit.

He installed a 'door' by using a foot pedal and later attached a second exercise - a pulldown - to the same frame, creating what may have been his best tool, if not his favorite - the Super Nautilus Compound Pullover and Torso/Arm Machine. "It is a machine," said Arthur, "'without compromise.'"

Jones then did the same - combined two exercises on one machine - for shoulders, legs and chest, upping the ante on intensity. In the end, he recommended one hard set of each 'double' machine per week as the best way to make the elephants grow.

## APRIL 21

### Sergio Comes Clean

Arthur Jones was the least likely of candidates to enter the bodybuilding scene in 1970: "I did not compete, seldom worked out in a commercial gym, did not associate with other people who were training, never wore short-sleeve shirts, and took very few pictures of myself; in those days, most people still believed that you were crazy if you lifted weights, so I went to great lengths to avoid any notice of my exercise."

His reception was cold for another reason. "I tell the truth, and it shocks people. I am against fraud, against deception." There were plenty of both.

"Quite frankly, most of the people involved in exercise disgusted me, and I clearly understood that a very large percentage of them were either fools or frauds, or both. A situation that has changed primarily in the direction of becoming more widespread."

Joe Weider was then at the top of the heap (and still is). If you wanted to make it, you had to hook up with him or pay the price - as did Cuban, Sergio Oliva.

Oliva first visited Arthur Jones months before the 1971 Mr. Universe competition in London. He had the first over-20-inch arm Jones had ever measured - despite Weider's claim of Arnold's 22½" - and the first arm larger than its owner's head.

Oliva's muscle bellies (size determinants) were so long that the combined mass of his forearm and biceps limited his ability to contract. It led Jones to suggest, "It might well be that Sergio's arms would measure more than they do if they were actually a bit smaller - if this reduction came in the form of 'shorter' biceps and/or 'higher' forearms."

Ellington Darden witnessed Oliva's first workout with Jones. Sergio performed a leg press with 460 pounds for 17 repetitions, a leg extension with 200 pounds for 16 reps and then headed for a 400-pound squat. When his knees unlocked, he "went to the floor like he had been knocked in the head." His second attempt was the same; he finally completed seven repetitions with 300 pounds.

In an interview with Brian Johnson (2002), Oliva praised the system that got him into the best shape of his life. "You keep going until you can no longer move," he said. "And when you think you're going to rest, he (Jones) has you going to another machine! By the time you get to the other machine, you feel like you're going to die, pushing yourself to the maximum again. When you finish, all you can do is lay down on the floor."

He also commented on bodybuilding politics. In 1970, he finished second in the Mr. Universe contest in London where, "Everyone knew I beat those guys." From there, he flew to Paris for Mr. Olympia where Weider denied his entry due to his participation in the non-IFBB-sanctioned event in London. He was allowed to do a posing exhibition.

The next year in Essen, Germany (Mr. Olympia), Sergio arrived in such good shape that Weider tried to dissuade Arnold from competing. The result? "Even Arnold himself said he didn't win, that it was nothing but politics, but they gave it to him," reported Sergio. "After that contest, Weider put the promoter out of business because (he) did not want to run the contests the way Weider wanted to, with placings predetermined."

Oliva's opinion of Arthur Jones was different. "Anything I have to say about Jones is good," he said. "He is the only honest man I met in bodybuilding. If he says 'I'm going to pay you so much,' he does. If he says that next year you're going to look a certain way, then you will look that way. He's the type of person you like to deal with since he won't screw you or use you. And everyone who went down to Florida knows that."

... everyone but Arnold, who became a major critic of Nautilus® thanks to Joe.

## APRIL 22

---

### The 'Apollo' Moonshot

I was a fish out of water, didn't know a hook from a crook as a first-year college basketball coach, which ultimately led to my being hooked by a crook. A salesman slid in on practice one day, and I bit.

The bait was a gadget that could "effectively condition the entire team" with a slew of resistance exercises for the major muscle groups, including the action of running. Since I had no control of the school budget, I purchased one for myself. It was lightweight, portable and fit a hectic schedule.

The "Apollo® Exerciser" was a cylinder with a rope entering and exiting at one end. Its outer case twisted to modify the tension on the rope (from one ounce to 600 pounds) within the cylinder. A strap at the other end attached to a door or platform. I read the instructions, selected the most appropriate movements and used it - when needed - for about five years. If it was good enough for astronauts, it was good enough for me.

Little did I know.

Around that time (1973), Nautilus® inventor Arthur Jones wrote several articles about current forms of resistance. In one, on page 11, I found the picture of "a highly advertised friction-based device (isokinetics)," the Apollo.

According to Jones, the device provided positive-only (lifting) resistance, no lowering resistance, which the manufacturer hailed an 'advantage.' Jones saw it otherwise.

"Such machines use a 'speed limiting' device," he said, "an arrangement which permits a movement at a pre-set speed only. There is no actual 'resistance' in the true sense of the word - but if you pull as hard as possible, then you will (in theory, at least) be encountering maximum-possible resistance during a large part of the movement."

The salesman claimed the work was full range. Jones disagreed: "Actual full-range movement against resistance is utterly IMPOSSIBLE with anything except a rotary form exercise machine."

The slickster downplayed the role of negative work (lowering weights) on the basis that it could make you sore. Arthur would have mooned him on the spot.

"It is the negative resistance that pulls a muscle into a fully extended, 'prestretched' position. The position that almost all muscle physiologists agree is required for best-possible results from exercise." He then added, "There is NO resistance provided in the contracted position - the ONLY position in which it is possible to involve all of a muscle in any form of exercise."

But that wasn't the worst of it. The instructions urged a maximum effort through a full range of motion, to which Jones replied: "If you are silly enough to follow such poor advice then don't be surprised if your blood pressure rises so high that you start spurting blood out of both ears like a two-spigot fountain. And don't be surprised if you yank your muscles clear loose from their attachments."

A maximum effort on every repetition denied the muscle the 'warm up' normally provided by the performance of several sub-maximal efforts before it fails.

"I suppose it is only natural," Jones concluded, "to expect people who have large green horns growing out of their heads to consider such horns 'beautiful' - and advantage of some sort - but it remains to be demonstrated that horns are an actual advantage to modern man."

It's nice to know you're as dumb as the boys from NASA.

# APRIL 23

---

## Average Genetics, a Little Luck and Chicks to Boot

Curiosity, a stroke of genius, average genetics and a bit of luck led to the formation of the most influential company in the history of exercise, Nautilus Sports/Medical Industries®.

It all started in a hot and dirty basement - probably a YMCA afterthought - in Tulsa, Oklahoma in 1948. There was no air conditioning or staff to keep the place clean. Few cared; even fewer noticed. The dungeon was for 'weightlifting' and - at temperatures exceeding 100° and humidity at 100% - might have been ideal for a modern Yoga class, if anyone had thought.

But there was little thought those days, just lifting. At least that's the way it appeared when a young man named Arthur showed up three times a week and trained for four non-stop hours. Three gallons of water later, he emerged only partially satisfied. His arms and legs grew, but his torso did not. He wanted to progress on every exercise, every set, every session - to be as strong as he could be. He read and consulted the experts of the day, but no one had answers.

Arthur set out to find his own.

"If I had been one of those few and fortunate individuals who find it easy to build all of their body parts, then Nautilus would never have happened. Because, in that case, I would almost certainly have been convinced that I already knew the secret to success, and thus would not have been inclined to seek a better method of exercise. Or, if I had been one of those few but unfortunate individuals who find it difficult to build any of their body parts, then Nautilus would never have happened. Because, in that case, I would probably have quit in disgust, wrongly convinced that exercise offered nothing of value."

Fortunately, Arthur Jones was, in a genetic sense, disgustingly average.

He realized that rapid results were possible because of the response of his legs and arms, but he suspected something was wrong because that same rate of progress was not apparent in other parts. He blamed his exercise program and changed everything about it. Nothing made much of a difference.

He then looked at the equipment and began to build "the first really serious attempt" at something that would better stimulate his lagging torso. Everything happens for a reason.

Jones went to Tulsa to be recruited for the Jewish-Arabian war. He wanted to fly a jet fighter in combat and didn't care on which side he fought, but he wasn't dumb. He didn't trust the recruiters on either side, and rightly so. "Some of my friends", he said, "fought on one side, some on the other side...a few got killed, even fewer got paid."

One day, Jones met a fellow pilot in the dungeon, a Senior Captain of American Airlines®, Percy Cunningham, a man interested in exercise and young ladies. "And since," according to Jones, "he assumed that I knew something of value on the subject of weightlifting, and since, he had an almost limitless supply of young and very attractive girls, stewardesses for his airline, it rather naturally followed that we became friends."

Jones got the better end of the deal. "The very firm opinions that I then held on the subject of exercise," he said, "left a great deal to be desired, while the girls that he knew left little if anything to be desired."

Cunningham funded the materials used to build the first Nautilus machine, an attempt that failed, but a start "in the direction of a logical approach to exercise."

By 1968, Jones understood the problems he was trying to solve. The rest is history.

## APRIL 24

### Not Exactly

I witnessed a pathetic site involving a healthy, teenage basketball player and a trainer with a 'special' work visa because of superior credentials.

You be the judge.

It began with the trainee asking about speed of movement on a leg curl machine. After a vague reply of "fairly fast," he performed 15 repetitions in the same time it took me to perform three on an adjacent machine. He then rested a minute and repeated. During my second exercise, the youth sauntered toward a one-legged wall squat where, following an effort of medium intensity, he rested and repeated. By then, I was several exercises along and engrossed in my own efforts.

The teen finished his routine (two sets of chest flys) as I began my last exercise and walked by talking about his next session - with no visible signs of discomfort. As he left, the trainer hollered, "Good job, see you tomorrow."

I coached college basketball in Virginia from 1976-1980. From opening tip-off to final buzzer, there was no rest. Stop, start, accelerate, decelerate, shift laterally, up, down, sprint, back-peddle, jump, muscle an opponent, move without the ball - I'd compare basketball to any sport in regard to physical demands. Soccer (which I also coached) comes close - but only close. You can disappear on a soccer field and not affect the game. There's nowhere to hide in basketball.

Physical preparation for high-level competition should address the major components of fitness: strength, cardiovascular condition, flexibility, improved muscle-to-body-fat ratio and injury prevention. Only proper strength training accommodates them all:

- Perform each exercise to a point of muscle failure (where you can no longer continue with a full effort, where movement is no longer visible). Nautilus® inventor, Arthur Jones often warned that completing a set of exercise with anything less than a full-out effort warrants staying home. Benefits are realized only when work is HARD, which means most trainees need to be pushed, not babysat.
- Perform each exercise with a slow speed of movement. Slow strength training (where the weight is felt every inch of the way) ensures good form, full-range strength, a flexibility gain and protection from injury (both during and after). Slow also elicits a greater heart response because, you guessed, it is HARDER.
- Move quickly from one exercise to another. When possible, prepare the next station so you can begin within seconds of completing the last. If you perform sets: move to another exercise (instead of rest) and return later; or, select a complimentary movement and alternate AB, AB before moving to the next pair. If you think you won't make it through the workout that way, remove exercise from your program - too much prevents you from working HARD. Minimum time between exercises increases both intensity and cardiovascular response. You can't rest on the court.
- Perform each exercise through a full range of motion. This ensures a stretch at the end of the movement and triggers a 'stretch reflex' that increases muscle fiber recruitment during the lifting phase. The first improves flexibility; the second, strength.

What I saw that day fueled my own efforts. The more they floundered, the more quickly I moved from station to station. The more they rested, the harder I worked; the harder I worked, the greater the toll. About that workout the next day?

If you work HARD, you'll want to stay home tomorrow.

APRIL 25

---

## Building a Biceps Machine

How could a man who captured crocodiles, elephants and poisonous snakes for a living be stopped in his tracks by something as simple as a human biceps? This was definitely a cry for "HELP!"

Arthur Jones sought to build an exercise tool that activated as many muscle fibers as possible in the biceps of the upper arm. Despite the fact that his arms grew like weeds, standing curls with a barbell were frustrating. They provided no resistance when the muscle was in a fully contracted position.

That wasn't the only problem. The major function of the biceps was to supinate the hand (rotate it to a thumbs-out position); the secondary function, to raise the hand to the shoulder, what Jones called the 'contractile' function. The two had to be maximized and combined, which proved a greater challenge.

"Given the balanced strength curve for isolated contractile function of the biceps, as well as the balanced strength curve for isolated supinational function of the biceps," he pondered, "how do you double balance the perimeters of two separate spiral pulleys, each of which provides the required variation in moment arm for separate sources of resistance, when the supinational resistance source is driven by a flexible shaft which is affected by the contractile movement, which movement imparts 158.4 degrees of rotational movement to the round pulley which drives the supinational-resistance source spiral pulley on a common axis?

Since the act of contracting the arm increases the contractional strength, and since the act of supination also increases the contractile strength, it is - for the purposes of building an almost 100% effective compound curling machine - necessary to double-balance the two separate sources of resistance provided each arm.

In effect, if the two sources of resistance (actually three sources of resistance, since there is only one, common source of contractile resistance for both arms, and two, separate sources of supinational resistance - one clockwise, one counterclockwise) are double balanced (balanced in relation to each other), then it is literally impossible to make significant movement in either direction without almost exactly corresponding movement in the other direction. You would find it impossible to 'bend' the arms without also 'twisting' the forearms - or vice versa; because, unless you supinated in similar degree, and simultaneously, you would not have the strength to contract and vice versa."

Jones took the problem to physiologists and mathematicians, but concluded, "Up to this point, without single exception, they have declined to even offer an opinion. And I am fairly certain that several of them remained glassy-eyed for several days after first hearing the problem." Ironically, his plea for help surfaced in a bodybuilding magazine, when he had yet to meet a bodybuilder who knew the major function of the biceps.

I have used five different models of his biceps machines over the years: Omni Biceps (with a foot pedal for negative work); Multi Biceps (independent arms); plate-loaded Biceps/Triceps; Compound Position Biceps (best contracted position); and MedX® Biceps. On most, he fixed elbows to pads (which provided stability) but wrestled with hand position. Some models featured one grip choice; others, multiple; but in the end he opted for a less-supinated hand position because of the stress of full supination on wrists. It seemed a compromise, and Jones did not like compromise.

I don't think the problem was ever solved to his satisfaction.

## APRIL 26

### Realistic Expectations – Arms

The reported size of arms in today's bodybuilding magazines is grossly exaggerated. According to Nautilus® inventor Arthur Jones, a man with an arm as large as some claim would have to weigh 800 pounds and be ten feet tall. The largest arms he measured through 1982 belonged to Cuban bodybuilder, Sergio Oliva at 20 ¼," with honorable mention to Arnold Schwartzenneger at 19 7/8."

Jones hadn't met Ray Mentzer.

Ray showed up for a workout at the Nautilus complex on January 5, 1983 weighing 253 pounds with an arm measurement of 19 ¾." Jones pushed him to failure on eight exercises - the duo-squat machine in two modes (including the brutal akinetic position), lower back, chin-ups, dips, pullover, pulldown, arm-cross and decline press - and then instructed him to repeat the workout twice a week. Mentzer returned on February 21st with an arm that measured 20 1/8." By July 9th, it was 20 3/8."

The arms of Oliva, Schwartzenneger and Mentzer dwarfed anything Jones had seen.

The chance of developing a 'Mr. Olympia' arm according to Ellington Darden, Ph.D. is probably about one in a million, if not less. Therefore, of the

150 million males in the United States, approximately 150 have the potential for a 20" arm.

The major factor that contributes to the ultimate size of an arm, according to Jones, is the length of the muscle bellies of the triceps and biceps, a factor entirely determined by genetics and one that can be measured.

To determine the potential size of your biceps, strike a double biceps pose (upper-arms parallel to the floor, at 90° to forearms and hands supinated - thumbs out). Have someone measure the 'gap' between the inside edge of your biceps (where the muscle begins) and the crease in the skin on the front side of your elbow.

To determine the potential size of your triceps, hold your arms by your side with elbows straight and contract your triceps. Have someone measure the distance from the tip of the elbow to the top of the inside of the horseshoe formed by the medial and lateral heads of the muscle (the length of the long portion of the flat tendon).

In both cases, the shorter the (tendon) measurement, the longer the muscle belly. Use the chart below to determine your potential for arm size.

| Measurement of: | | | |
|---|---|---|---|
| **Biceps Gap** | **Triceps Tendon** | **Muscle Length** | **Size Potential** |
| ½" or less | 3" or less | Long | Great |
| ½" – 1" | 3" – 4" | Above Average | Good |
| 1" – 1½" | 4" – 6" | Average | Average |
| 1½" – 2" | 6" – 7" | Below Average | Poor |
| 2" or more | 7" or more | Short | Very Minimal |

Another method of determining potential arm size for the average trainee was reported by Joe Roark - multiply the size of your wrist (in inches) by 2.3. That is, if your wrist is seven inches in circumference, your arm has a potential of 7 x 2.3 = 16.1 inches.

According to Darden, "Almost without regard for starting condition, size of bones, length of muscles, or even age, you should be able to build a level of muscular size and strength that will amaze most people. A few individuals can attain a muscular size that would amaze anybody."

Set realistic training goals. Most arms aren't the 'freaks' we thought they'd be.

APRIL 27

---

## Pumping Up

Muscular work places a demand on the body that is met by the heart and circulatory system in the form of increased blood flow to the working area. The added circulation transports needed fuel to the working fibers and assists in the removal of excess waste.

If the demand is low and the muscle allowed to continue for a while, the inflow of blood and subsequent outflow reach a balance that results in a slight enlargement of the working muscle. Studies have shown that a contraction below 20% of a maximum voluntary effort has no effect on blood flow.

If the demand is high, however, as during heavy strength training, the circulatory system cannot keep up. With contractions as high as 50-60% of maximum, there is no blood flow whatsoever in the working muscle. The congestion can cause a muscle to swell to astonishing levels, a phenomenon known as muscle pump or pumping.

Its effect is threefold:
- A pumped muscle feels heavy because of increased fluids within.
- A pumped muscle feels stiff because of a temporary loss of flexibility.
- A pumped muscle appears less defined.

Only two factors influence the degree of pump - the number of repetitions performed and the intensity of effort. While most exercise is discontinued well before a noticeable degree of pump is produced, prolonged activities such as walking are distinct. Calf muscles, for example, are much larger in the evening than in the morning. The difference does not indicate that walking was productive or properly performed, just prolonged. According to Ellington Darden, Ph.D., "It is possible to produce an extreme amount of pump from exercises that do nothing to build either size or strength." A long walk (high repetition, low resistance and restricted range-of-motion) produces a muscle pump without providing a stimulus for growth.

In contrast, a few sets (8-12 repetitions) of a full-range exercise carried to fatigue will produce the same degree of pump and provide stimulation for growth. The arm routine developed at the Nautilus® Research Center in the 1970's - biceps curls immediately followed by negative chin-ups and a 30-second rest; then triceps extensions immediately followed by negative dips (three sessions of less than five minutes each) - guaranteed a half-inch of growth in a week.

Enter the bodybuilders.

Most serious trainees believe that the longer they exercise the greater the pump, and the longer it remains. In reality, a HARD workout produces an upper-arm pump of approximately half an inch. Two hours later, the measurement will be slightly smaller than it was before the workout. Twenty-four hours later, the size will return to its pre-workout measurement or slightly larger, if growth was stimulated.

Muscle size varies under daily conditions. Upper arms, for example, are larger than normal first thing in the morning, slightly smaller an hour after a large meal, larger on hot days and smaller on cold days. The ideal time to take measurements is *after* a workout because it provides information as to future growth. According to Nautilus inventor Arthur Jones, muscle pump precedes growth. If a muscle that normally shows a ½-inch increase after a workout registers ¾ of an inch after the same type of workout, it is ready to grow to the pumped size within 48 hours.

The bad news? Unlike the pump itself, bodybuilders might now stay forever.

## APRIL 28

---

### Keep It Simple

If not for the 'thud' behind, we would have missed it.

I was first to glance back as college teammate, Paul Sinclair and I left the final green, putters in hand. "Look," I uttered as a ball bounced and rolled toward the hole from about 25 feet. Paul turned as it struck the pin and dropped. We looked down the fairway to identify the protagonist and saw a lone golfer with a squeaky pull-cart emerge from behind the 150-yard bush. When the ball disappeared, he stopped, threw his arms in the air and hollered, "PAR."

His good fortune was the highlight of our day.

One of the peculiarities of golf is just that - a high-handicap player can hit a shot a tour pro would be hard-pressed to repeat. Luck plays a role, yes, but a factor of far greater importance is at work - ignorance. Beginners and youth approach the game with a minimum of clutter.

I was reminded of that last month when I played with a pair of novice golfers. Both encountered success on difficult shots around the green because they approached each as if it was nothing more than the next shot. "Here's the ball, there's the hole. Let's play." It was something I'd forgotten.

Golf was fun as a teen. Yet, by the time I reached a level of competition that would have forced me to eat peanut-butter sandwiches the rest of my life, my score was linked to self-worth, mood and state of mind. What pride remains occasionally provokes a renewal of that misery, which is why it is always a joy to see the game played, as it should be, from a simple perspective.

In his book, *Golf is Not a Game of Perfect*, Dr. Robert Rotella links poor performance on the course to an over-emphasis on mechanics and swing thoughts - clutter appropriate for the practice tee. Playing should involve reacting to a target with a mind free enough to allow the body to do what it already can. As with many things, the less you know, the better off you are.

Strength training is no exception.

If you ask 100 trainers, you get 100 opinions about exercise, which is why most people who have trained with weights for any length of time accumulate some "far-fetched" ideas along the way. According to Arthur Jones (one of the few intellects in the field), hardcore trainees are the worst. He claimed that he *never* met a bodybuilder who knew the major function of the biceps and often challenged their ideas about training the inner, outer, upper and lower regions of the chest muscle. For a group that deifies both biceps and chest, it was apparent to Jones that the more you lift weights, the more your ears seal to common sense.

With that in mind, avoid the gym rats with all the gear. They take their activity (and themselves) too seriously, despite the fact that their work ethic becomes suspect toward the end of each exercise. Bodybuilding has lost most of its physiological roots and become little more than a social event.

Strip your strength training down to essentials: train harder (with more intensity), slower (in regard to speed of movement *during* exercise) and briefer (in reference to the length of each workout). You'll be three steps in the right direction, and four ahead of the guys with the gear.

As in golf, ignorance can be a blessing.

APRIL 29

## Hammer Time

Anna entered the gym with purpose: at 38, she wanted to regain the shape she had before two children. Using an efficient high-intensity strength training program and cardiovascular exercise, she trained hard, never missed and eventually exceeded everyone's expectations.

Anna was so thrilled with the results that she threatened to one day drag her husband in. Months later, Jose arrived with his own brand of training. He refused to increase the weight from its modest start and put up more resistance at the door than inside.

Following months of so-called "exercise," Jose was searching for his workout card and came across that of his wife. He scanned it, took it to a few machines and then approached me with a bewildered look.

"Is my wife *really* using this much weight?" he asked in reference to several exercises.

"Sure is," I replied.

Jose was stunned. He immediately increased his resistance to her level on *every* machine, raised them again the next time in, and monitored the situation for the rest of his membership.

It's comforting to know that you are stronger than your wife.

More recently, something similar happened when the son of a man many consider "the greatest golfer of all-time" entered our facility. The young man was the undisputed long-drive 'king' of the family, but was not as physically imposing as I was led to believe. Nonetheless, he had played golf that afternoon with a gym member who had trained for years and who, on a par-four hole, out-drove the king's 'best' by a margin of 50 yards. The runner-up took a sudden interest in our services.

Sometimes it takes a little buckshot to tune up the band. A blow to the ego, a stern medical warning or an occasional insult often provides a greater stimulus for action than the traditional avenues of encouragement and education. In plain English, if the hammer hits hard enough, you respond.

I once dealt, as a gym owner, with the problem of attracting and retaining clients whose priorities were anything but exercise. Mondays were typically packed with those repenting weekend sins. Fridays were empty. Any sniff of a holiday or weekend made most people vanish days before *and* after. Short of hiring nude instructors or offering free whisky for anyone who made 12 repetitions on Fridays, I developed a handful of techniques (of which I am not particularly proud) that worked:

- I told conservative members that, for the time they had been training, their weights were pitiful, and encouraged them to progress as often as they could (with repetitions and weight) within the confines of good form and physiology.
- When a member blatantly ignored form, I countered with education and common sense to improve safety and results. If that didn't work,

I resorted to, "I can't believe you're paying me to do *this*," or, "I wonder what you'd look like if you did *anything* right." It opened more ears than minds.

- When a member continued to ignore gym guidelines, I'd ask, "How much did you pay me?" and write a check on the spot. No wonder one guy repeatedly inquired when he entered, "Where's the German?" It wasn't hair color.

Create your own motives for exercise, but be forewarned - success takes discipline, something many of us only pretend to have.


## APRIL 30

---

### One Step in the Right Direction

"If you want to find out something about strength training," said Nautilus® inventor Arthur Jones, "write down all the questions and take them to the nearest gym. Find the biggest guy there, ask him everything and record *every* word he says. Then take it home and do exactly the opposite. You'll be one step in the right direction."

Jones believed that the training regimens of the majority of bodybuilders were not efficient or effective, and that less exercise would produce a better result.

Mike Mentzer listened.

Mentzer first met Jones at the Mr. America competition in Culver City, California in 1971. Although he placed tenth, he was so impressed with the victory of Casey Viator (who had trained with Jones 11 months prior to the contest) that it prompted a visit to DeLand, Florida two years later.

According to *The Nautilus Bodybuilding Book*, Mentzer claimed that he was in the best shape of his life during preparation for the 1978 Mr. Universe competition (when he performed only three 25-minute workouts per week, as advocated by Jones). At the same time, his contemporaries spent hours in the gym and refused to believe that a small amount of exercise could produce such size and strength.

Despite Mentzer's claim, fans thought he peaked at the 1980 Mr. Olympia contest in Australia where he looked awesome beside major competitors, Tom Platz (famous for his massive lower body) and Arnold Schwartzenegger (making a comeback after seven years of inactivity).

The crowd "booed" when Arnold took the stage - he wasn't nearly as 'ripped' or as 'big' as he was in his competitive days - but they couldn't get enough of Mentzer. No one had seen him look that good. When the final judgment came down, Mentzer took fifth, Schwartzenegger first.

The crowd booed the judges out of the building. Menzer broke the trophy over his knee and scrapped with Arnold in the locker room. Days later, Mike was arrested wandering the streets of early-morning California and committed to an institute.

Months later, upon his release (or escape), he flew to Orlando, Florida and convinced a taxi driver to take him to Ocala to visit his 'father' (Arthur Jones), who he claimed would pay the fare. Somebody called Jones who had the taxi intercepted by the police.

Mike (and his brother Ray - Mr. Universe, 1981) continued to train body-builders in their MedX®-equipped center in California. He also wrote intellectual books on high-intensity training. His writing, like that of Jones, was based on logic and physiology - and beyond the comprehension of most.

It was not a popular stance.

Months ago, Ray Mentzer found his brother dead of a heart condition in his home in Arizona. Days later, Ray died in the same house of the same cause.

Jones withdrew from the exercise scene years ago. The system he advocated was sound and effective, but to its detriment, brutally hard. Many refused to accept it; others simply couldn't do it. To most, it was a bad memory.

Yet, as with pioneers in any field (and as Mentzer put it), "If you want to lead the orchestra, you have to turn your back on the crowd."

For a fleeting moment in 1980, he clearly led the orchestra.

# MAY

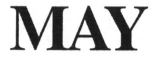

"Now the same people who brought you one outrage are going another great step in the same direction...but this time they have gone way too far; ruining a few thousand knees is bad enough, but destroying a few million already-injured lower backs is going just a bit too far. You can live with a ruined knee...but you might not be able to live with a ruined lower back."

Arthur Jones

# MAY 1

---

## A Little Help from My Friends

I must have had an identity crisis in college. I wore saddle shoes when it wasn't fashionable, a freshman beanie in every class for the entire year, and saved a cheerleader from makeshift villains on weekends in a *Superman* outfit at 'Home' football games.

Things weren't much different as a runner. I'd heard so much about the challenge of a marathon that its very mention teetered on the ordinary. With a personal best of only 10 miles, surely Superman could run *more* than a marathon.

So, I borrowed a car and set out from the school parking lot through the streets of Hamilton, Ontario, with one eye on the odometer. The trip ended at a mailbox in the town of Stoney Creek, an exact distance of 15 miles. A non-stop run to the mailbox and back would either up my bragging rights or leave me in a dumpster. I wasn't sure which.

To start, I extended my runs from seven to ten miles three times a week and consulted two professors: exercise physiologist, Digby Sale; and Britain's former Olympic track-and-field coach, Geoff Gowan. Both warned of potential risks and spoke of the latest trend, carbohydrate loading. Excitement mounted as the day approached, but it never happened. The added training produced shin splints that took weeks to heal.

I set a new date, the first Saturday in November.

Two days before the event, dorm treasurer Ned Jones tapped on the door. He asked if I would dedicate the run to a scholarship fund in the name of the dormitory (Whidden Hall) and the late Dean of Students, Ivor Wynne, who had passed away only days before. Despite my respect for both (the Dean's son was a golf teammate), I wanted a hassle-free run. We compromised: Ned organized, I ran.

The day was ideal - 50°F, overcast with a slight breeze - as I set sail with no fanfare or water. At 13 miles, I encountered what runners call a 'stitch in the side' that required several digging fingers for relief. It lasted two miles. When I reached the mailbox and reversed direction, I sensed adversity. The last half would be against the wind and, as I would later realize, uphill. But I wasn't done either.

At 18 miles, Ned and two friends showed up with oranges and water. They took turns running in front to cut the wind. When I was out of gasoline at 21 miles, they prodded. When I neared downtown, five miles from 'home', I'd had enough. They refused to let me stop.

Soon, the sight of familiar territory led to the brash belief of a final flurry; but my legs denied the request, eventually plodding a tired body across the line. I wobbled to the dorm on knees that popped up like a puppet's and legs that cramped as I bent to untie my shoes. I remained in motion and ended in a warm bathtub, feet firmly pressed on the wall above the spigot.

The 4-hour and 20-minute ordeal had done me in. I could barely walk for a week.

Some things are worth the effort if something is learned in the process. Note:

- Challenge yourself, but set realistic and reasonable goals. Training at 10 miles to run 30 is like practicing for a golf tournament by playing tennis. Planning is more valuable (and less painful) than enthusiasm.
- Find someone to push you to your limits. Even a motivated athlete, training alone, is capable of muscle failure on only a few exercises.
- Don't try the Superman route. It'll only get you 30 miles closer to a dumpster.

Thanks, guys.

## MAY 2

### Muscle Soreness

A line from an article written by Nautilus® inventor, Arthur Jones provided a potent reminder of what I felt for seven days. "When a muscle that has not been accustomed to heavy workloads is worked intensely - *or for a long period of time at a normal level of intensity* - then some degree of muscular soreness will usually result. In some cases, this can be literally crippling in its effects - for as long as a week."

The headline in *The Spectator* read "Memorial Marathon," the text: "Gary Bannister, president of McMaster's Whidden Hall which is aiding a fund created in the name of the late dean of students, Ivor Wynne is running 30 miles today from Hamilton (Ontario) to Winona and back with sponsors for every mile he completes." (November 3, 1970)

The goal of "not stopping my legs" lasted four hours and twenty minutes, and raised $650 to honor the Dean. A week later, I was still using my arms and the other banister to climb the cafeteria stairs.

It wasn't pretty, but I needed to eat.

The many theories (and lack of consensus) concerning muscle soreness become meaningless when we understand the cause/effect relationship.

A one-repetition effort, for example, rarely creates extreme soreness because muscles are not capable of a maximum input without a proper warm-up and time to recruit their working fibers. *Some* degree of soreness is produced, but only an 'awareness' that provides information about the effect of the training procedure.

In the late 1960's, Jones conducted a series of tests "to determine the effects of most types of exercise." When untrained subjects performed several sets of bench presses, they experienced soreness in the muscles of the chest. When they performed three heavy sets of one repetition each, they felt it in the front shoulder with little or no discomfort in the chest and triceps. The bench press, while not a direct exercise for any muscle, affected the anterior deltoids more than other groups.

Jones also tested the effect of a spectrum of upper-back exercises - regular chin-ups *alone*, behind-the-neck chin-ups *alone*, conventional pulldowns *alone*, and rowing *alone* - on untrained subjects. A few performed one heavy set of each.

Two days later, no one reported much discomfort in upper-back muscles - many, nothing - but all were sore in the arms, and some were unable to use them for days. In contrast, a group that used a Nautilus Pullover machine reported soreness in the upper-back muscles with residual discomfort in chest, trapezoid, abdominal and triceps groups.

Muscle soreness indicates the location and intensity of work. Because muscles adapt quickly to 'hard' exercise, soreness produced in an area that has trained for at least a week indicates that things were not hard enough - or lacked good form - initially.

Negative work creates more soreness than normal work because of greater intensity. Muscles are 40% stronger lowering than lifting. When lowering is carried to fatigue, a larger hammer hits the system and its ability to recover.

Most discomfort can be avoided by a 'break-in' period, as follows:

- Train every day for 4-5 days (20-30 minutes) during the first week. Perform one set of 8-10 exercises (8-15 repetitions) and avoid complete fatigue.

- Train every other day (3x) the second week, and work harder.

In the case of extreme soreness, more exercise is the only solution to restored function - especially when function involves the need to eat.


## MAY 3

---

### Guesswork at Best

Towing the line of physical trainer can be as tricky as Blondin crossing Niagara Falls on a tightrope. On one hand, first-time clients want a little muscle soreness to feel they've done something; on the other, they don't want the kind that cripples both function and return. When in doubt, the best approach is probably the first, conservative; but even at that, the best of trainers are guessing.

Most 'experts' agree on only one thing related to muscle soreness - that it's misnamed. According to Arthur Jones, "The contractile tissues (of muscle) do not have the type of nerves required to either record or transmit pain."

For that, some of the focus has shifted toward the connective tissue - a direction Jones calls "pure guesswork at best." Other speculation revolves around supposed microscopic tears that occur in muscle tissue due to training, a theory that Jones dismisses in reference to the first two workouts of an untrained subject: "If one hard exercise produced 'damage,' then two hard exercises should produce more damage and thereby make the soreness worse. But that does not happen (soreness dissipates after the second workout)... So I believe we can scrap the theory about damage to the muscle."

Without knowing what muscle soreness is - let alone when, where or if it will occur - it may be influenced by the following:
- The intensity of the exercise relative to the condition of the muscle. A muscle in 'poor' condition is more likely to get sore than one in 'good' condition.
- The frequency of workouts. Infrequent workouts increase the chance of soreness.
- The exercise itself. Some exercises produce more soreness than others.
- Change in sequence, number of repetitions performed and equipment used. "It appears that muscular soreness, whatever it is, results primarily from a change in your accustomed pattern of activity; in effect, the body is reacting to something new." (Jones)

- Style of performance. Negative work produces more soreness than positive work by providing the highest possible level of intensity during exercise, which, in turn, provides greater stimulation for muscle growth and a deeper inroad into recovery ability.

Performing a hard first workout after a layoff will produce muscle soreness the next day, and more the second. From there, if you do no further exercise, "the degree of soreness," says Jones, "will increase day by day for a period of five to six days, eventually reach a peak, and then gradually go away." It might last as much as 7-10 days. If you perform a second workout within a few days of the first, it will diminish.

The fact that some exercises make you sore while others do not remains a mystery. Your first set of leg-extensions, for example, left the impression that your thighs would melt and you'd *never* walk again. But you did, with minimal discomfort.

An untrained Jones once performed six sets of exercise on a prototype chest machine. "I wanted to get my pectoral muscles as sore as possible," he said, "believing that the resulting degree of soreness and location of the soreness would tell me how well the machine was working." His chest swelled for days, but it was not sore.

The muscle groups that produce the greatest initial discomfort are chest, inner thigh and calves. A gradual increase in work intensity over the first 10-14 days of training should help you survive the crisis, regardless of the 'change' you throw at your body.

## MAY 4

---

### Water

There are varying degrees of stupidity and attempting a 30-mile, non-stop run without water was high on the scale. Although it was fashionable among coaches at the time to forbid athletes water during football practice to 'make men,' my decision was born of another seed. I didn't want to drag a container around.

Water and I weren't exactly friends. At age five, I watched Dad rescue my brother as he was swept down the Welland Canal by the current of a passing freighter. I took little comfort in its midst throughout a lifesaving course in college. And, apart from the odd fishing excursion, a few water-skiers I trained, the golf balls I sacrificed to it and the times it boiled on the stove, my exposure to water was limited.

Still, I should have known better.

At the 18-mile mark, three students paid a welcome and unexpected visit. They brought oranges and water, ran in front of me to block the wind and played Knute Rockne when I was about to quit at 25 miles. I credit their urging for my success, but the truth was evident: without water, I would not have made it.

I never understood that lesson completely until three years later in Danville, Virginia. Frustrated by the rejection of a female, I set out at noon on a hot, sunny day to run 23½ miles without a shirt and, of course, without water. At 21 miles, I hit what distance runners call "the wall." Dizzy, light-headed and out of energy, I straggled into a Burger King®, doused my head and drank. I stumbled home in three hours and 10 minutes - left, right, left, right, left, right. It was the first and only time I stopped during a run (for the record, I did stop for funeral processions).

It was the last time I attempted a run of more than 20 miles.

Nautilus® inventor Arthur Jones once said, "If you want to discover the function of something, don't focus on what you can do with it. Focus on what you can't do without it." I could run 21 miles without water, but not much further. Lack of water during prolonged exercise can lead to heat exhaustion, the major reason they cart athletes off during "Ironman" competitions.

The human body is composed of approximately 70% water, most of which enters through the mouth. During activity, water is expelled as sweat through pores in the skin (the body's way of regulating temperature) and exits the nose and mouth in the breathing process.

How much water do you need during exercise? Much depends on the activity itself. According to nutritionist and runner, Brenda Hilcoff:

- Drink 2-3 large glasses of fluid two hours prior to participation in physical activity and another 1-2 cups (8-16 oz.) 10 minutes before start-time.
- Drink at least 8 ounces of water every 20 minutes during the event.
- After the event, drink to quench your thirst and then drink more (2-3 cups within one hour after the event).

Water requirements during strength training are different - or should be. If you work hard, your workouts must be brief. If you need water during training, ingest a small amount only. Too much can create nausea - the feeling I get when I see someone ingesting water after *every* set of *every* exercise, as if they deserve a reward.

If a trainee can't finish a hard, 20-minute workout *without water*, I'll send him off to Danville, throw in a cool day and the girl to boot.

## MAY 5

### Recreation or Exercise?

Would a well-conditioned athlete consider the walk of an elderly person around the block exercise? Would an armchair quarterback classify the performance of his hero as recreation? Would the quarterback agree? Many people indulge in recreation in the firm belief that it is 'exercise;' while others engage in exercise and would label their efforts as anything but 'recreation.'

The confusion between the two is born of the fact that they share elements - the most prevalent, movement. Because of movement, some recreational pursuits produce benefits common to exercise, such as an increase in cardio-vascular fitness or a loss of body fat. Unfortunately, it has led to the belief that any movement has 'exercise' value; and worse, that exercise should, or can be fun.

Exercise and recreation are miles apart:

**One.** Exercise is designed around a logical, strategic and systematic attack upon the body's muscular functions. Its purpose is to stimulate change by sending a signal to the body. If the signal is strong enough (that is, has enough 'shock' value) and accompanied by adequate rest and nutrition, the body will make the appropriate modification. If the signal exceeds the amount required for stimulation, it can prevent results by consuming valuable recovery energy; and if it is accompanied by bad form, may result in injury. The elements of intensity, duration, frequency and form inherent in proper exercise lead to measurable progress.

Recreation, on the other hand, is instinctive and governed by personal whims. I like to play golf, for example, in my spare time - a personal choice. The philosophical difference was clarified by Nautilus® inventor Arthur Jones: "If you followed your instincts, you would do quite a few things. But you wouldn't exercise."

**Two.** Exercise is based on the universal concepts of biology, physiology, structure and function. Therefore, an exercise program for an athlete might not differ much from that of a pregnant woman or rehabilitation patient. If a muscle needs strength, the approach is the same regardless of how that strength is used. Recreation is personal, not universal.

**Three.** Exercise is general in its application and effect. It results in overall physical improvements that contribute to any skill, sport or recreation. Improved cardiovascular condition, for example, helps you play better soccer, hockey and golf. Recreation is specific in that it involves the use of skills specific to the activity practiced. If you want to improve at basketball, work on skills related to basketball.

**Four.** Exercise stimulates physical changes in the body that can lead to psychological changes as a side effect - a reward at the end of the rainbow. For the most part, recreation is performed for the mind and for the pleasure that participation brings.

**Five.** Exercise is not fun. It pits intellect against instinct, resulting in internal tension. On the other hand, fun is the major criterion for choosing recreational activities.

The following is a recommended approach to balance the two:
- Identify and accept the risks involved in any form of recreation.
- Prepare for those risks by performing exercise for the muscular systems involved, and accept exercise for what it is - HARD WORK. Don't pretend to enjoy exercise other than the satisfaction derived from progress (in strength, flexibility, endurance, body leanness and resistance to injury).
- Then, participate in the recreation of choice with your new physical tools.


MAY 6

———


### Bodybuilding Magazines


Don't be fooled by what you read in bodybuilding magazines. And you might.

Today's publications are long on ads and short on articles - which is good, because most articles are what Nautilus® inventor Arthur Jones called "worse than worthless."

Among other things, trainees are led to believe:
- If they lift weights, they will look like the guy in the photo (few have the potential for such size, regardless of how they train). If I bounce a basketball, will I grow tall enough to play in the NBA?

- That they can buy success, find strength in a bottle or eat their way to muscular size. Fifty years ago, there was little mention of nutrition in bodybuilding publications. Today, there's nothing but.

The first thing that slaps you in the face about the magazines is the fact that the exercises are the same as last month, last year, last decade - just a new star re-shuffling the old deck. According to Jones (who wrote in *Ironman* in the 1970's and 1990's), "Weight-training publications ran out of anything significant to say over 20 years ago - and having said the same things in 1,000 different ways, the publishers are understandably quick to give attention to almost anything that might be considered new or original; but originality is no proof of validity."

The second thing is the bias. Several years ago, "Collegiate Mr. America," Ellington Darden, Ph.D. submitted a nutrition article to Weider's *Muscle and Fitness* that advocated the use of no food supplements (a balanced intake based on experience and research). It was rejected for philosophical reasons. Months later, the magazine published an article on the Bulgarian training system that featured Darden's bibliography at the end. The error went unnoticed.

The third relates to reader requirements - where a degree in chemistry would make a good start. The ingredients of advertised supplements (that somehow pass government tests) are mixed with enough other elements to make the effect useless or unknown at best, and dangerous at worst. In no time at all and with few exceptions, they are replaced by a better ill-tested formula - which only confirms my belief: "If it can't be pronounced, bodybuilders will buy it."

A degree in math might also come in handy. "Most bodybuilders have followed so many different routines by the time they attain a point of recognition," says Jones, "that they really have no slightest idea regarding 'which routine produced which result' - but they invariably think they do." The reported workouts of today's stars resemble complex formulas (example: 120lb. [3x20] X 5) that, properly performed, would kill an adult gorilla...and destroy any trace of quality.

Lastly, the reader requires a sense of humor. According to Jones, "There was a time when most (trainees) read the magazines strictly for laughs. But now, quite a few take everything they read in the muscle magazines at face value - primarily, I think, because they want to; because the publishers have learned just what their readers want to hear and are very careful not to give them anything else."

If you insist on muscle magazines, take my advice: first, skip the sexy cover and the nutritional ads, and then ignore the rest. If you want something refreshing, unbiased and educational, read an article by Arthur Jones. He hits the nail on the head, tells the truth and provides plenty of humor in the process.

May 7

---

## Physical Culture

"He was poor; he was sick; he couldn't hope for much schooling. So, of course, he didn't have a chance. **But look at him today!** He's a man of sixty, with the body of a man of twenty - a man of extraordinary vitality; of broad education; of immense wealth." And more. The adjacent photo was worth a thousand words. Bernarr MacFadden - "the foremost physical culturist of all time" - had hair like Don King.

I recently scoured a May 1930 issue of MacFadden's *Physical Culture* magazine to glimpse bodybuilding's past. The focus on 'Health, Happiness and Beauty' and the cover's feature articles reflected an era when resistance training was not in vogue: "Be at your Best at 65," "How to be a Good 'Mixer' and Prosper," "Prolonging your Life by Sunshine," "Banish Cold Hands and Feet," and "The First Essential of Right Eating."

The cover was misleading.

MacFadden firmly believed that strength training was the path to 'good' health. In 1921, he sponsored the first bodybuilding contest in the U.S. and declared the champion "The World's Most Perfectly Developed Man." His commitment surfaced in articles and ads, some featuring his products and services (mainly books and courses); others, those of his mail-order competitors - Earle Liederman, the Jowett Institute of Physical Culture, the Strongfort Institute, Siegmund Klein and Charles Atlas.

The ads were few, the articles plenty. Of 137 total pages, 114 (83%) were articles or information-oriented. Most of the 23 ad pages (predominant or complete) were bunched at the front of the magazine. In the last 114 pages, there were only five full-page ads and approximately 45 pages with traces of drawings, pictures and advertisements. Once the articles began, it was pure text.

In contrast, I scoured a May 2002 issue of Joe Weider's *Muscle and Fitness* magazine - 72 years had passed.

Weider's publication had 248 pages, of which 207 (83%) were ad pages (predominant or complete). The majority dealt with nutritional supplements or 'growth' products, which came as no surprise with survival at stake, and when valid drug testing would surely hand the trophy to the nearest janitor. Approximately 33-50% of the 41 pages dedicated to articles or 'information' was laden with pictures. But the cover made it a bargain: "8 Complete Routines," "31

Exercises to Get You Ripped," "6-Week Fat-Loss Plan," "Great Glutes – 20 Fast Fixes," and "9 Solutions for Puny Pecs."

The only thing puny was the text.

One article was a reminder of Ellington Darden's comment in the *Nautilus Advanced Bodybuilding Book*, 1984. "The author urges the reader to train as hard as possible, and then lists a workout schedule that makes hard training impossible... Almost any one of the published workouts (over the past 30 years) would kill Hercules himself."

**Week One, Day One:** eight sets of an exercise using a 14, 14, 14, 12, 12, 12, 10, 10 repetition scheme and an intensity level of 45%, 45%, 50%, 50%, 50%, 45%, 45% and 45%; plus 10 other exercises averaging seven sets each (similar reps and effort); plus two sets of four distinct 'plyometric' movements.

**Week One, Day Three and Five:** different exercises, similar repetition patterns and intensity levels – approximately 1,000+ explosive repetitions followed by eight sets of bone-crushing jumps on stairs, times 12 weeks. Enough to make your hair stand tall.

Oh, *Physical Culture!* At least it was culture.

## MAY 8

### Hunting and Searching

Golf is a mystery. When you hit a bad shot, you can pinpoint the cause; when you hit a great one, you have no idea how it happened. Two or more wrongs can make a right; a right and wrong can make a right or wrong; and two rights can make a wrong. As they say, "Anything's possible on the PGA Tour."

To add to the mystique, two of the greatest ball-strikers in the history of the game, Ben Hogan and Moe Norman, never took a lesson. They believed the game could not be taught, only learned. Both hit balls to discover what worked and forged swings that were, by modern standards, unconventional. Neither cared about beauty nor the 'why' behind a successful shot. It was all about results.

Arthur Jones was the same with exercise. The Nautilus® inventor never questioned the fact that less exercise produced more results and spent years reducing the amount in his own program before he actually understood 'why' it worked. That muscles could lower more weight than they could lift, he applied in a number of practical ways before he understood 'why' - 17 years later. The same occurred when he used light work (instead of rest) immediately after heavy exercise to facilitate recovery. Some things made no sense - but they worked. Jones took them at face value and forged on.

It was something he learned from his hunting days in Africa.

"Capturing animals by running them down in broad daylight with a vehicle would appear to be a very dangerous method of capture - since it obviously involves very strenuous and sometimes long-extended efforts on the part of the animals; while capturing the same animals at night, using the element of surprise, would seem to be the easiest method - and the least damaging to the animals, since such captures can normally be made with no chasing at all. But, in fact, quite the opposite is true in both cases."

"An animal captured at night with no chasing," he explained, "stands a very good chance of dropping dead shortly afterwards, apparently from shock - while an animal that might appear to have been chased almost literally to death in broad daylight will seldom suffer any bad effects and will usually do quite well in captivity afterwards. There is, of course, a limit to just how much chasing an animal can stand - but within reason, such chasing actually seems to reduce the chance of shock from the capture."

"In a similar vein," he continued, "an animal that is shot by surprise will frequently drop dead from a wound that would not have bothered him much if he had been warned of danger in advance of the shot. While an animal that is aware of danger prior to the shot will sometimes continue frantic efforts with a wound that would seem to make any movement impossible - there are many accurate reports of large animals killing hunters after having their hearts destroyed by heavy bullets."

Jones applied those observations to exercise.

"It is obvious that a certain amount of time is required for a muscle to prepare itself for intense exertion - without which preparation, damage may result; secondly, it is also obvious that a muscle so prepared is then capable of working at greater intensity."

Muscle preparation can occur in different forms:
- The anticipation of exertion, which triggers the nervous system.
- Performing sub-maximal repetitions before full-out efforts (as in a 'normal' set).
- A general warm-up.

Why horses are walked after a race may never be fully understood, but it works.

MAY 9

---

## Have You Finished Yet?

It was a beautiful day for world-class water-skiing, but it wouldn't last. With two titans of medicine sitting side-by-side for the first time, I knew it wouldn't be long before the 'big' question was asked - the one that would ruin the day if you were near.

So, where was I? Near.

Dr. Fulton, medical physician for the U.S. ski team and orthopedic surgeon for Nautilus Sports/Medical Industries® (Lake Helen, Florida) sat to my right; Dr. Bajares, orthopedic representative for the Venezuelan team, beside him. Both were there for support. As conditioning coach of the Venezuelan team and owner of a training facility in downtown Caracas, I was all set to view the Latin-American Championships.

Once medical duties and an exchange of pleasantries were covered, the topic of exercise rolled in like a dark cloud. Dr. Fulton was the first to drop the bomb.

"Well, Guillermo (Dr. Bajares), what do you do in your exercise program?"

The 20-year bodybuilder began a dissertation I thought would never end. He detailed the number of sets and repetitions he performed, his frequency of training, his sequence, his rationale, his stance, his grip - everything but his shoe size.

All the while, competitors fell, crowds cheered, champions were crowned and lunch was served. Bajares carried on.

By some miracle, Dr. Fulton retained his ability to stay awake until the final word, at which he responded, "Well, Guillermo, I guess we're going to have to invite you to Lake Helen and show you how to train."

Fulton had witnessed some of the most intense workouts in the history of exercise, workouts supervised by Nautilus inventor, Arthur Jones. They were brutal (by necessity and design) and brief - so brief that they were criticized by the bodybuilding community as inadequate. They were anything but.

In 1971, 18 year-old Casey Viator performed three, 25-minute, whole-body workouts each week for 11 months and won Mr. America hands-down. In 1983, former Mr. Universe, Boyer Coe, reduced his training from 12 exercises, three times a week to eight exercises, twice a week (one set, 16 total minutes) to increase his size and strength. Mike Mentzer produced his best results with three 25-minute sessions a week when he captured the Mr. Universe title in 1978. And Mr. Olympia, Dorian Yates, adhered to brief, hard workouts in his successful years.

Bodybuilders aren't the only ones over-trained in quantity and under-trained in quality. Months ago I met a golfer who told me how much he trained to avoid muscle size. Hour after hour, set after set - he could have attained the same lousy result using one tenth the time and effort.

It is difficult to conceive of, let alone perform, less exercise when your workouts are long. In the early days of Nautilus, the rejection of 'less' was common - and understood. The concept came from a man with little compassion for bodybuilders. Most lasted only a few minutes before they collapsed to the floor with Jones in their face.

Things are no different today. Hard workouts, well within the grasp of everyone, are not on anyone's agenda - which doesn't change the facts. Best results from strength training are still within reach by what Jones called "outright hard work."

Don't look for ways to make exercise easier, faster and longer; look for ways to make it harder, slower and briefer. Then spend the time you save doing something you enjoy.

## MAY 10

### Dad

I left a trace of salt on a pillow last night, thinking of a man who passed away in November of 1984, a man who deserved more than 65 years, but you never know. When I glanced in the mirror next morning, I saw a mini-version - same build, shorter, lighter - with one glaring difference. The mini took 40 years of strength training to get there; Dad didn't exercise, at least in any formal sense.

Jack Bannister was abandoned by his mother in England, sent to Canada at the age of three and raised by relatives. He played football in high school - a 180-pound center on a team that competed for the provincial championship - and was an accomplished distance swimmer. The lumbering, rhythmic stroke he displayed when he took his boys to the Welland Canal or to a northern lake during vacation was something to behold. When we turned five, he introduced us to hockey, a game he played and coached. He always encouraged participation in sports.

Years later, Al and I reciprocated by introducing him to golf, a game that led him to abandon the post of Deacon in the local Anglican Church. He soon got Mom involved and established Sunday as 'family day on the links.' By then, his boys were champions. Al attended college on a scholarship, I won a few club championships, and Dad wasn't far behind. He lowered his handicap to 10.

Golf was a welcome addition to the family.

One Sunday morning, Dad shot a three-over-par, 75. On another, he carried my bag to victory in the Champion of Champions tournament at Lookout Point Golf Club (Fonthill, Ontario) in 1970. Years before, I caddied for him in a match in which, two down on the 15th, he 'boomed' a tee shot about 15 inches. In 1971, we shot 77 in an alternate-shot Parent-Child tournament through a rainstorm that forced most of the field off the course and threatened to cancel the event. Dad spoke up and proudly displayed the trophy on the mantle. The laughs at the dinner table on Sundays were often aimed in his direction, but he never complained - only the laughter counted.

I remember Dad in non-golfing times. The night he carried a vomiting son from the bedroom to the bathroom, straddling the splash beneath. The night he delivered deserving blows to a son who stole a bag of chips from the corner store. The time he paddled his boys for smoking - I was in grade two. The day he threw his lunch pail into the Welland Canal upon retirement. The pleasure he derived from maintaining the best lawn in the neighborhood and from performing chores around the house, always with his shirt off, always sweating, always whistling.

I remember how he handled his final months. Cancer had attacked his vital organs and made him so weak that he collapsed on the way to and from the bathroom. Lack of mobility was frustrating. He never moaned.

In the end, he refused treatment - why prolong the inevitable? I last saw him two months before he passed away and it was the only time that I was physically larger - and pure deception to think that I could ever be. The night of our good-bye, we shared a love and respect he had always shown, and a courage that was present until the end. There were no tears, but they weren't far away.

Now when I look in the mirror, I see a mini-version of the man I miss - same build, shorter, lighter - and that glaring difference.

When it's my turn, I'd like someone to think that I at least filled half a shoe.

# MAY 11

---

## The Last Word

In 1970, Arthur Jones opened Nautilus® headquarters in Lake Helen, Florida where Ponce de Leon once sought the Fountain of Youth. This time, however, hundreds of bodybuilders and athletes who came 'to learn about exercise' were left searching for a way to complete the brutal workout. If nothing else, they learned who was in charge.

From the start, Jones was adamant about maintaining standards high above the drug-infested situation that 'Muscle Beach' had become. His invitation was open "so long as your attitude is reasonable and your actions are acceptable by our standards; but keep it clearly in mind that they are 'our standards' - and since we are offering cooperation and help on a free basis, we can certainly continue to dictate standards, and we will."

By the time I toured the facility (1980), his 'hobby' had grown but his standards and Lake Helen remained the same. The shabby façade of the first gray building housed the world's largest television studio, 170,000 square feet of 'sets' and equipment that made NBC's "look like an outhouse" (according to NBC officials). With 1½ studios built, Nautilus Television Network operated three eight-hour shifts, five days a week and produced two half-hour video tapes every four hours and 200 weekly hours of programming for cable networks. By 1982, Jones planned nine studios and 1,000 weekly hours of programs (six times that of anyone). "When the real video revolution comes," he said, "we'll be the only one in town that can do something about it."

The plan was grandiose. Jones, RCA's largest purchaser of commercial videotape equipment, aspired to produce shows "on any and every subject you can think of including how to skin a catfish, speak Swahili with a Northern Rhodesian accent, and rear a child." He planned educational tapes for elementary and high schools, universities and hospitals, and a satellite hook-up to send tapes to his health clubs - not to homes, and no major broadcasting. "We're not insane enough to let the federal government have anything to say about what we do."

Around this time, The Beach Boys contacted Nautilus to install a line of machines in a transport truck for use on cross-country tours. Someone on the Nautilus staff came up with the idea of having the group perform a concert in one of the studios while they were there. During the negotiations, the group sent a list of 'demands' for the proposed performance. General Manager Jim Flanagan read them to Arthur, who interrupted, "Jim, tell those...uh...Beach

Boys to shove their $50,000 check (you know where). When they're here, it's my rules."

The TV studios provided an opportunity to fulfill another dream. From the beginning, Jones knew that his exercise philosophy would be at odds with the establishment, and it was. "And while it isn't quite true that I live on an island in a lake full of crocodiles," he commented, "I probably would if I could."

The "Crocodile Lounge," a 30,000 square-foot room (under construction) contained a half-million gallon fish tank filled with large crocodiles and thousands of tropical fish. It would soon host Jones' own talk show, "Younger Women, Faster Airplanes, and Bigger Crocodiles." Experts from the field of science, medicine and education would be lowered into the tank on a glass-encased living-room set and Arthur couldn't wait.

"We're going to make it a super '60-Minutes,'" he said. "Where they insult people, we're going to crucify them."

It wasn't exactly the 'fountain' that Ponce de Leon had in mind.


## MAY 12

---

### The Most Significant Discovery in the History of Exercise - Part 1

In 1986, the Chairman of the Board of Nautilus Sports/Medical Industries®, Arthur Jones, published an article in the *Athletic Journal* titled, "Exercise...1986, The Present State of the Art... Now a Science." The 'Now a Science' addition referred to the recent completion of a series of tools that totally isolated muscle function and allowed him to accurately identify four new physiological factors in exercise.

Arthur called his breakthrough, "The most significant discovery in the history of exercise...a discovery that will send shock waves around the world, a discovery that will change exercise forever, and change it for the better."

In theory, he was right.

The first of his 'discoveries' established the existence of at least two distinct responses to exercise. Some people (designated TYPE S) demonstrated "an almost totally specific response to exercise," while others (TYPE G) demonstrated a "general" response.

Figure 1 shows two curves that represent full-range tests taken less than six minutes apart to determine the strength of the muscles of the front thigh. The first test (Curve #1) was conducted just before an exercise; the second (Curve #2), immediately after. The exercise was performed with both legs to

Gary Bannister, B.A., B.P.E., M.Ed.

momentary exhaustion using a resistance that was based on the subject's start-ing strength (one that would allow approximately 10 repetitions). But it was *not* full-range. The exercise was restricted to the first half of the movement (right side of chart) and the ***effect*** or immediate consequence of the exercise appeared in, and was limited to, that same range of movement. There was no effect where exercise was not performed - a typical TYPE S response.

Jones confirmed other parameters related to TYPE S subjects:

- The ***effect*** was similar in magnitude when exercise was performed in the last half of the movement only (left side of chart).
- The response was similar with long-term exercise. TYPE S sub-jects produced *results* or long-term benefits only where they worked and few, if any, where they did not.
- "Approximately 72% of a random group showed a TYPE S re-sponse to exercise."

In contrast, Figure 2 shows two curves that represent the effect of exercise with a TYPE G subject. The same full-range pre-exercise test (Curve #1), half-range exercise (performed on the right side of the chart only) and post-exercise test (Curve #2) produced an effect so unique that Jones suspected an error. But there was no error. In the end, 28% of a random group of people showed a TYPE G response to exercise - the same magnitude of ***effect*** in the unworked as in the worked range.

Did TYPE G subjects produce long-term ***results*** in both ranges by per-forming partial-range exercise? Jones didn't know at the time but thought they would, based on the observation that a large group of untrained TYPE G indi-viduals had flatter strength curves than their TYPE S counterparts. They (TYPE G) were approximately 22% stronger in their weakest position near full exten-sion (left side of chart). He suspected that the strength was a "carry-over from the normal activities that produced their strength in the peak position...a carry-over that TYPE S individuals apparently do not get."

TYPE S individuals are weaker in their weakest position relative to their peak strength and benefit from exercise only in the range they work. Type G individuals receive full-range benefits from partial-range exercise. The impli-cations for strength training and rehabilitation are evident; the case for full-range exercise, established.

216

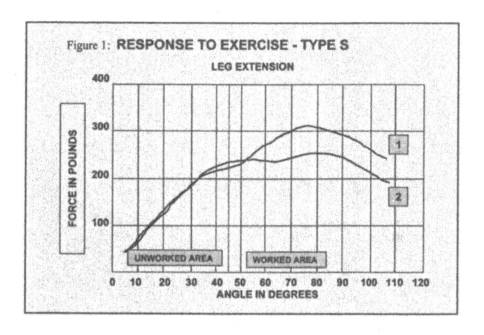

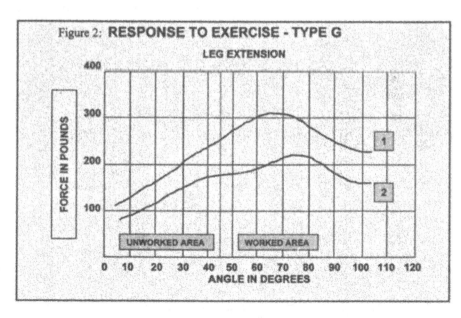

MAY 13

---

## The Most Significant Discovery in the History of Exercise – Part 2

"What may well be the single most important discovery in the history of exercise" remained a mystery to its discoverer even after the fact.

"Nobody in their right mind even claims to know what gravity is either," said Arthur Jones, "but we can measure it, and we can use it to good purpose, and we can avoid the problems associated with it even though we don't know what it is."

In 1986, Jones unveiled four new physiological factors in exercise that revealed vast genetic differences among people. The second really got him going.

"On a scale of zero to one-hundred," he said, "if the first factor (TYPE S and TYPE G response to exercise) is a four, then this second factor is at least a ninety-nine, and almost certainly a hundred... Now we know why some people can, and why some people can't, why some people do, and why some people don't; and we now know what is required to take advantage of at least some of the advantages provided by this factor, and we know how to avoid at least some of the problems associated with this factor."

The factor in question was the relationship of positive (lifting) strength to anaerobic endurance, more commonly known as muscle fiber-type or rate of fatigue.

For more than 40 years, Jones realized that his strength and local muscular endurance had a fixed relationship. If he could lift 100 pounds once, he could lift 83 pounds exactly 10 times - not 9 or 11 - 10. When his strength went up or down, his anaerobic endurance fluctuated "to exactly the same degree" - regardless of strength level, style of training, equipment or the amount of exercise performed.

He was enraged when he encountered a man who performed only four repetitions with 80% of his starting strength level, and surprised when another performed 23 repetitions under the same conditions. Their ratios were different.

Figure 1 demonstrates the *effect* of a limited-range exercise carried to a point where movement was no longer possible. The subject performed a pre-exercise test (Curve #1), seven repetitions to fatigue, and a post-exercise test (Curve #2). Despite the high level of intensity involved in the exercise, the magnitude of the effect (strength loss) was small - 3.05%. According to Jones,

"Such an effect will produce little or nothing in the way of benefit, regardless of the length of time devoted to such training."

Figure 2 demonstrates the *effect* of another subject who performed exactly the same test and exercise procedures. This individual performed only six repetitions to failure, an effort that reduced his initial strength by more than 44% (14 times that of the previous subject; a difference of 1,447%).

In a different testing procedure, Jones encountered subjects who performed a series of maximum-effort repetitions at or above their initial level of strength.

"Exercise always produces an effect, an immediate consequence," he said, "but it certainly does not always produce a result, a long-term benefit. Too little in the way of an effect will not stimulate a benefit, and too much effect will literally prevent a benefit."

Jones later determined that an effect of 20-25% (a combination of weight, repetitions and intensity that lowered starting strength by 20-25%) produced optimal benefits.

How much exercise is enough? By quantifying this factor, trainers and therapists can now design a program for an individual based on logic and fact instead of superstition, "with the ability to measure both the effects and results of such a program."

It's about time.

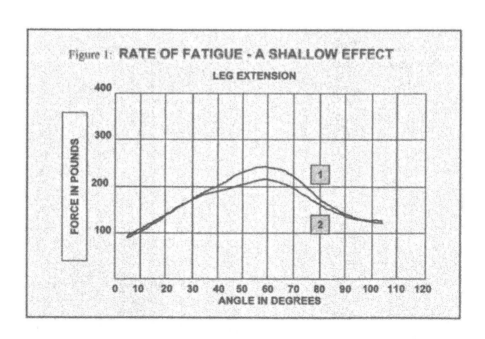

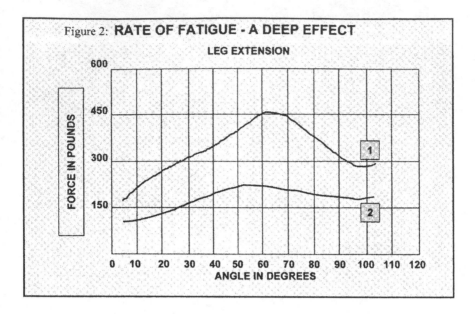

Figure 2: **RATE OF FATIGUE - A DEEP EFFECT**

MAY 14

---

## The Most Significant Discovery in the History of Exercise – Part 3

Arthur Jones was so excited about the second of four physiological discoveries that the third seemed anti-climatic. But it was no less important.

The third factor dealt with tolerance to exercise and recovery ability. Some people possess a high tolerance and recover quickly, while others demonstrate a low tolerance and recover slowly. Those with a low tolerance must be handled with caution.

Figure 1 shows what Jones called a 'recovery' test. Curve #1 represents a pre-exercise test, the test of a subject's fresh strength. Curve #2 represents a post-exercise test, a test conducted *immediately after* exercise. Curve #3 (dotted line) represents a 'recovery' test conducted approximately 45 minutes later. The exercise, a leg extension, was limited to the first half of the movement, the right side of the chart.

A comparison of Curves #1 and #2 indicates that the subject elicited a TYPE G response from the effort - a full-range effect from limited-range exercise. It also indicates "a greater magnitude of effect than normal," a factor Jones thought may be related to muscle fiber-type (noting emphatically that his 'speculation' was weaker than an 'opinion'). Despite the magnitude of the effect, the recovery from exercise was rapid: approximately 84% in the worked area (right side of chart); and 64% in the unworked range (left side of chart).

Figure 2 shows the same recovery test with a distinct result. This subject demonstrated the same TYPE G tendency as the previous subject but less of a magnitude of effect from the exercise. Despite that, his rate of recovery was dreadfully slow. Two hours and three minutes after the post-exercise test, he had recovered only 8.39% of his strength.

"A loss in strength may result," said Jones, "if this subject is exercised in the usual manner."

In contrast, Figure 3 demonstrates a subject with a TYPE S response to exercise and a remarkable rate of recovery. Approximately 58 minutes after the post-exercise test, the subject had regained 106.9% of his exhausted strength. He was stronger than his pre-exercise-test level - had already gained a benefit from the exercise.

Jones tested approximately 100 subjects to determine the range of differences reported above and suspected that further testing would increase that range.

It did.

One strong, healthy gym owner from Gainesville, Florida produced a unique magnitude of effect. Every time Joe Cirulli exercised to a point of failure on a MedX® Lumbar Extension machine (a low-back device), he lost approximately 85% of his strength regardless of the weight used or number of repetitions performed. The huge loss peaked Arthur's interest to measure his ability to recover.

Figures 1 and 2 demonstrate that the ability to recover from exercise is unrelated to the magnitude of the effect. The subject in Figure 1 lost more strength as an immediate consequence of the exercise than did the subject in Figure 2. Yet, his rate of recovery was faster.

Cirulli took "weeks" to return to pre-exercise levels. His pattern of recovery was so predictable that Jones only needed to glance at his watch to say, "Well, it's been about four and a half hours. He's still down 78%."

The implications are clear. Some people can't stand much exercise; others can. And exercise prescriptions should take into consideration what can now be measured.

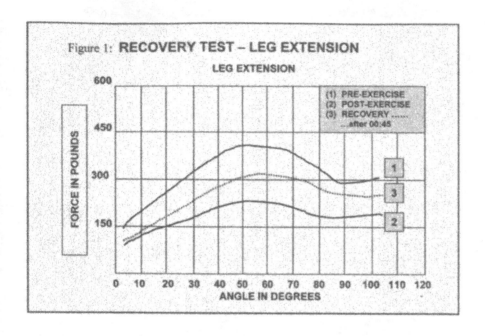

Figure 1: **RECOVERY TEST – LEG EXTENSION**

LEG EXTENSION

(1) PRE-EXERCISE
(2) POST-EXERCISE
(3) RECOVERY ......
...after 00:45

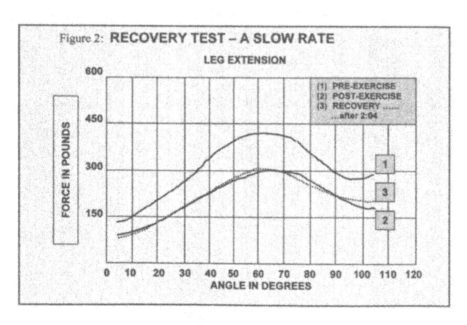

Figure 2: **RECOVERY TEST – A SLOW RATE**

LEG EXTENSION

(1) PRE-EXERCISE
(2) POST-EXERCISE
(3) RECOVERY ......
...after 2:04

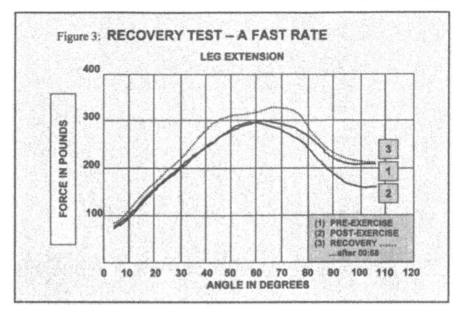

Figure 3: **RECOVERY TEST – A FAST RATE**

MAY 15

---

**The Most Significant Discovery in the History of Exercise – Part 4**

'Pride comes before a fall' was on his mind as he pondered the implications of a discovery that would have "no less that stunning consequences in the field of medicine."

"If, on a scale of zero to one million, everything else that I have ever accomplished in my life is equal to only five, then the discovery of this factor is something on the order of ten million." The man who had already accomplished a lot in life was excited again.

It began with a 1972 research study to determine the effects of negative-only exercise (lowering weights). It continued with a 1976 article entitled "The Metabolic Cost of Negative Work" (*Athletic Journal*, January) in which he speculated that the difference in output between positive and negative work was the result of internal muscle friction.

By 1986, Arthur Jones had proven himself correct.

Figure 1 shows the relationship between "three distinct levels of strength." The lower curve on the chart represents positive or lifting strength; the upper curve, negative or lowering strength; and the bar graph, static or holding strength.

223

The tests were conducted, in order: positive, negative and static. The positive and negative curves were produced by a dynamic test at a slow speed of movement. Static strength was determined by a series of isometric tests conducted throughout the range.

Jones spent $3 million building a dynamic testing tool (superior to anything before) simply to prove that the technology was futile. Nonetheless, as imperfect as the curves are in Figure 1, they serve to compare the relationship among the three levels.

Positive strength (the ability to move against resistance while muscle contracts) always measured lowest. From there, muscles were 20% stronger supporting a weight (static strength) and 40% stronger lowering (negative strength).

The ratios were established by thousands of tests over years, but Jones was quick to point out that they were only valid for fresh muscles. The relationship changed when a muscle fatigued. On one occasion, Jones reduced a subject's initial positive strength by 97.9% only to see his negative strength diminish by 18.9% - a result that could only have occurred because of an increase in friction during exercise. The subject's initial negative-to-positive-strength ratio of 1.4 to 1 quickly became 57 to 1 with fatigue. In the end, when his positive output was only 3, his negative output was 173.

The implications are of special importance to rehabilitation. A muscle too weak to lift a weight can still be exercised in a meaningful way, by lowering weight. A muscle too weak to produce a measurable force could produce a surprise if tested in a negative fashion. "A limb that is hanging in an utterly useless manner," said Jones, "can still be exercised with negative work...and if the nerve is still alive, it will respond."

"A thousand years after I am dead, and long forgotten," he continued, "millions of people who will never have heard of me will be helped beyond measure by the understanding of this factor." To spread the word, Jones launched a fleet of airplanes from his private jetport in Ocala, Florida to fly medical doctors to his home.

"I will not live long enough to see the final consequences of these discoveries (all four factors) ...but of one thing I am very sure, the benefits will be enormous in scope, literally beyond calculation. Medical benefits, health benefits, and benefits that are almost beyond price for anybody that is interested in exercise for any purpose."

Almost 20 years later, I have yet to meet a trainer even vaguely aware of *any* of the four 'discoveries' - let alone an idea of how to measure and use the information.

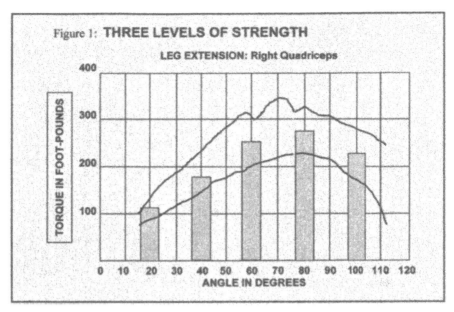

Figure 1: **THREE LEVELS OF STRENGTH**

LEG EXTENSION: Right Quadriceps

TORQUE IN FOOT-POUNDS

ANGLE IN DEGREES

MAY 16

---

### The Most Significant Discovery in the History of Exercise – Part 5

The most significant discovery in the history of exercise was not a broom-stick - but you'd never know it. I worked in several rehabilitation centers that boasted little more. Then, as now, owners could bill the same with a broom-stick as with the Concorde®, which allowed them to clean up more than a few floors along the way.

A broom is a broom but, before 1986, the 'Concorde' was a motorized testing and exercise tool with a technology (*isokinetics*) that one man found worthy of attack.

"Standard of the Industry...indeed. Reliable data...indeed. The only thing they (proponents of isokinetics) have been able to establish," said Arthur Jones, "is the simple point that Barnum made famous over a hundred years ago...there is a sucker born every minute and two to take him."

After 15 years of slaying the dragon to no avail, the MedX® inventor be-came enraged when isokinetics was applied to low backs. "Now the same people who brought you one outrage," he said, "are going another great step in the same direction...but this time they have gone way too far; ruining a few thousand knees is bad enough, but destroying a few million already-injured lower backs is going just a bit too far. You can live with a ruined knee...but you might not be able to live with a ruined lower back."

By 1986, there was light at the end of the tunnel.

"Finally, after I have been pointing out the fact that these tools are utterly worthless all during those years, at least a few people did get around to conducting the simple tests they should have conducted years ago; tests that clearly establish the fact that these tools are even worse than I could possibly make you believe."

He went on, "This whole field (medicine) is knee-deep in fraud, phony claims, faked research and assorted other outrages; which situation led us to start on the thirteen year project that we have just completed, the project that finally developed the tools that are required to conduct meaningful tests, accurate tests, repeatable tests."

That they were. Accuracy? "Almost 100%, so close that no measurable degree of error exists. For the information of any skeptics, I will point out the fact that anything in excess of an effective straight drop of one-half inch will result in a hard landing in an airplane...with a straight drop of one and one-half inches, things start breaking in an airplane...with a straight drop of four and one-half inches almost everything breaks. Yet it is possible to land an airplane without breaking things...my point being that you can produce very accurate and very repeatable results, given the right tools."

The right tools were not available, so he built them.

As proud as Jones was of the four new physiological discoveries about which he wrote in 1986, his equipment was the greatest discovery in the history of exercise. The consequences of the information gleaned have already vaulted the fields of exercise and rehabilitation into the next century. In specific, his low-back machine has proven itself the only meaningful way to access the muscles that extend the lumbar spine.

As Arthur would have said, "Put a value on that, Gideon."

Years from now, when tools are available to isolate the function of the major muscle groups, proper testing will identify the exact range, amount, frequency, intensity and duration of exercise for healthy living, sports performance and the treatment of injuries.

You can't weigh yourself with a kettle or fix a back with a broomstick - but, according to too many, you can keep trying.

226

MAY 17

———————

## Strength Gain and Strength Loss

Muscle can't sit still. At any point in time, it is busy reacting to one of three signals: one that increases its strength; one that decreases its strength; or one that maintains the status quo. By the age of 30, I had experienced all three.

At 16, two years of lifting weights made it clear that a muscle could increase its size and strength if the demand upon it was greater than usual. Larger arms, legs, chest and back were proof.

From 22-30, without counting the few occasions I was motivated to seek a higher level of conditioning, I learned that a muscle could easily maintain its strength if the demand was normal.

At age 30, I witnessed what I had always read - that a muscle begins to lose strength approximately 72 hours after its last stimulation, regardless of how much time it has trained. I watched the results of hard work disappear as I lay in a hospital bed recovering from back surgery - my first exposure to inactivity in 16 years.

Nonetheless, common sense dictated that response to the three signals was mutually exclusive. If a muscle was losing strength, it could not be gaining or maintaining strength *at the same time*.

So we thought...

In the late 1980's, MedX® inventor Arthur Jones tested thousands of front-thigh (quadriceps) muscles and discovered something new. He first tested for strength through a complete range-of-motion (ROM) on a computerized version of a leg-extension machine, and then performed one of two procedures:

1. He exposed the subject to a limited-ROM exercise (either 0-52°, upper range or 52-104°, lower range) using a resistance based upon the initial test. He then re-tested through a complete ROM (0-104°) to determine the immediate effect of the partial exercise and the muscle's rate of fatigue. OR...

2. He exposed the subject to a limited-ROM exercise (as above) two or three times a week for several months, then re-tested through a complete ROM to determine the long-term results of partial exercise.

Jones found that people exhibited either a *Specific* or a *General* response to limited-ROM exercise. A *Specific* response established fatigue (1, above) and a strength increase (2, above) in the "work" area, but no fatigue or result in the "non-work" zone. A *General* response exhibited a near identical fatigue

(1) and strength increase (2) *throughout* the ROM, regardless of where work was performed.

Jones took it a step further. He selected a subject who had demonstrated a Specific response to exercise and trained him in the lower ROM (52-104°) for 18 weeks (17 total exercises). The man increased his strength more than 60% in the worked area. He then trained him exclusively in the upper ROM (0-52°, a previously non-worked area) for five weeks. A re-test revealed a strength loss where he once exercised (lower ROM) and a strength gain where he was currently exercising (upper ROM) - *at the same time*.

A simultaneous increase and decrease of strength in the same muscle was, in fact, common. Approximately 72% of 10,000 test subjects responded to quadriceps exercise in this manner (80%, in the case of low-back muscles).

The implications are clear. Perform full-range exercise during workouts to insure full-range strength. After all, half an exercise is likely to produce half a result.

MAY 18

---

### Muscle Recovery From Exercise

Muscles recover from exercise at different rates - rates that were only estimates until the advent of tools that could isolate muscle function and measure the parameters involved.

In an article published in the *Athletic Journal*, "Exercise...1986: The Present State of the Art...Now a Science," Nautilus® inventor Arthur Jones heralded four new physiological factors unveiled by research with his latest equipment. He had tested more than 100 subjects and presented the 'extreme' differences in a muscle's ability to recover from exercise.

The test procedure was as follows:

*One*, a pre-exercise test of strength; *Two*, an exercise; *Three*, a post-exercise test of strength; and *Four*, a later test to determine the extent of recovery. At one extreme, Subject A lost 28% of his strength while performing a leg extension exercise to fatigue. Two hours and three minutes later the muscle had recovered only 8.39% of its strength - a slow recovery. At the other end, Subject B lost only 10% of his strength performing the same exercise. Fifty-eight minutes later he had recovered 106% of his strength - a fast recovery.

Between the extremes, Jones saw everything. Some subjects lost a lot of strength during exercise, but recovered quickly; others lost little, but recovered slowly. The implications were clear: Some people have a high tolerance for exercise; others do not. Those with little tolerance "must be handled with great caution if bad results are to be avoided," said Jones, "bad in the sense that a loss in strength may result if exercised in the usual manner."

By 1993, he presented an update in the form of a book - *The Lumbar Spine, The Cervical Spine and The Knee* - and the range of differences was even greater. "Some subjects recover from fatigue caused by exercise in a matter of minutes," he said, "while some do not even start to recover for a period of several days." A gym owner in Gainesville (Florida) consistently lost more than 85% of his low-back strength when exercised to fatigue and took several weeks to fully recover. Jones tested him so frequently that he would often consult his watch to determine the state of the muscle's recovery. It had an established pattern.

Jones also discovered that "recovery from fatigue is selective in regard to position." That is, a muscle recovers at different rates throughout the range of motion. In one case, recovery was nearly complete in four hours except for the final degrees of both extension and flexion. When the same subject was given less time to recover, he showed total recovery in the middle third of the range but large deficiencies at both ends.

Jones established a protocol. He tested 'recovery' about five hours after the pre- and post-exercise tests because most subjects showed complete recovery by then. Those who had not were re-tested two days later. If they still had not recovered, they were deemed 'low tolerance' and most such subjects possessed a high percentage of 'fast-twitch' (fast-fatigue) muscle fibers. Jones advised them to train not more than once a week with few repetitions (8-10).

He observed other trends: "Subjects that do best on a schedule of one exercise every second week are common...and some few will not make gains in strength if exercised more frequently than once every third week."

If your exercise results are not up to par, do less - and train less frequently.

## MAY 19

### Kick Sand in My Face?

At 14, I was as close to the proverbial 90-pound weakling as one could get. What saved me from that end was, in part, a comic-strip ad that featured a bodybuilder who kicked sand in the face of a "skinny" guy at the beach. The victim had two choices: vacate, or train and win the girl. Somehow, it motivated me to take up strength training.

The ad claimed that a powerful body could be built without the use of barbells and dumbbells, and the public went for it in a big way. The new method, "dynamic tension," and a man named Charles Atlas made thousands of dollars in what turned out to be the most successful fraud in the history of exercise.

It all began around 1921, when a wealthy man interested in promoting exercise, Bernarr MacFadden, held what may have been the first physique contest in history. He rented Madison Square Garden and spent a lot of money promoting what turned out to be a flop. A year later, he tried again with the same result. Among the out-of-shape competitors - strongmen, wrestlers and football players - was an Italian immigrant (the eventual winner), who, for the next half-century, became known as Charles Atlas.

By any reasonable standards, his physique was pitiful. Yet, because MacFadden had copyrighted the term "The World's Most Perfectly Developed Man" and never conducted another contest, Atlas claimed to be "the winner and still holder of the title" for 50 years.

Recognizing that there was no profit in selling barbells, Atlas developed a 'secret' method of training that ignored tradition. Training with weights (then called 'weightlifting'), he claimed, was dangerous and of no value.

He was eventually sued by a manufacturer of barbells and denied, under oath, that he ever used weights for the purpose of exercise. When finally questioned by the judge, he admitted that he had indeed used them - but only "to test his muscles."

"How often do you test your muscles, Mr. Atlas?" inquired the judge.

"Three or four times a week."

"How long does it take to test your muscles?"

"Two or three hours."

The sand kicking stopped for the moment, but fraud had just begun.

Today, fraud in the field of exercise is common, with nutritional supplements, low-back strengthening, rehabilitative testing and 'isokinetic' exercise leading the way.

Thirty years ago, there was little mention of nutrition in any bodybuilding publication. Now, there's nothing but. The floodgates opened when the supposed benefits of massive amounts of protein were announced in the early 1950's. Nautilus® inventor Arthur Jones summed it up when he said, "Bodybuilding is 100% nutrition - but only if you don't eat. Just try going without food for a week and see what happens to your body."

In 1986, University of Florida research confirmed that low-back muscles are not strengthened if the pelvis rotates during a backward movement of the torso. Yet, every major equipment manufacturer promotes a 'back' machine that allows pelvic rotation.

For the past 20 years, rehabilitation clinics have used motorized equipment that provides dynamic (vs. static) strength testing and isokinetic exercise (a constant speed of movement) - neither accurate nor safe. Yet, the medical community continues to make health decisions based upon the data provided by these technologies. And insurance companies keep paying and paving the way.

With big money at stake, there's enough sand ahead to make even Atlas look puny.


## MAY 20

---

### Verticality

Our Grade-9 Latin teacher made it interesting. Between conjugating verbs under pressure to singing such steadfast favorites as "Gaudiamus Igatur" and "Three Blind Mice," Alex Prokich kept it fun. He didn't deserve our abuse.

Mr. Prokich competed in the 1936 Olympics for the Yugoslavian soccer team - good preparation for the pressure provided by a handful of hooligans that ridiculed teachers. For him, we'd jog down the hall, look over a shoulder and holler in broken English, "You'll never catch me, Jesse (in reference to Jesse Owens)."

Things have a way of coming back around.

By Grade 11, Mr. Prokich was our math teacher - his specialty, not mine - and I don't recall what sparked the incident other than my typical behavior. Suddenly, the calm of the classroom was interrupted by a loud **"Get out!"** aimed in my direction. As I gathered things at an inappropriate pace, he about tore the wood off the corner desk trying to get down the aisle where he issued a second, much louder, **"GET OUUUUUUUT!"**

Talk about vertical leap: I had it that day. He spewed me into the hallway and worked on a few soccer techniques he hadn't tried in years.

The importance of verticality, however, took longer to sink in than the leather. I first recognized it in college, in events like the long-jump, high-jump and hurdles (with their combinations of vertical and horizontal displacement), and in sports such as basketball and volleyball where jumping ability was prime. But I never related it to strength training, where its importance is perhaps greatest.

According to Nautilus® inventor, Arthur Jones, "For all practical purposes - in the field of exercise - we can (and should) ignore anything except vertical movement of the resistance; it makes no slightest difference in which direction we are pushing or pulling, and the 'total amount' of movement is of no importance - what matters, and all that matters, is the vertical movement of the resistance."

Take a standing biceps curl. The first third of the movement pushes the weight from the body in a horizontal plane. The middle third lifts vertically; the last third, horizontally - and the hardest part is obvious. It's tougher to lift your car than push it.

Logically, the most demanding sports are those that require vertical displacement of resistance. Enter the vertical jump.

Philadelphia Hall-of-Fame player and coach, Bill Cunningham once told me that the 76'ers tested a gadget to increase vertical ability - leaping against bungee cords fixed to a platform and the player's waist. After a multi-week trial, Bill lost six inches of jumping height. His ability returned when the project was scrapped.

A research study conducted by Jones at the US Military Academy (West Point, 1975) compared, among other things, the effect of two Nautilus Hip and Back machines - the 'Super' (both legs at once) and the 'DUOsymmetric-POLYcontractile' (one leg at a time) - on the vertical jumping ability of 22 members of a volleyball team. The 'Super' fashioned an increase of 2.25% in six weeks (less than 60 seconds of exercise, 3X/week), while the 'DUO' produced a 6.57% increase. If other jumping muscles had been strengthened to the same degree, the subjects might not have landed.

What do I think of sports performance programs? Not much, but they're fun. So much fun, they're a joke. And the best advice I have for participation in such nonsense is this: **"GET OUUUUUUT**, and don't look back over either shoulder."

MAY 21

———

### Operation Elephant

One minute a herd of elephants grazed peacefully across the parched African plain. The next, it lay in a heap of gray and bloody flesh - male, female and young, lifeless all. They called it 'thinning out the herd,' someone's job. It looked downright brutal.

The incident was orchestrated and filmed by the soon-to-be Nautilus® inventor, Arthur Jones. Like his exercise philosophy, the event had to be specific, brief and hard:

"In order to kill an elephant quickly with a .600 Nitro-Express rifle, you must hit him in the brain, with a 900 grain bullet delivering an impact force of about 8,000 foot pounds - but you can shoot an elephant 10,000 times with a .22 rifle delivering a total of both grains of bullet weight and foot-pounds of impact force many times as great as the totals from the .600 and still not kill him, and certainly not quickly, if at all."

Despite his expertise, the act weighed heavy on his mind.

Jones was a brash renegade who liked to keep the world informed of his ideas - once, too often. When he was about to expose the Rhodesian government's lies about the commercial slaughter of elephants in 1969, he was expelled from the country.

Down, but not out, he embarked on a humanitarian mission in the summer of 1980 that caught the attention of another TV show, 20/20. He stripped down one of three newly acquired 707's and flew from his home in Ocala (Florida) to the Hwange Game Reserve in Rhodesia (now, Zimbabwe). The goal - to save the African elephant from extinction. According to Jones, "There won't be any left by the year 2000."

When he landed on the remote runway, time was tight. He had to fly out in daylight to clear the trees at the end of the strip and had a limited number of hours to move 63 baby elephants up a slippery ramp to the jet. At the same time, he had to keep them hydrated, fed, entertained and alive. The crew hustled about as Jones oversaw the loading, papers in hand. The last elephant waddled on board at sunset.

"Tell them I want it brought here **NOW!**" he snapped in reference to a portable starter needed to crank the plane. His wife, Terry, jumped about two feet high and landed the same time the engines kicked in. It was only the start of Arthur's problems.

With everything on board, the door at the top of the ramp wouldn't close. It had been sabotaged by someone on the ground wanting to ruin the effort or extract more from Jones' pocket (as if $1 million wasn't enough).

But Arthur was no fool. He had one hand firmly on his wallet and the other on a stash of weapons he brought to "shoot his way out, if needed." Besides that, an escort of what appeared to be interested spectators (armed to the hilt in Jeeps®) was 'on call' beside the runway - just in case. They finally jimmied the door shut and taxied down the dirt path.

The 22-hour return was rewarded when all 63 babies, tired and disoriented, scooted down the ramp to their new home, an outdoor area shaded by large trees.

During the first night, the elephants destroyed some of the foliage in an effort to feed, which prompted Jones to place heavy wiring around each tree. When the animals repeated the behavior, Jones installed high concrete walls around everything edible.

He should have installed them around the TV host who commented during the show, "There are some people who say that you could put your money to better use."

Arthur looked up with a stare that would have given Count Dracula the heebie-jeebies and slowly uttered, "Roger, I made that money...and I'll spend it any way I want."

Next segment, please.


## MAY 22

---

### Barbells, Machines and Mud

My first contact with mud as resistance occurred during a high school cross-country meet. The route started on the track and ran through a half-mile of grassy fields to a set of railroad tracks at the end of the property. It then followed the tracks for about a hundred yards, turned left across a ditch through a farmer's field and eventually funneled to a narrow path in dense woods. You had to establish position early because there was no way to pass anyone beyond.

The starter's gun went off at 3:00 PM despite an all-day rain.

My skill at running the railroad tracks left me in good stead as I crossed the ditch and jumped the fence. About 20 steps into the field, however, my shoes sounded like plungers each time they resurfaced from the quagmire. The mud crept up my calves and sucked energy from every step. Suddenly, a white sock appeared. I quickly pulled the shoe from its hole, scrambled for the path in the woods and glanced back at what resembled an Easter-egg hunt with cursing. Mud had done us in.

Years ago, I read an *Ironman* article written by 1972 Collegiate "Mr. America," Ellington Darden. It described the use of mud as resistance and featured pictures of the author immersed in a mud-filled tub. While Darden described some of the potential benefits of mud, he also identified its limitations.

If you move a body part through air, the resistance encountered is minimal. If you move it through water, greater resistance is provided by the denser medium. If you move it through mud, resistance is further increased: The thicker the solution, the greater the resistance. Therefore, water stimulates the body better than air, and mud better than water, which is not the only reason the medical community recommends exercise in liquid mediums. The buoyancy of liquid is gentle on joint systems and allows arthritic patients to move without discomfort.

Despite the positives, there are several drawbacks to exercise in liquids:

- Buoyancy may contribute to a loss of bone mass (as in a weightless environment).
- Negative work, the most important part of exercise, is void. The controlled lowering of resistance triggers greater muscle-fiber activation in a contracted position and improved stretching in an extended position. With *negative only* work, better muscle isolation and exercise form are ensured.
- It is difficult to measure resistance and progress.
- Liquid mediums are low on the totem pole of resistance 'quality.'

A better choice would include:

- *Partner-resisted exercise* - provides superior resistance due to higher intensity.
- An *adjustable barbell* - provides improvements in fitness due to its ability to increase resistance with ease (though resistance is not rotary, balanced or direct).
- A *Universal*® gym - allows a safe, convenient alternative to barbell movements.
- A *Nautilus*® machine - provides resistance that satisfies the needs of the muscle throughout its range of motion (also the *hardest* form of exercise).

Mud may kill bee-stings, preserve archaeological finds, cover faces for aesthetic purposes and provide hours of solitude on a golf course when no one else is dumb enough to be out there. But that's where it ends.

If exercise is judged by the quality of resistance and the quantity of the range of motion (as it should), mud doesn't have much value at all.

## MAY 23

### Letting It Happen

I set out at noon one day from Averett College in Danville, Virginia on a routine seven-mile run. My body echoed its usual protest until it shifted into second gear at the half mile. The pace was brisk (as it was every now and then) but left little indication of anything out of the ordinary.

By the time I rounded the curve that marked the last mile, however, things had changed. The pace was effortless. I accelerated and abandoned thoughts of conserving energy for a final burst. My weightless feet sprung from the asphalt like never before. The faster I ran, the easier it seemed. With no downhill or breeze behind, my windpipe felt like an 8-lane highway, my lungs endless. The easier it seemed, the faster I ran. Easier, faster. Faster, easier. I was barely cognizant as I passed in front of the school library. I saw no buildings, no people, just blur. My legs refused to stop as momentum carried what was left of my skeleton down the street. The bones, it seemed, were enjoying the ride. Eventually, somewhere downtown, far from the learned halls, I crashed in a heap of exhausted joy.

I sought the same exhilaration during the runs that followed - certain that it required effort. No go. I then tried to 'make it happen' to no avail. The intensity of what struck that day was unique. I don't know where it came from or where it went to, but the feeling never returned.

Timothy Gallway talked about similar experiences in his book, *The Inner Game of Golf.* He believed that "getting into a zone" (if that's what happened) was a result of allowing your body to free itself from the confines of the mind (self-doubt, criticism and pressure) and perform in a way that it already knew. Getting out of your own way allowed for optimum performance through what he called "relaxed concentration."

I had enjoyed a few out-of-mind experiences in golf, when the senses were keen and things flowed without effort. After each, I sat back and wondered, "Where did that come from?" My conclusion, "It just happened."

Running and golf have provided a glimpse of the *Promised Land*, but strength training has not. Nor will it. To produce maximum results from strength training, you must first 'make it happen' before you can 'let it happen'

In the early 1970's, Nautilus® inventor Arthur Jones used both in his approach to bodybuilding. He first asked candidates how they trained and, regardless of the reply, drove their over-trained bodies to a hotel on a remote beach far from the temptation of exercise. Days later, he'd fetch them. Their response to his training was exceptional for obvious reasons - it was *hard* work, yet provided adequate time for recovery. When plateaus were encountered, Jones invariably cut the *amount* of exercise performed and increased the *intensity* of what was left. The results were immediate - and superior to anything that had been tried before.

If your exercise expectations are not up to par, ask yourself:

- Are you 'making it happen' by taking each exercise to momentary muscle failure, where a 100% effort does not produce a complete repetition in good form?
- Are you 'letting it happen' with enough rest and recovery between workouts?

In strength training, hard work and rest equals success. If you first 'make it happen' and then 'let it happen,' who knows what might happen.

Most hardcore trainees are afraid to leave the gym long enough to find out.

## MAY 24

### It's Never Too Late

Several years ago, I played golf with a man whose artistic talent as a painter was overshadowed only by his prowess with a putter. Over the course of an afternoon in which the temperature surpassed his age, Phil Beamon sunk more than his share of putts and made it look easy in the process. His only complaint in the stifling heat was the length of his backswing.

"I can't seem to make a turn," he grumbled.

While Phil pondered golf's Royal & Ancient move, I thought, "The only turn I'll make at his age will likely come from someone else's input."

Phil was 90, and lifted weights for 30 minutes three times a week.

Resistance training is the best exercise choice for seniors. Although the consensus is that people die from more-prominent causes, a close look reveals that lack of muscle strength may be a significant underlying factor.

The body needs movement and the only thing capable of producing movement is muscle contraction. With age, the loss of muscle mass and flexibility can have a devastating effect on mobility. When movement declines or the body goes unused, a vicious cycle of muscle atrophy is initiated which slowly shuts the body down. Leg strength no longer supports body weight, making it difficult to get out of a chair, and eventually, out of bed. In the end, the reported 'heart failure' (or cause of death) may have been due to a lack of muscle strength and mobility.

Fortunately, movement can reverse the process. While any physical activity provides some benefit for those in poor condition, cardiovascular exercise (tennis, swimming, walking) is the most popular choice among seniors. But cardiovascular activity alone fails to build or even maintain adequate levels of strength and flexibility because of its inherent low resistance and mid-range movements. Proper resistance training, on the other hand, improves muscle strength, flexibility, cardiovascular condition and the performance of any physical activity.

In a 1999, 14-week study by Westcott, Reinl and Califano, 19 nursing-home patients demonstrated significant physical changes from strength training. The brief protocol (one set of 6 exercises, 8-12 repetitions at a slow speed of movement, twice a week) decreased body-fat percentage, fat weight and the incidence of 'falls' among participants. At the same time, it increased lean muscle mass, overall strength, joint range-of-motion, mobility distance and functional independence. The average age of the participants was 88.5 years.

In a 1996, 8-week study with 1,132 sedentary adults and seniors, Westcott found that an older group of subjects (61-80) produced results that matched middle-aged (41-60) and younger (21-40) groups. Starting with similar bodyweights and body-fat percentages, the three groups produced comparable results in bodyweight loss, body-fat reduction (in amount and percentage) and lean weight increase. The study concluded that the "older exercisers replaced muscle at the same rate as younger participants" (2.3 and 2.4 pounds, respectively).

Westcott noted another interesting phenomenon. Unlike the younger subjects, more than 90 percent of the seniors continued to strength train after completing the program.

Adults lose approximately one pound of muscle per year through the aging process. That pound can be easily replaced in a month by proper strength training.

MAY 25

———

### Tales from the Crypt

After more than four decades of strength training, I might be lead to believe that strength is unrelated to muscle size. About as strong as I can be, I'm far from filling a closet, let alone the free-weight section of a gym. The finest methodology and a fair share of toil produced little more than an athletic build, good health and no regrets.

Did I miss something more than a 'push' along the way?

According to Nautilus® inventor Arthur Jones, I probably did.

"A recently-arrived trainee," uttered Jones from headquarters in DeLand, Florida (1971), "asked me how long it would take him to get as big as Sergio (Cuban bodybuilder, Sergio Oliva): 'Will it take me a year?'

'At least,' I told him; but he will, eventually, be just like Sergio - in a hundred years, or so, they will both be skeletons and then nobody will be able to tell the difference between them. But in the meantime, it is possible to tell the difference - and in that particular case, a year one way or another probably won't do much in the direction of reducing that difference."

Like most, I missed the 'big' limb on the family tree.

In May of 1974, Jones wrote an article in *Ironman* magazine, "Average Expectations From Training," in which he predicted the final measurements of a high-school football team "if they stayed in training for a period of 18 months." More than half had participated in a weight-training program the year before and were physically above average (compared to a random group). His predictions appeared as follows:

| Body Part | Starting | Expected after 18 mo. | Gain |
|-----------|----------|-----------------------|------|
| Body Weight (lbs.) | 167.19 | 195 | 27.81 |
| Normal Chest (in.) | 37.5 | 45 | 7.5 |
| Rib Box (in.) | 33.25 | 37.5 | 4.25 |
| Waist (in.) | 32.2 | 32.5 | .3 |
| R. Thigh (in.) | 21.73 | 25.5 | 3.77 |
| L. Thigh (in.) | 21.98 | 25.5 | 3.52 |
| R. Calf (in.) | 14.93 | 16.75 | 1.82 |
| L. Calf (in.) | 14.88 | 17.0 | 2.12 |
| R. Upper Arm (in.) | 12.96 | 17.0 | 4.04 |
| L. Upper Arm(in.) | 12.67 | 17.25 | 4.58 |

The numbers are group averages and meaningless from the perspective that response to exercise depends on many individual factors. But they are interesting in another way.

With the exception of the thigh, Jones expected the weak limb to surpass the strong in size. The reason: the weak side has to work *harder* to lift the same weight the same number of times and will normally catch up to, if not surpass, its counterpart.

His expectations were lofty otherwise. A 4-4½ inch addition to the arm of a teen is significant; 28 pounds of bodyweight with only .3 inches destined for the waist, ambitious; and an increase of 7-8 inches at the chest, a tailor's dream. But as great with numbers and as honest as he was, Jones was demanding as hell. If the average player had trained with him for the duration, few would have doubted the outcome - or forgotten the effort - had they survived to tell the tale.

One day we'll all look like Sergio, if we're patient enough to wait.

## MAY 26

### Defending the Cam

Arthur Jones realized that effective involvement of the entire muscle mass during exercise required an ever-changing resistance.

"As you move any part of your body from one position to another position in relation to other parts of the body," he said, "you change your strength, either become stronger or weaker; there is no movement of any part of the body wherein your strength remains constant throughout a full range of movement."

It took him a long time to put the idea into practice.

"In a first attempt to provide that requirement for the most productive form of exercise," he explained, "I welded hooks to a barbell in 1939; hooks which enabled me to add chains to the barbell in an attempt to vary the resistance during the exercise. This was not a practical solution, but it was a start."

He set out to build a tool that applied a variable resistance directly to his upper back. The development of a 'pullover' machine is history, and best described by Jones:

"In the starting position, the elbows are forced back well behind the head, and in this extended position the lats are quite weak; if heavy resistance is employed in this position, then it would be impossible to start the movement. Thus the resistance must be variable; it must be light in this position, and heavier in other positions. In order to effect this variation of resistance, we have employed what we term the 'Nautilus System' of spiral pulleys; the large, spiral shaped pulleys located on each side of the machine.

In this starting position, the radius of the pulley is quite small, and thus the resistance is low. Later in the movement, the radius of the pulley is greater and the resistance is increased in proportion. At the finishing position of the movement, the radius of the pulley is at its greatest and the resistance has reached its highest point as well.

Or, at least this is true in general terms, although, in fact, while it is constantly changing, the radius of the pulleys (and thus the resistance) does not always increase; in some cases, the resistance increases up to a certain point and then decreases, as it must in order to remain in balance with changing strength levels produced by changes in involved body parts positions.

While it is perfectly true that the strength of a muscle constantly increases as the body parts move from an extended to a flexed position, it does not follow that this increase takes form in a straight-line fashion; that is to say, the increase in strength is not constant at a given rate of increase.

Second, changing positions bring about greater and lesser degrees of involvement of other muscular structures, and thus 'total' strength may be decreasing while the strength of a particular muscle is increasing; for example, most of the effort is provided by the latissimus muscles, but the movement is assisted during part of the range of movement by the pectorals, the abdominals, and the trapezoids, as well as by several smaller muscular structures. Thus, while the strength of the latissimus muscles increases during the entire movement, 'total' strength for the movement (the strength total provided by all of the involved muscles) actually decreases near the end of the movement.

So, in order to remain in balance with this total strength level, the resistance must increase up to a point, and then decrease slightly, and this variation in resistance is exactly provided by the variation in the curve of the spiral pulleys."

Jones' competitors are still scratching their heads.

MAY 27

---

### The Long and Winding Road

The high-school cross-country meet in St. Catharines, Ontario always generated a flood of nervous energy - the car ride, the warm-up, the last call - that culminated with a gunshot and rush of human flesh. We were away.

The route began in a sub-division but took a sudden turn from pavement to a dirt path that descended deep below a bridge. I scrambled to the bottom along the riverbank and matched strides with teammate, Les Selby.

We were not expected to do well, and it soon became apparent. As we ran up a small hummock, the entire field appeared before us. Les and I were well back and couldn't keep up. We glanced behind and spotted a runner as far from us as we were from the pack - and laughed until we recognized the green and gold of the alma matter.

As I said, we weren't expected to do well.

On we pressed over a stretch of flat terrain, falling further behind at every stride and dreading the remnant of the Niagara escarpment that lay ahead. As we approached, the loose surface of the cliff was strewn with bodies; the air with profanity. I decided to grind it out to the summit and passed 30 runners clinging to whatever they could find - and more at the top with two miles to go.

To make a long story short, I finished in 15th place.

We weren't expected to do well.

Many face the same when they enter the realm of resistance training. With a high dropout rate among novices, trainees are not expected to do well.

Here's how to handle it:

- Nervousness and uncertainty are part of the deal. Accept it for what it is and move on. If you are in poor physical condition, remember that most start under the same umbrella. If you think you're behind the pack, glance around - there's bound to be someone worse off. Don't fall into the trap of comparing yourself to others (in looks, progress, strength or otherwise).
- Seek a professional orientation at the starting gate (the basics of progression, form, overload and intensity).
- After months of numerical progress, you will meet an escarpment in the form of a plateau. Rather than quit, take the approach of Nautilus® inventor, Arthur Jones. Increase the intensity of exercise to stimulate change *and* decrease the amount or frequency of exercise to permit change. "A child may increase their height by as much as an inch overnight, literally in a few hours," he said. "I noticed the same thing in regards to gains in muscular size. Size increases do not occur gradually, but, rather, occur suddenly, so quickly that I was never able to determine just how little time was actually involved." Progress is rarely linear but commitment must be. Persist with patience.
- Strength training is hard work, but it pays. You'll feel better in a month and see results in three. Why? Initial gains from strength

training don't appear in the form of hypertrophy (muscle size); they appear as nervous system changes. Gains in size and strength follow. Focus on each step but think long term. You may surprise yourself.

One day, I plodded along the Niagara escarpment and suddenly grew. Forty years later, when I face plateaus in my exercise program, my legs keep churning.

## MAY 28

### Pancho

Coach Michael Sanchez-Vegas pulled the eager athlete aside. The Venezuelan water-ski team stood one jump away from the world championship.

"All we need is a jump of 150 feet," he said, "a distance well within your range."

Instead of petrified, the kid couldn't wait to show the world.

Mike had his hands full.

"We're not looking for a world record," he repeated, "just a solid jump."

He may as well have been talking to the boat.

A confident 'Pancho' San Miguel set out for the final effort, determined not to disappoint. Mike crossed his toes and headed for a vantage point along the shore.

Pancho cut wide-left behind the boat then crossed the wake to the far right where he lingered for the assault on the ramp. The moment he cut, Mike knew it was late.

The kid whipped into the slot and approached the ramp at 75 miles per hour, about as fast as you could muster on a pair of jump skis. He hit the ramp with fire in his eyes and a mountain of heart. His knees buckled, but he held on - Pancho San Miguel didn't do things halfway. This jump would show the world. Upward he soared but, unlike the eagle in his dreams, quickly descended in a heap. The mighty effort had blown a knee and the hopes of a nation.

Years later, the bushy-haired redhead knocked on my gym door with the rest of the Venezuelan contingent to prepare for the Latin-American championship. Pancho hadn't changed. He flicked a cigarette at the door and entered.

We talked about intensity. He could handle it. We talked about muscle failure. He was ready. We talked about gradual progress (we had two months to prepare). I may as well have been talking to the boat.

He pushed and pulled, grunted and groaned, and never backed down. It didn't take long. The out-of-shape skier promptly ended in a familiar heap in a corner of the gym, with nothing but a blown ego. But that was far from the end of Pancho San Miguel. He came back, time after time, until he abandoned that corner. The kid was tough and, despite the smokes, possessed a cardiovascular ability as high as anyone. At least he wouldn't allow anyone to believe otherwise.

I have always encouraged trainees to work as hard as possible. I'd rather see someone go full out on an exercise and lay on the floor for five minutes between efforts than tip-toe around, doing a little here, a little there. Hard work is essential to the production of best results from strength training, and pays quicker dividends than low-intensity work.  But it has its time and place.

If you adopt a conservative approach, you will likely stimulate a conservative result and quit in frustration. If you hit the gym at 75 miles per hour, you might produce an injury or a degree of muscular soreness that will force you to quit. You must start slowly and increase your intensity gradually. But make no mistake - you must, at some point, learn to work hard.

Intensity is defined as a percentage of momentary ability, and is a relative term. For an elderly woman, it might mean getting out of a chair. In strength training, it means performing an exercise to volitional failure (where a 100% effort no longer produces a complete repetition).

High intensity is a physiological must and should be a long-term goal. Seek it to soar.


MAY 29

---

### Fast Food


I'm not into food, but I am into fast, which is why I waited 30 minutes only once to enter a restaurant - when McDonald's® opened its first facility in Venezuela.

A month after the grand opening, I drove to Chacaito (a suburb of Caracas) to savor the quality of the effort and was pleasantly surprised. The food was better than expected and the service, outstanding.

There were 12 cash-register lines and 54 - count them - young, hustling employees. The frenzy created by the arrival of fast-food was unlike anything I'd seen, including the current lawsuit against McDonald's for "making America fat."

In the early 1980's, the optimum diet for health was 55-58% carbohydrate, 30-35% fat and 12-15% protein. The average American consumed 3,400 daily calories consisting of 45% carbohydrate, 43% fat and 12% protein. Recommendations included a reduction in the consumption of calories, fat, refined sugars and protein (then, more than 100 grams per day).

"The most popular fast-food meal (hamburger, fries and shake from McDonald's)" reported Ellington Darden, Ph.D. in *The Nautilus Nutrition Book* (1981), "contains 59% carbohydrate, 28% fat, and 13% protein" - the 'optimum' recommended for athletes. Only fresh fruit and an occasional serving of liver were required for balance. The meal was rich in protein and ideal, not high, in fat. Darden wasn't alone.

Twelve years before, Dr. Howard Appledorf, Food Science Professor at the University of Florida claimed that a hamburger, French fries and milkshake were the nutritional equivalent of a small steak, baked potato and salad. "A hamburger dinner is really meat, bread, and potatoes," he said, "only in a different form than a steak dinner." The fast food version lacked only vitamin A - a want easily corrected by ketchup on the fries. Although some fast foods were high in calories and fat, Dr. Appledorf found (through chemical analysis) that most foods sold in fast-food restaurants were "highly nutritious."

Dr. Judith Stern and R.V. Denenberg evaluated the following fast-food meals with regard to the US recommended daily allowances for vitamins and minerals:

1. Super-burger, regular fries and vanilla shake.
2. Three pieces of fried chicken, roll, coleslaw and potatoes.
3. Half of a 10-inch pizza and iced tea (with two tablespoons of sugar).
4. Fried-fish sandwich, regular fries and vanilla shake.

They found the meals ample in vitamins B1, B2, B12 and niacin, but low in vitamins A, C, B6 and folic acid; adequate in calcium, phosphorus, sodium, iodine and zinc, but low in copper, iron, magnesium and manganese. They recommended adding green leafy (or yellow) vegetables, fruits, nuts and liver - an occasional trip to the salad bar.

Some meals were poor choices. A fried chicken dinner or fish sandwich provided approximately half of its calories in the form of fat. A typical meal (burger, fries and shake) provided nearly half of the daily caloric requirement of males (and more than half for women and children). Three such meals per day would increase a waistline.

Obesity is caused by many factors - genetics, lack of exercise, environment, caloric intake and socialization. In the end, it's the number of calories that count, not whether they come from McDonald's.

There are too many opinions and calories out there, and too many lawyers waiting to take a large bite.

## MAY 30

### Food – A Two Way Street

I have most, if not all, of the Nautilus® literature from 1970, the MedX® literature from 1986 and "The Arthur Jones Collection" (an autobiography and an unpublished 16-chapter article, "The Future of Exercise") on order. What I don't know, I soon will. But I am certain of one thing - there is, and probably will be, little mention of nutrition.

Other than the times he plunged into exercise after a prolonged absence, Arthur Jones didn't have eating habits, unless reaching for tidbits along the way were considered. His documented black-coffee and burnt-toast breakfasts and a handful of lunches and dinners I witnessed were proof enough.

Arthur was about education, not food. During meals, he spent more time pushing air out than shoving food in. His ears were open to anything that had merit, but his mouth was sealed whether the chow had merit or not.

A French-fry here, a leaf of lettuce there; a stab of meat, a jelly-bean - meal after meal - it was hard to believe he could survive an 18-hour workday.

Many thought he didn't understand nutrition or was against it, but not so. Jones thought it was much simpler than its portrayal in bodybuilding publications.

"For more than 20 years," he said, "I was closely and directly involved in the importation of a very wide variety of delicate wild animals - keeping such animals alive and healthy in captivity is primarily a matter of diet, one missing ingredient can be the difference between a death rate of 90% or one of less than 1% - so I learned long ago that a proper diet was of utmost importance. I also learned that there are three distinct requirements in the way of a proper diet - these are, (1) a proper variety of foods, (2) a proper amount of food, and (3) the 'quality' of the foods."

In a move that some wrongly viewed an attempt to bolster his grasp on the subject, Jones hired Ellington Darden, Ph.D., who had just mended years of supplement taking with doctoral studies in nutrition. His boss kept him on a sane path.

Jones was a pilot most of his life and applied the experience to weight training. He knew that an over-rich mixture of fuel-to-air, for example, reduced maximum power production in flight. "(Your body) like an engine," he said, "requires a proper chemical mixture in the fuel itself; if the mixture is changed - in either direction - then the result will be a reduction in power, NEVER an increase, ALWAYS a reduction."

At one time, Jones believed that a diet slightly rich in protein was possibly "an advantage during periods of rapid growth," but there was a limit (established at .4 to .8 grams per pound of bodyweight). Most trainees, he claimed, were 'playing it safe' by overloading with protein, a mistake in every case.

The most important nutritional factor for bodybuilding was 'amount.' Whenever he returned to exercise after a layoff, he maintained his caloric intake for three months, during which time he gained 12-15 pounds without adding body fat. From there he gradually added calories (100 per day to start) until he reached his goal.

"The subject of diet," he said, "is probably the most completely understood factor involved in physical training - but not by bodybuilders, who have been brainwashed into spending hundreds of millions of dollars on products of little or no value."

Jones knew his indifference would enrage those with a commercial interest and those, like bodybuilders, who thought his stance was born of ignorance.

A "simple statement of the facts" was a chance Jones was always willing to take.


## MAY 31

---

## Settling

Brevity has been a selling point of fitness programs for years. Yet, those who first embraced it were forced to modify their philosophies to accommodate clients with time restraints. After all, only hard-core trainees had the time to hang around for the marathon sessions that most perceived a 'requirement' for success. The introduction of Nautilus® machines supposedly changed all of that - but it may have only added fuel to the fire.

When Arthur Jones introduced his hard, brief training method that he claimed produced best results regardless of equipment (1970), most accepted the idea of intensity, but few believed that such brevity could ever be productive. Surely, something was lost in the process.

The system was hammered from all angles. Some bodybuilders tried it - more claimed they did when they really didn't - and dismissed the concept. Others perceived it as just what the doctor ordered for an ailing industry - a commercially viable, 30-minute strength-training program. Jones stood firm - brevity was an "absolute requirement" for best results.

The system was a supervised circuit that represented, by far, the most difficult and efficient way to attain maximum muscle size, strength and cardio-vascular exercise - but it was not commercial. Properly performed, it was so hard that it turned people away. The free-weight crowd boohooed the whole thing, claiming that it didn't live up to its hype, that it was lousy for size, strength and cardiovascular exercise, that it better suited executives and was nothing but commercial.

As a gym owner back then, I found it difficult to keep members motivated and just as difficult to retain their trust in what was proposed. I bombarded them with updated information, conducted seminars and created routines that emphasized body parts or muscles used in specific sports. I chained makeshift 'books' of routines for any and every purpose to the walls and concrete pillars throughout the gym. They were for members only, not for our competitors.

Other gyms approached the problem of providing variety in different ways. The Gainesville Health and Fitness Center set rows of machines in lines so members could perform Routine #1 in one line and Routine #2 in another. Many gyms allowed members to use the equipment as they saw fit, without order or supervision. In both cases, trainees settled for what they liked and rarely changed.

People are creatures of habit. We settle for things regardless of what they are or how beneficial it may be to modify them in minor ways. My workout, for example, has rarely changed in the past several years: leg extension, leg curl, hip abduction, calf raise, chest press, pulldown (or chin-up), lateral raise, row, triceps extension and biceps curl. One set, approximately 10 repetitions, 15-20 total minutes - properly performed, I can barely make it.

The other day, a new chain of fitness studios opened, featuring a 30-minute circuit for women. Someone, I thought, had finally seen the light (although the light is 10 minutes more than what it could or should be). My curiosity fizzed when a member told me that, other than the first few sessions, the program was unsupervised and that you were allowed only 30 seconds at each station (when 60-90 is ideal). One peek in the front door confirmed all doubt. The gal running the show weighed about 300 pounds.

I think I'll become a dentist. At least you see a result when you pull teeth.

# JUNE

"Anybody dumb enough to use plyometrics will probably get just what they deserve, hurt."

Arthur Jones

## Leg Extension – A Case Study

In the early 1990's, Arthur Jones tested thousands of subjects using a prototype knee machine that isolated the muscles of the front and rear thigh (quadriceps and hamstring). The tests determined strength, muscle fiber-type, fatigue and recovery rates, the effects and results of exercise, and a ratio of quadriceps-to-hamstring strength. They also revealed a range of individual differences greater than anticipated.

Jones delighted in unusual physiology but focused on things of value to the average trainee, as in the following case study.

Figure 1 displays two strength tests of a subject's isolated quadriceps muscles. The bottom curve (A) depicts his strength before an exercise program; the top curve (B), his strength 18 weeks later; and the area between the curves, the increase produced by the program. The exercise performed was limited to the first half of a leg extension movement (right side of chart). In this 'worked' area, strength increased an average of 60% with a gain of more than 80% in one position. In the 'unworked' area (left side of chart), an increase of 13% was attributed to a test of fresh and exhausted strength before and after each session, a procedure that exposed the quadriceps to 'some' exercise. Nonetheless, the response was what Jones called 'Specific' - results where work was performed; none where it was not - typical of approximately 72% of tested subjects.

The need for full-range exercise was apparent, as was the need for *infrequent* exercise. The gains in Figure 1 were produced by an amount of exercise that many consider inadequate - 17 sessions of one set each, in 18 weeks.

Following the program, the subject continued to exercise once a week for 12 more weeks and produced no further gains. He then tried two sessions a week to see if additional exercise would result. His strength remained the same.

At that point, Jones measured his strength (Figure 2, Curve A) and initiated a program of exercise restricted to the *last* half of the leg extension (left side of chart). Curve B represents the subject's fresh strength following a one-set-a-week regimen for five weeks. Figure 2 reveals, as before, strength gains where the muscle worked, yet simultaneous decreases where the muscle performed no work, this time, the right side of the chart where *no* testing or exercise was allowed.

"Only the leg extension exercise," affirmed Jones, "is capable of producing full-range increases in strength in the quadriceps muscles; and then only if a full range of possible movement is used. But again, according to the 'experts' the leg extension exercise is evil, dangerous, of no value, to be avoided like the plague. Sure."

The so-called 'experts' - trainers and therapists - advocate the use of compound (closed-chain) exercise, such as squats and leg presses for quadriceps work at the expense of single-axis (open-chain) movements such as leg extensions. Compound movements may work more muscle mass but just as certainly eliminate the possibility of full-range exercise for *any* of the involved groups. They also provide a maximum overload for *only* the weakest link in the chain, the muscle that will ultimately fail. Accordingly:

- Leg extension exercise is a 'must' for maximum quadriceps strength and size.
- Full-range exercise is essential for full-range strength.
- Not much exercise is required to produce good results.
- More is rarely the 'answer' to training plateaus.
- Advice from 'experts' should be avoided like the plague.

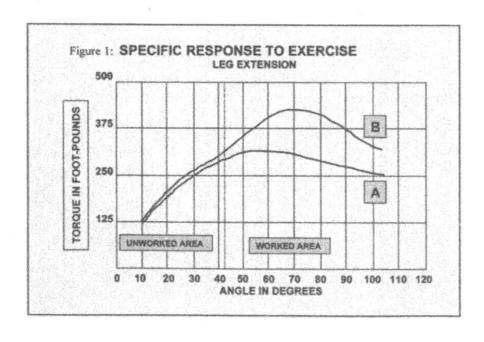

Figure 1: **SPECIFIC RESPONSE TO EXERCISE**
**LEG EXTENSION**

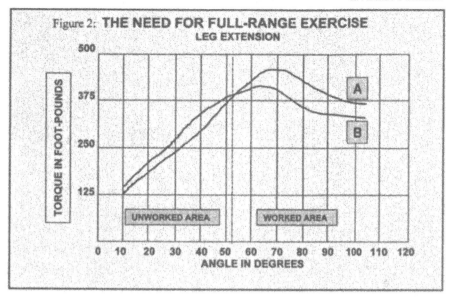

Figure 2: THE NEED FOR FULL-RANGE EXERCISE
LEG EXTENSION

JUNE 2

## Danger

The first 'game' for the Averett College men's soccer team in the fall of 1972 was full of surprises. The moment we arrived, the opposing coach announced that he had only 10 players to our 11. We decided that both coaches would play, which was no problem - running 25 miles a week left me in good stead.

As the team kicked the ball around, I stretched my upper and lower body and joined them on the field. The warm-up wasn't enough.

During the execution of a simple push pass, my groin suddenly 'popped.' I ignored the fact that I couldn't plant, cut or deliver a pass and faked about five minutes of play before announcing my retirement.

I was strong from training but had no access to exercise for the muscles of the inner thigh. They were flexible, but strength is more important than flexibility when it comes to injury. They were also accustomed to straight-line (non-lateral) running and once injured, could barely tolerate the minimal resistance offered by a slow-moving ball. Each touch felt like it added a day to the recovery.

The experience echoed the words of Nautilus® inventor, Arthur Jones. "It is not the resistance that causes injury, it is your attempt to move (or restrain the movement of) the resistance that causes injury." The attempt must be careful, but rarely is.

Most trainees throw rather than lift weights, which results in momentum - the tendency shown by a moving mass to continue movement and, more important, by a stationary mass to remain stationary. Any attempt to move a stationary mass such as a barbell imposes a 'jerk' on connective tissues and, to a lesser degree, on muscles.

Fortunately, "Connective tissues do not perform work," says Jones, "they have a level of resistance to pull which remains constant throughout an exercise. If it can withstand 100 units of pull on the first repetition, it can withstand 100 on the tenth...but the 'danger factor' certainly does NOT remain constant." In a 100-pound barbell curl, the force "would be approximately 1,000 pounds in the first repetition and about 80 pounds in the tenth repetition - a ratio of about 12 to 1 - and the 'danger factor' would be calculated by squaring the force ratio, or twelve times twelve, 144."

The first repetition is far more dangerous than the last.

As such, most injuries occur during the first repetition - not because a muscle is cold, but because the potential to produce force (strength) is highest at that point. The 'danger' is best reduced by performing several slow repetitions before the maximum efforts demanded by the final repetitions, as should occur in a normal set. The performance of a warm-up set with a lighter resistance - a common practice among trainees - is a poor idea because it *adds* exercise to the workout and can ultimately interfere with recovery.

The best way to increase the strength of connective tissue, according to Jones, is by "supporting heavy weights in a variety of positions with little or no attempt to actually move them suddenly." Tendons and ligaments are not subject to much in the way of growth, but the attachments can be injured if too heavy a load is imposed upon them. And the attachments can be strengthened if they are exposed to gradually increased loads, in the same way that muscular strength is induced by exercise.

If you can't find time to 'support' weights, do the next best thing, move them slowly to produce maximum strength and to protect the supporting cast from unwanted surprise.

JUNE 3

---

## The Logic and Dynamics of Muscle Contraction

It took only a few games of golf and soccer, to realize that **"a chain is only as strong as its weakest link."** In golf, there was always something to prevent a best score - a putt, chip or drive. In soccer, the disparity of talent on our team was so vast that the better players were reluctant to pass to the poorer ones for fear of losing the ball.

It took only a few games of both to realize another adage, **"function dictates design."** In golf, I avoided half-swings by design. In soccer, the selection and placement of players was dictated by function, as was the way they played to their individual strengths.

It took more than a few years to realize the importance of **"both"** to strength training.

Nautilus® inventor Arthur Jones was fascinated with the shape of skeletal muscle, "a lot like a catfish with a tail on both ends," and equally curious about function. The shape of a muscle, on the surface, seemed out of sorts with its function. It wasn't.

"It has been stated, and generally believed," he said, "that the strength of a muscle is in direct proportion to its cross-section; but nobody ever explained just which cross-section they were talking about: the relatively large cross-section near the middle of the muscle or the much smaller cross-section near the end of the muscle?"

If a muscle, he questioned, was strongest in its thickest part (its middle), how could a high level of strength be used if the muscle was limited by the strength of the smaller cross-sections at the ends? Remember the chain?

Jones addressed the issue with logic and a few questions of his own.

"Muscular contraction is progressive," he said. "When a muscle is fully extended (in its longest position), then no contraction has occurred; and full contraction can occur only when the muscle is in its shortest position. So the obvious question then is: just what part of the muscle has contracted when the muscle's length is halfway between its longest and shortest lengths? And, which part of the muscle has not contracted in that position?"

The shape of the muscle provided the answer.

"Muscular contraction," he said, "starts at the ends of the muscle and progressively moves towards the middle as contraction and resulting movement continue."

If a muscle is half contracted, the contraction occurs partially up the cross-section of the muscle (from both ends) and its output is limited by the girth of that cross-section. It then becomes obvious: to exercise all of a muscle, the muscle must reach - and encounter adequate resistance in - a full-contracted position. "If not," claimed Jones, "we are exercising only part of the muscle, and the smallest part at that."

In addition, strength gains are greatest in the range of motion where work is performed (vs. the range where no work is performed) which clarifies the need to focus on the last inch of contraction, and to 'squeeze out' a pause, once there. In the case of the standing biceps curl that does not provide an adequate resistance in a full-contracted position, try the following *immediately after* a hard biceps exercise:

- (1) Fully supinate your wrists (thumbs-out); (2) fully bend your arms (hands toward shoulders); and (3) fully raise your elbows straight above your head.
- Then, do all of them (1, 2, & 3) together, as far and as hard as you can, in one static contraction. (Because you've never been there, the muscle may cramp).
- Hold and squeeze that position twice for approximately 15 seconds each.

The above information was first featured in an article by Arthur Jones in *Ironman* (January, 1997). He kept us in the dark for more than 30 years.

## JUNE 4

---

### The Process of Elimination

It may sound negative, but you can discover what works by discovering what doesn't.

I was attracted to physical activity at an early age - played hockey at five and enjoyed success in playground activities. By 13, I wanted to be an athlete or, at least, a role model by leading an athletic life. It was a matter of making the right choices.

I began by eliminating things that might hinder progress. I chose not to smoke - it was rumored 'bad' for performance. I chose not to drink - the loss of control evident in peers and the fact that peers were doing it at all turned me away. I chose running and weight training as fundamental to the eventual focus - golf, where I launched the same process.

Starting with lessons, I worked diligently on the swing and soon realized that an emphasis on mechanics tied me down. So, I turned to results and tried to establish the cause-and-effect relationships between ball-flight and impact. More importantly, I began to *feel* that certain movements produced certain results, and recognized that correction reverted to basics.

I tried the same with strength training, but the rules were different. Where ball-flight provided instant feedback in golf, workouts provided nothing of the same. Results were far from instant, cause-and-effect difficult to determine, and Joe Weider's wall-charts provided no indication I was on the right track. Fortunately, almost everything worked back then. But I learned:

- Only one result from exercise was *instant*, injury - once by a jerky movement, once by exceeding the range of motion. The cause and effect was clear: The force imposed on the muscle was higher than it could handle.
- Only one result from exercise was *direct*, injury. Size and strength gains were indirect, with the body as middleman, which is why things took their sweet time.

The Nautilus® inventor underwent the same process to arrive at a state of what he called 'negative knowledge.' "People have been asking me for more than 50 years," he said, "just what they should do in attempts to improve their results from exercise, but I have never been able to answer their questions; what I can tell them, instead, is a few things that they should not do, things to avoid, things that will not help them and may hurt them. It took me a very long time to learn just what worked best for me, and even longer to learn that the same things were not always best for other people."

The other day, an amateur golfer was singing the praises of her instructor who was working toward a swing change that both agreed would take a year to perfect. If people, I thought, put as much energy and thought into the form of their workouts as they do their golf swings, the world would be a better place. But they don't have to. Where it takes a year to make a major swing change in golf, and months to effect a minor change, a change in exercise form can be instant and last a lifetime. It deals with basics.

The basics of exercise proposed by the Nautilus inventor reach far beyond goals or philosophy - a slow, controlled speed of movement, proper set-up and posture, little rest between exercises, constant tension on a muscle during exercise, pauses in contracted positions, full-range movement and muscle failure.

Basics deal with quality, not quantity. And when the quality of training improves, (1) the quantity is automatically reduced (must be for continued progress), and (2) results improve. What more is there?

As with everything - better input means better output.

JUNE 5

### Conditioning for Golf

Legendary golfer Moe Norman never lifted weights or believed in 'fancy.' He carried one wedge - "If you have more, you never learn to hit any of them" - and wasn't alone. Most pros of that era (early 1960's) had only heard of strength training through Gary Player or Frank Stranahan - the guys with the 'odd' approach.

Times have changed.

Many of today's pros are involved in conditioning, with cardiovascular (which has little to do with golf) and flexibility exercise at the helm. Strength training, for the most part, has been replaced by sports-specific training and functional activities, leading many to believe that strength potential can be reached *without* "lifting weights."

In 1995 and 1996, Wayne Westcott, Fitness Director at the South Shore YMCA in Quincy, Massachusetts conducted three studies to investigate the role of strength and flexibility in golf performance.

|  | Study 1 | Study 2 | Study 3 |
|---|---|---|---|
| Fat Loss | 3 pounds | 4.8 pounds | NA |
| Muscle Gain | 4.1 pounds | 4.3 pounds | NA |
| Blood Pressure | -5 mm Hg | -6.4 mm Hg | NA |
| Flexibility | +24% (overall) | no change | +23% hip flexion +25% hip extension +8% shoulder abduction |
| Leg Strength | +55% | +58% | NA |
| Clubhead Speed | +5 mph | +3 mph | +5.4% |

Study 1 examined the effect of strength and flexibility exercise on 17 recreational golfers (mean age 57.8 years) who were assessed for bodyweight, body composition, blood pressure, hip and shoulder flexibility, lower-body strength and clubhead speed. They performed 30 minutes of strength exercise and 10 minutes of stretching three times a week for eight weeks (one stretch each of hip flexors and extensors; shoulder rotators and protractors; and trunk rotators and extensors on a StretchMate®).

Study 2 investigated the effect of strength training only (without stretching) on 31 recreational golfers (mean age 51.7 years). Torso rotation and forearm exercises were added to the strength routine.

Study 3 investigated the effect of flexibility exercise only (using the same stretches as Study 1).

Similar and significant differences in body composition, resting blood pressure and muscle strength were produced in the first two studies, regardless of whether stretching was performed. However, when stretching was included (Studies 1 and 3), significant improvements were made in flexibility and clubhead speed.

"The strength training programs in both studies (1 and 2)," mentioned Westcott, "were designed for overall muscle conditioning rather than sports specificity." The exercises included (in order): leg extension, seated leg curl, leg press, chest cross, chest press, pullover, lateral raise, biceps curl, triceps extension, back extension, abdominal curl, neck flexion and extension, and weight-assisted chin-ups and dips. Each exercise was continued to a point of momentary failure - 1 set, 8-12 reps, 5% increase in weight; 2-second lift, 4-second lower - exactly what Arthur Jones proposed 20 years before.

Golfers are special people. They don't need special exercise.


## JUNE 6

————————

### High-School Baseball

The high school I attended was not far from the US border. It was small - 230 students spread over five grades - but alive with sports. The only activity I was forced to do at home was lift weights because there was nothing at school...or so I thought.

One day while chasing down a stray ball in PE class, I uncovered a bench and a few barbell plates stuffed in a dark closet near the boy's locker room. By the end of the day, I had established a "Weight Training Club," sponsor and all. Twice a week, I dragged the equipment upstairs to Room 203 and hosted what became a dismal failure. Other than a few hardened thugs who trained "to incite racial riots in Buffalo on weekends," there was little interest.

Twenty years later, I owned a set of Nautilus® machines in a business that lacked exposure. So, I hooked up with a physician who worked with the Douglas High School baseball team in Parkland, Florida and spent two hours a week supervising workouts in *their* facility, a far cry from Room 203.

The place was the size of two classrooms and housed a squat rack, leg press, hack-squat, Olympic benches for chest exercise, a leg extension and leg curl machine and a variety of stations for free-weight work. The walls were lined with dumbbells, barbells and storage-racks for plates.

I collaborated with Coach Fred Michael on the design of the program. The coach knew baseball but was uncomfortable with strength training. I made a brief presentation to the players, distributed a few handouts and we were on our way.

Things soon ground to a halt. The junior and senior varsity teams trained together during tryouts, which resulted in too many players (75-100) and too few exercise stations. My role was reduced to keeping people 'busy' and to correcting poor and dangerous form. Once the teams were selected, the player-to-equipment ratio became manageable, but not ideal.

There were some lessons learned.

I had coached at high school and college 20 years before under the same conditions - not enough equipment to go around. But it wasn't all negative because it revealed the character of individuals. If I had to chose the Douglas team based on performance in the weight room, there would have been a few 'stars' on the bench. Some worked hard from the moment they entered. Others hid like a barbell in a dark closet and performed only wrist curls when pressured.

The surprise came when I watched them play. Only a few of the better players were the 'workers' in the gym. They 'got by' on raw talent and knew they wouldn't be cut for poor exercise habits. They also felt no pressure from teammates who, in their opinion, needed to work hard to catch them. Some of the stars were lazy, while others were convinced that strength training would hurt them. It confirmed what Nautilus® inventor Arthur Jones often reiterated: "The great athletes are the ones who have the most to gain from strength training...and are the most unlikely to use it."

At the end of the second season, I donated three refurbished Nautilus machines to the school - a Leg Extension, Leg Curl and Multi-Exercise device. The addition allowed the players to complete the three exercises I should have made mandatory from the start - chin-ups, dips and squats.

Wrist curls just don't cut it.

JUNE 7

---

## Big John

There was a buzz in front of the scoreboard, and justifiably so. The "Early Bird" at the St. Thomas Golf Club was the first tournament of significance each year on the amateur scene in Ontario and, for that, drew a great field...and lousy spring weather.

As the media scanned the board, one question recurred, "Who is this Krickovich guy?" He had fired a 1-under par 35 on the front nine.

All doubt was put to rest when a fellow competitor, his playing partner on weekends, stepped up. "Just head out to the thirteenth hole," he pointed, "and look for the guy with the 17-inch wrists. That's John Krickovich."

Big John held a number of course records in the Buffalo (NY) area and crossed the border to play our club on weekends. His gentle demeanor was nothing but façade. When he ripped into a golf ball, things happened: it started low, rose like the pros, never wavered, and increased the size of his caddy's arms replacing sod.

John's great talent, legendary divots and timely humor were overshadowed by only one thing - the size of his forearms. You didn't shake hands with him *before* play; you patted him on the back and prayed you were on his team.

Large forearms are highly desirable among men. Their ultimate size is a product of genetics, hard work and good form - the last of which is rare.

The contraction of forearm muscles can produce movement in seven directions: flexion (wrist curls, palms up), extension (reverse wrist curls, palms down), supination (twisting clockwise), pronation (twisting counterclockwise), bending toward the thumb, bending away from the thumb, and gripping. Of the seven, only the first two can be performed in a meaningful way with a barbell; and only if the muscles are isolated.

The correct starting position for wrist curls is seated on a bench with hips higher than knees, feet separated about four inches at the ankle and elbows wedged into upper thighs so that only the wrists protrude beyond the knees. The torso and head should be bent well forward over the thighs to allow their weight to 'lock' the forearms in place.

This position provides isolated full-range exercise and a resistance that, according to Arthur Jones, "varies in close proportion to the changes in strength that occur as the hands move from the starting extended position to the finishing flexed position." The range is short (approximately 90°) which makes it easy to 'miss' exercise due to speed. When working forearms, move *slowly* and pause in the contracted position.

The muscles used in reverse wrist curls are more difficult to isolate. They require a bench that allows placement of wrists *higher* than elbows (by a slope of approximately 35° in relation to the floor, a slope that also makes the resistance close to 'ideal' throughout the range of motion). The muscles on the top of the forearm are smaller than on the underside, a fact that should reflect in the weight selection.

Forearm supination and pronation can be performed with a dumbbell weighted on one end; movement toward and from the thumb, with a dumbbell held at the side moving in a 'thumbs-up' motion or the reverse. Gripping requires a special apparatus.

Forearms are lucky. They harvest a 'spillover' effect from upper-arm exercises. Nonetheless, they should be trained *after* arms. Small muscles fail before large ones.

Big John's legacy was more. He never practiced before play - just sat on a bench and watched. When asked, he'd tap a forefinger to his temple as if to say, "Thinking about it."

It's something trainees might try before workouts.

## JUNE 8

### Of Dumb Thumbs and Wrist Twists

People do dumb things with dumbbells despite the fact that it doesn't take a genius to figure out what's right and what's wrong.

The first factor is gravity. If you jump off a building, you don't go up; you go down, straight down. The force of gravity is straight down, which makes 'vertical' movement the most productive part of a lift. If you lift a weight straight up, as in an overhead press, chest press or squat, you lift directly against gravity. But how it *feels* is tempered by another factor, the leverage of the joint systems.

"Put 1,000 pounds on the back of an untrained man," remarked Nautilus® inventor Arthur Jones on the dynamics of a squat, "have him bend two inches at the knee, and he will *not* hit the floor." The mechanical advantage is enormous in that part of a squat.

Fortunately, muscles have sensors that can distinguish hard from easy. An overhead press, for example, feels *difficult* in the mid-range of movement, but *easy* near the end of the lift where arms approach extension. If elbows become locked at the top, the bones (not the muscles) support the resistance. The same occurs in a chest press, where locked elbows represent a rest. Therefore, the common practice of rotating wrists at the end of a chest or shoulder press performed with dumbbells adds *nothing* to the exercise. There is *no* effective resistance in that position, but it sure looks good.

A chest fly with dumbbells on a flat bench is much the same. While it is important to finish with upper arms close to each other in the contracted position, there is no resistance at that point (due to arm position and gravity). Again, twisting dumbbells to where palms face each other for a 'clang' high above the chest adds *nothing* to the exercise. But it sure sounds good.

Biceps curls present a different yet related set of problems. Unlike presses, properly performed arm curls rotate around a single axis, the elbow. As such, the weight *feels* easy at the start and end of the movement, and heavy only when forearms are parallel to the floor (due to the direction of gravity). Since the major function of the biceps is to rotate the hands to a thumbs-out position (supination), it is imperative that hands are in that position when forearms are parallel to the floor. Yet, most trainees lift the weight through that critical zone in a thumbs-up posture and rotate thumbs outward only when the dumbbell is at chin height, too late to be effective.

A few suggestions about biceps curls:

- Perform dumbbell curls with palms facing up (thumbs out).
- Perform them from a seated position to minimize lower-body involvement and to better isolate the working muscles.
- Avoid alternate dumbbell movements (one arm first, then the other) unless you seek variety. They allow one arm to rest, promote body sway and 'cheating' when things are difficult, and take twice the time to reach fatigue.
- Perform barbell curls with a straight bar. An 'easy-curl' bar (one that appears bent where you grip it) does not allow full supination or total biceps involvement. Anything 'easy' is always less productive.

A suggestion about dumbbell chest presses and flys, and shoulder presses:

- Don't 'linger' (because of the rest you get) or rotate your hands when you reach a theoretical position of contraction.

Save your wrist twists for creative escapes on the Smith machine.

Gary Bannister, B.A., B.P.E., M.Ed.

JUNE 9

---

### Experience

The other day, I parked in the lot of a restaurant adjacent to the immigration office in West Palm Beach and was told (by INS) to return in the PM. I decided to run some errands, but my vehicle wouldn't cooperate. The clamps on the tires took two hours and $65 to remove. I parked it correctly upon return.

Somebody once said, "Success comes from good judgement, good judgement comes from experience, and experience comes from bad judgement." We're supposed to learn from our mistakes.

Arthur Jones believes that we don't.

"To this very day most of those utterly stupid opinions (on the subject of exercise)," he said, "are still believed by many people who should now know better, should know better, but generally do not know better."

Some people get so involved that they fail to see the big picture. Whether with work or sport, total immersion can become as much the problem as the solution. Its victims generally fall into one of two categories: they believe everything, regardless of source; or they believe nothing due to their own preconceived notions.

Neither situation is healthy.

According to Jones, "It is neither necessary nor desirable to devote your entire life to any one subject; on the contrary, if you do so, you will almost certainly limit your ability to learn anything of value." In that regard, he made it clear that the interests that labeled him *eccentric* - capturing exotic animals and flying airplanes - were an advantage.

"From my hands-on experience with flying," he said, "I gained a clear understanding of many of the simple laws of basic physics that are involved with exercise: What is torque? What is moment arm? What are the results of impact force? What happens when you suddenly change direction of movement?

From my study of animals I became aware of the fact that very little in the way of exercise is required for building enormous levels of strength and muscular size. How do you like the muscular size of a gorilla? Or a lion? Yet, both gorillas and lions perform almost no exercise or hard physical activity. But when they do work, they work very hard...but very briefly, and not very often. An adult male lion can get over a 10-foot-high fence with a 500-pound cow in his mouth. At a bodyweight of more than 500 pounds, a gorilla can perform a one-arm chin up so easily that he appears to weigh nothing."

He then added, "I strongly suspect that if you exercised a lion or a gorilla as much as many bodybuilders train, you would probably kill them, and it is certainly obvious that they do not 'need' that much exercise."

Jones learned something else from his days of thinning herds in Africa. "It has been firmly established that when the population (density) of any type of animals exceeds a certain point...the animals seem to go insane. In my opinion, that state of affairs now exists among people."

The solution? Learn from the mistakes of history, from the mistakes of others and from your own mistakes.

"And," he concluded, "if you are interested in exercise, base your opinions on your own experience, stop paying attention to any of the current crop of supposed experts. Few, if any, of whom could find their own ass if given 20 attempts with a bright light and an arrow on the target and with an Indian guide leading them by the hand."

JUNE 10

---

### Pre-Exhaustion for Emphasis

Many people exercise 4-6 times a week with routines that emphasize only one or two muscle groups at a time. Their workouts consist of identifying *every* exercise in the gym for those groups and then performing them in a haphazard sequence.

*"Is there anything I missed?"*

On 'chest' day, for example, they follow one chest exercise with another and another. Between efforts, a long, seated, prevent-others-the-pleasure-of-performing-this-exercise-on-my-day, hard-earned rest prevails. *"Who would want to rush to the next ten chest movements anyway?"* The next day, it's the same thing with a different muscle.

"Dumb," says Arthur Jones.

"The human body is a unit - and must be treated as such; you do not feed your body in sections, and you sleep the entire body at the same time - yet most current weight-trainees are firmly convinced that a so-called 'split routine' is an absolute requirement for producing the best rate of progress. While the weight of all available evidence clearly supports the contention that more than

three weekly workouts will result in a condition of overtraining - in all cases."
*Nautilus Training Principles, Bulletin #2, 1972.*

There are many ways to emphasize a muscle group *without* training more than three times a week. One is the use of 'pre-exhaustion.' A compound movement, such as a chest press, involves the large muscles of the chest (pectorals) and the small muscles of the back of the arms (triceps). During maximum efforts, the weak link (triceps) fails before the stronger chest muscles. 'Pre-exhaustion' fatigues the chest muscles immediately before the press, making the smaller triceps muscles temporarily stronger than the chest muscles. When the press ultimately fails from its weak link, 'pre-exhaustion' will have forced the larger chest muscles to a greater state of fatigue.

Pre-exhaustion sequences start with the isolation and exhaustion of a large muscle group *immediately* before a compound exercise that involves the same muscle and a 'fresh' helper. Perform no more than three of the following *per* workout:

- Legs: Leg Extension - Leg Press; Leg Extension - Squat; Calf - Leg Curl.
- Chest: Arm Cross or Fly - Chest Press; Arm Cross or Fly - Dips.
- Back: Pullover - Torso Arm or Pulldown; Pullover - Chin-Ups.
- Shoulders: Lateral Raise - Overhead Press.
- Arms: Biceps Curls - Chin-Ups; Triceps Extensions - Dips.

The Director of Research for Nautilus Sports/Medical Industries®, Ellington Darden, Ph.D. took the concept of pre-exhaustion a step further when he sandwiched an isolated exercise between two compound movements. The combinations were performed as part of a 10-to-12-exercise machine workout for the entire body. He later created *double* "pre-exhaustion" sequences with free-weights in a 14-exercise workout. An example of a chest workout (from *Massive Muscles in 10 Weeks*, 1987) follows:

- **Emphasis Phase:** *no-rest* Chest Press-to-the-Neck/Bent-Arm Fly/Negative-Only Dips - *brief rest*, then - *no-rest* Chest Press/Bent-Arm Fly/Negative-Only Dips/Push-Ups.
- **Whole-Body Phase:** *brief rest*, then Leg Press, Leg Curl, Leg Extension, Calf Raise, Pullover, Biceps Curl and Triceps Extension.

Seven chest exercises followed by seven full-body exercises satisfy both the desire for emphasis and the need for whole-body work.

Properly performed, it will keep you away from the gym tomorrow.

## JUNE 11

---

### My Favorite Gym

I drove around the block a second time. The area was laden with two-story structures that looked more residential than commercial - no signs, few numbers. The clutter on the front porch of one I selected led me to a narrow stairwell on the side of the building where a homemade sign with an arrow signaled victory, "**Gym➜.**" It was hard to believe this place was listed in the yellow pages.

"How could you get a set of exercise machines up here?" I thought as I ascended the wobbly wooden structure. "It's too narrow and rickety. No way."

I opened the screen door and knocked. There was no reply. I pushed my way in.

The floor creaked with every step through the musty odor. A stream of light from a lone window settled on a pair of physique pictures on the unpainted wall in front. The photos were unfamiliar, though I would soon learn about the great John Grimek. Beside them, a shower stall complete with plastic curtains stood like an outhouse in an open field. I can only assume it had water. Seventeen original Nautilus® machines, a squat rack, a set of dumbbells and three Olympic barbells completed the decor. The place was as empty as the shower, but a hand-written sign near the door at the back of the room turned things around in a hurry, "**Ring Bell for Help.**"

I rang, then heard a grunt and shuffle. The door popped opened and the owner emerged amid a waft of burnt toast. A hunched yet sprightly little demon looked at me with a glint in his eye and introduced himself. "Benny."

The 84-year-old weightlifter was intrigued that I owned a similar facility in Venezuela and that I had spent time with Nautilus inventor, Arthur Jones. Each workout, we shared tidbits about Jones and his philosophy.

Benny and Arthur had a lot in common. Both had been involved in the field of physical training long enough that neither had a kind word left. As a young man, Benny had a dispute with Weider of Canada® over the quality of a purchase, his first and last. He also refused John Cardillo, a "Mr. Canada" who hailed from the same hometown (St. Catharines, Ontario) access to his gym because he had a police record. Jones could have added plenty to that conversation. Both recognized the superiority of Nautilus machines over traditional exercise and were advocates of full-range strength. Both were meticulous about equipment. Arthur took years to develop it; Benny took the time to maintain it better than most. His 'old' machines were smoother than mine.

In the mid-1980's, a few of my Venezuelan gym clients toured facilities in the U.S. in search of ideas for a sports club they later established. They had their best workout in a basement gym found by chance in New York City. It housed a handful of Nautilus machines and trainers who believed in anything but 'easy.'

A small but growing number of gyms dictate training philosophy (such as super-slow). Although they fail to satisfy clients who claim to know what they're doing or who refuse to be pushed (too many to count), they definitely improve the results of the average trainee, provided the philosophy is safe and logical.

I had some great workouts in that musty little room, always training in fear that the owner might suddenly appear to blow the whistle on the time he allowed per visit.

Benny didn't accept anyone who stayed "more than 30 minutes," and retained only 30 members - enough to pay his rent.

It's surprising 30 people could find the place.

JUNE 12

_____

### Keeping It Off

A typical day in the Venezuelan gym business was flattering. Once word got around, members dropped by at noon or after work with a potential client, a friend who was curious or in need. The curiosity was nurtured by the arrival of Nautilus® machines, the latest exercise craze. The need stemmed from the fact that most 'friends' had not participated in exercise for years. It showed.

"Hey, Chico," laughed one man as he rolled back his suit to expose a large, protruding stomach, "How long will it take to get rid of this?"

"How long did it take to get it?" I asked.

"Ho. Ho. Ho," he blurted and answered something vague.

"With that discipline, it will probably take twice as long."

Only my Spanish was worse than my humor.

Reducing body fat is the first step in the disciplinary process. The exercise and diet sections of bookstores provide a variety of solutions that lead to nothing but confusion. To date, the most efficient and effective program belongs to Ellington Darden, Ph.D. - author of numerous Nautilus books in the 1970's and 80's. Darden's research consistently demonstrates fat losses of 10-12 pounds in six weeks with women and 12-18 pounds in one month with men. His plan - a decreased, balanced caloric intake combined with brief, high-intensity strength training. Once a satisfactory body-fat level is reached, the body can increase its intake *without* further gain because of an improved muscular state (women gained three pounds of muscle; men, 3-4). The new habits (of exercise and diet) make it easier to 'keep it off.'

Statistics, however, show otherwise. According to Dr. Jim Hill, University of Colorado, only about 5% of those successful at losing weight are able to maintain the new level. Dr. Hill tracked a group that had experienced success *for at least five years* to discover what they had in common. The results:

- They *expected* failure but vowed to keep trying.
- They didn't deny themselves (food had become an emotional crutch they used).
- They weighed themselves often and kept track of progress.
- Nine of ten performed exercise (about an hour a day, ranging from brisk walking to becoming an aerobics instructor).
- They added bits of physical activity to their daily routine (such as walking up stairs or parking further away from buildings).
- They ate a high carbohydrate, low-fat diet (Darden advocates approximately 50% carbohydrates, 25-30% fat and 20-25% protein in his balanced approach).
- They ate five meals a day (on average). Many nutritionists advocate spreading out the total caloric intake to avoid hunger and binge eating.

There are other factors at work. A special presentation of CNN (July 8, 2002) made it clear that many are dealt a poor genetic hand. One study showed that some children were heavier than others despite identical metabolic rates. Research in the pharmaceutical field is currently being directed toward the alteration of genes through drugs.

Nonetheless, through all the mud, exercise that increases the body's muscle-mass-to-body-fat ratio is the best choice. Strength training not only increases metabolism during exercise, it burns a significant amount of calories when the body is inactive.

A great second choice is anything that keeps you coming back.

## JUNE 13

---

## A Lifestyle Change

When I entered high school, my brother Al urged me to run cross-country. He had experienced success with it and his designated intramural squad, "Alfa" (of which I was now a part) needed recruits. It was a great fit - I had been successful in running activities in grade school.

So, I woke up one morning at the age of 14, a cross-country runner.

There were things about it I liked - the exhilaration, the solitude, the camaraderie of belonging to a team and the conditioning it provided for other activities. But there was one thing I did not - getting sick.

With a short season and limited preparation time, I donned the team colors every day after class and headed down streets and paths that always led to the same end - the edge of the track. There, hands on knees, I provided the school's lawn a much-needed service. The sound alone scared the weeds into submission, but the message was loud and clear: "A N O T H E R...S U C C E S S – F U L...R U N."

That, sad to say, was the extent of my success the first season.

The second was much the same. Though my love of running had grown, I was disappointed when I didn't work hard enough to make myself sick; yet, despised the process of getting sick. The solution was simple - run year-round.

For the next 15 years, I ran three times a week, refused to don my shorts for less than seven miles, logged approximately 25,000 miles and *never missed once*.

Call it what you will, I made a lifestyle change, an easy decision at the time. It wasn't until I became a gym owner that I realized its ease was the exception, not the rule.

Once word spread (1980), Venezuelans flocked from every corner of Caracas to check out the famous Nautilus® machines the 'gringo' had brought to town. *"Now-tee-loose"* (with an emphasis on the tee) became the buzzword among those who exercised. Anybody who was 'a somebody' joined what came to be known as Gimnasio Multicentro. When they discovered that *"Now-tee-loose"* meant nothing but 'hard' work, the novelty soon wore off.

It was a lesson in human behavior.

Typically, a new client would enroll for a month, get excited about the program, enlist a friend and then disappear. Months later, he or she returned with an excuse and repeated the process. Delinquent members I encountered on the street often preceded their greeting with a confession, while many returnees insisted on using the same weight, making themselves sore enough to warrant further absence. Everyone, it seemed, was *into* being a member, but few were *into* exercise (my apologies to those who were and thanks to those who weren't).

Making a commitment and following through are major problems in the pursuit of personal fitness (and the reason why gyms survive). Here are two cold, hard suggestions:

- *Make time for exercise.* Two or three times a week: 20 minutes of proper strength training, 20 minutes of cardiovascular training. More may be counterproductive.
- *Keep making time for exercise.* Seventy-two hours without training leads to a decline in strength and cardiovascular condition, regardless of exercise history.

You don't have to live in a gym, run 25,000 miles or moisten lawns to enjoy the benefits of health.

## JUNE 14

### Carrying the Torch

The buzz of the crowd begged an outlet as we huddled on the corner of our childhood stomping grounds - far from Athens, Greece. The long-awaited Olympic torch, en route to Calgary for the 1988 Winter Games, was only minutes from passing through Fonthill, Ontario, Canada in the hands of a former high-school classmate.

The 'torchbearer' was selected from thousands of applicants across the country, an honor that prompted an article in the local newspaper. It praised his athleticism and love of sports, but left a few heads scratching. The only thing we ever saw him do - because he was hard to distinguish in a cloud - was smoke cigarettes under the tree across the street from school. During cross-country runs in P.E., he and others from the 'Smoker's Club' would start out in the pack, stretch out under a tree far from sight and smoke the pack hidden in their socks. When we returned, they'd join in - fresh and green.

Furthermore, the 'torchbearer'...OK, so I was jealous.

Self-proclaimed experts exist in every field. Their opinions and antics have all but ruined exercise and may soon repeat in sport's final sanctuary of sanity - golf. Spurred by the brilliant play and superior conditioning of Tiger Woods, the new interest in golf fitness is fast falling prey to the commercial whims of so-called 'experts.' As MedX® inventor Arthur Jones put it, "There are some people arrogant enough to call themselves experts, and many people dumb enough to believe them."

Several years ago, Dominion Fitness Concepts® marketed the Butch Harmon Golf Fitness Program® through MedX Corporation (in the post-Jones era). The program consisted of using a MedX Stretch and Rotary Torso machine as an integral part of a complete workout to increase the strength and flexibility of golf muscles. The cost of the new equipment was $8,285. The cost of using Butch Harmon's name was $14,400 *for the first three years*. To add insult to injury, the program failed to include the most important piece of equipment for golfers, the MedX Lumbar Extension machine - a device that isolates and strengthens the muscles of the low back. Thanks, but no thanks.

A few days ago in a 2003 post-tournament interview, the champion (a man who has been around for a while) spoke of discussing the relevance of fitness to golf performance with Mr. Harmon. Had he never heard of Gary Player or Tiger Woods, or read Jones' 1970 comment that, "A stronger athlete is a better athlete?"

A year ago, the same player commented on a fellow golfer's back problem by saying, "Oh, he just needs to do a lot of sit ups." The champion needs to do a lot of reading and seek a source that can at least distinguish a barbell from a truck.

As Jones once put it, "The blind leading the stupid."

If I were to follow someone in golf fitness, I would hitch up with Mike Malaska, often seen on *The Golf Channel* with instructor Jim Flick. We tested Mike at our facility in Jupiter, Florida two years ago and found him as fit as anyone we'd seen - strong, flexible, in great cardiovascular condition - and knowledgeable. He also demonstrated what Flick described as "the best swing of anyone *not* on tour." At least Jim was smart enough to pass the torch to a guy who had *exercise* expertise. Golfers should stick to golf.

In what amounted to '*Non-Smoking's Finest Hour*,' our athletic, sport-loving, flame-bearing classmate did not round the corner with a torch-lit cigarette in his mouth. And, as miracles go, he did not keel over.

Some people will sell their grandmother for a nickel.

JUNE 15

---

## Arthur's Articles

Arthur Jones first entered the field of exercise intending "to publish the results of his experimental work without taking credit under his own name." A friend convinced him otherwise.

"If you don't take credit under your own name," claimed Bill Pearl, "somebody will try to steal the credit for anything worthwhile that you have produced."

So, in the first few pages of his book, *Nautilus Training Principles: Bulletin No. 1* (1970), Jones introduced himself. It didn't take long to warm up.

"In Bulletin No. 1, several chapters were removed at the last moment before printing - chapters that I felt were perhaps too controversial; but I have promised myself that such will not occur again - this time (Bulletin #2) will include portions that may be offensive to some people, but which I consider necessary for a full statement, a true statement."

The runway was clear.

From 1971 to 1997, he filled the airways with books and articles, no holds barred. He wrote in *Ironman*, a bodybuilding magazine whose Editor, Perry Rader, allowed him to publish 'as is.' He self-published other works so that every word was controlled. Jones would have it no other way; nor would his readers.

He attacked the lunatic practices of bodybuilders, the mythical beliefs of coaches and the training routines of athletes who learned dumb things from both. He attacked the self-perpetuating air and dishonest research of scientists, and the acceptance of dangerous and inaccurate tools by therapists. He attacked the medical community whose understanding and practical application of exercise reflected little education. He questioned the exercise and rehabilitation tools of the day. Nothing escaped his scrutiny.

Jones backed his jabs with a logic that made people think, as in the following:

"I find it necessary to write an article such as this simply because it seems that almost nobody has ever made a serious attempt to apply the basic laws of physics to the field of exercise; instead, many people have blindly (if in many cases honestly) stumbled around in the dark in search of a source of illumination while holding the light switch in their hands all the time, and a few other people have produced a small candle in a large cave of ignorance and falsely proclaimed that it was the sun."

Jones crafted his first efforts out of boredom, "most articles being along the lines of the famous telegram, 'Screw you, strong letter follows.'"

"My God, Arthur," commented Pearl on one submission, "you can't print things like that; you have insulted everybody just short of the Pope and Jesus Christ."

"Not to worry, Bill," replied Jones, "I'll get around to both of them in a later article."

In his final attempt (*Ironman*, December 1997), Arthur hammered on politics, lawyers, the corruption of society, the end of civilization and other things he disdained.

"So, you might ask," he concluded, "just what does any of this have to do with exercise? Just everything, because the field of exercise is certainly no exception to our currently existing state of national insanity... If a solution exists, and that is a long shot at best, it must come from your own efforts; everything of any slightest value that is known about exercise, together with many other things of no value, has been clearly spelled out in my earlier articles. If you cannot, or will not, understand, or believe the things that I have tried to communicate, then, as the Chinese say, "Rots of ruck.""

The torch had passed hands.

## JUNE 16

---

### Your Turn, My Turn

We all make mistakes. It's how we learn. It's also why Arthur Jones was very careful to label opinions "as just that, opinions."

"Some of the opinions that I will express in this article (*Athletic Journal*, 1986) are almost certainly wrong...but like the professor in the old joke, I don't know which ones are wrong."

The joke he referred to was what a professor supposedly said to his class, "Only ten percent of what I am going to tell you is true, but the problem is that I don't know which ten percent."

Now, enter the gym scene and my opinion.

Approximately 10 percent of what the average trainee does in a gym is correct. The problem is, he or she doesn't know which 10 percent. And even a greater problem exists: Most trainers don't know which 10 percent.

A few months ago, I watched two enthusiastic males go through five sets of pulldowns on an exercise machine. They started with 75 pounds on the first set and increased the weight by about 10% on each subsequent set. First one, then the other. Your turn, my turn; over, and over. They then repeated the ritual on a seated rowing machine with a starting weight of 60 pounds, and later, on a biceps curl machine with 30 pounds. Their enthusiasm manifested itself in fast repetitions and general poor form.

What's wrong with this picture?
- Three exercises that involve biceps failure, in a row.
- What happened to the rest of the body?
- What happened to the use of seatbelts on pulldowns?
- Taking turns is an inefficient way to train - too much rest between exercises.
- Performing five sets is too much exercise and promotes poor intensity levels.
- They 'tied up' each machine for 15-20 minutes, something that might be an issue in the wrong gym at the wrong time.

What's right with this picture?
- Enthusiasm.
- Training buddy.

How would you change the scene?
- Include the upper back and biceps as part of a full-body workout.
- Perform two exercises for the same major muscle groups back to back only if you wish to emphasize those groups (not as part of a long, shopping list of exercises).
- Use seatbelts if they are provided. It's a 'must' on a pulldown if the resistance is heavy enough (which in this case it was not).
- Don't take turns with a buddy system. As with alternate work with dumbbells, it allows too much rest between efforts. A should train B totally; then B train A totally.
- Perform one hard set and move on. Your buddy should push you and have the next station ready, so that NO rest is taken.
- Focus on the intensity of each effort, not on the total amount of exercise you need to squeeze in that day.

If you want something other than my opinion, I'll say what Jones said to those who arrived to attack his theories, "I know nothing about exercise. What do you know?"

## JUNE 17

---

### Osteoporosis and Progressive Resistance Training

The aging process is unforgiving. Organs wear down, capacities diminish, structures deteriorate and the system no longer functions 'like it used to.' The decline eventually appears in the form of what Ellington Darden, Ph.D. suggested was the foremost indirect cause of death - lack of mobility. As the body becomes less active, it shuts down - and muscles are no exception.

From the age of 14 for women and 20 for men, the body loses approximately a half-pound of muscle and gains 1½ pounds of fat per year. The resulting loss of structural integrity is accompanied by a decrease in bone-mineral density, a condition known as osteoporosis. When the loss reaches levels that represent less than 25% of young, healthy adults, it is generally accompanied by fractures - which affect mobility. The entire process can be reversed by an increase in physical activity.

In a 2004 *Palm Beach Post* article on osteoporosis, the question "What kind of exercise is best?" was answered as follows: "Any kind of activity that causes you to move your body against gravity is good - walking, jogging, dancing, tennis, basketball. Lifting weights also helps keep bones dense." Nice try.

All of the suggested activities - except the after-thought of lifting weights - are aerobic and research shows that 'aerobic exercise' has little or no effect on an increase in bone mineral density (BMD). Too much, in fact, may result in lower BMD levels. To add insult to injury, all of the suggested activities expose the body to impact. Significant bone loss and participation in activities with inherent high levels of force invite injury.

Your best choice is the *Post* after-thought. Resistance-trained individuals consistently exhibit higher BMD values than subjects performing *other* forms of exercise.

In a 6-month study (Pollock, 1992), the average BMD of the lumbar spine of 35 subjects (60-82 years old) increased 14% after using a MedX® Lumbar machine (1x/wk., 1 set, 10-15 reps). Treadmill walking and stair climbing had *no* effect on the same.

In another study (Menkes, 1993), 11 subjects (59 year-old average) exercised three times a week for 16 weeks and increased their BMD levels by 3.8% in the neck of the femur (upper-leg bone) and 2.0% in the lumbar spine.

In a recent study conducted by Michael Fulton, M.D., BMD levels were increased by 4% with calcium supplementation, by 5% with resistance training, and by 17% with supplementation *and* resistance exercise.

The problem of bone loss is particularly devastating in heart transplant patients where steroid therapy increases the incidence of fractures in the long bones (44% of patients early in the post-operative period) and in the lumbar vertebrae (35% of patients). Furthermore, calcium supplementation, hormone therapy and all other agents have failed to reverse or prevent bone mineral loss after heart transplants. Yet, there's hope.

In a 1996 study by Braith and others, a 6-month program of resistance exercise (MedX® low back, 1x/wk.; whole body, 2x/wk.) restored BMD to pre-heart-transplant levels despite continued immune-system suppression with steroids. But the process was slow. Where muscle responded to training within weeks, bone required up to six months for an optimal training effect. The researchers also warned that advanced osteoporosis may be a contraindication for an aggressive approach to resistance training.

If you suffer bone loss, lift weights first - then add aerobic activity when it is safe. 'Movement against gravity' doesn't cut it.


## JUNE 18

---

### Multi-Tasking

One of the greatest ball strikers in the history of golf, Canadian Moe Norman drew the club back far enough for spectators to notice that there was no *P* or *PW* on the club's sole to denote "pitching wedge." It had been worn down to nothing.

"Here's one 11 feet high...22 feet high...33 feet high," he said as he struck three balls in rapid succession, each significantly higher than the next.

Moe was self taught but secured tips along the way from his childhood idols, George Knudsen and Canadian Amateur Champion, Nick 'The Wedge' Weslock. While the majority of professionals on tour carried several wedges to cover a variety of situations around the green, Moe carried one.

"If you have more than one," he said, "you never learn to hit any of them."

Without knowing it, Moe knew something about strength training.

Three major ingredients produce best results from training: progression, intensity and form - and now, a fourth, simplicity - and the reason is clear.

Golfers return to basics when they are 'off'; gym trainees gravitate to anything but.

The other day I witnessed someone in a shirt labeled *TRAINER* supervise a mobile set of lateral raises with one dumbbell, perhaps the smartest thing present. The client lifted the weight from her left side to shoulder height and simultaneously stepped sideways with her right foot as if to perform a hip-abduction exercise. It looked like a 2-for-1 sale at the dime store, only worse.

Stand in front of a mirror and step to your right (laterally) with a straight leg. Now, follow with a smaller left-foot step in the same direction and observe your shoulders - they move up and down with each step. If you place a weight in your left hand and lift it straight out from your side when your right leg lands, your torso tilts to the right. The added tilt helps the left arm 'cheat' on its task.

When possible, perform most dumbbell exercises (lateral raises, in this case):

- While seated (standing tempts the legs to cheat when it's difficult).
- With both arms at the same time (one arm at a time allows the non-working side to rest and encourages torso-lean away from the exercise), and...
- Without walking sideways (which magnifies the 'cheat').

Trainers must stay up nights creating new ways of performing the same old exercises. In most cases, they come up with something unique - not better, and often worse, just unique.

Moments later, the same *TRAINER* demonstrated a 2-pronged rope pull, one arm at a time in a rowing motion, from a high-pulley setting. First left, then right, then left - I don't even want to go there.

Functional exercises aimed at working several muscle groups at once suffer the same. They strengthen the weak link in the chain and produce fewer results because they lack isolation, and often focus. Movements on a Swiss Ball, for example, detract from the principal exercise (regardless of what it is) by shifting some of the focus to the muscles that keep you balanced. With compound movements, the *amount* of muscle-mass involved is key. If the muscle groups are large (a rarity on the ball) and the intensity high, the exercise can stimulate a significant strength response.

First things first. Isolate the large muscle groups and work them hard *before* you put them to task - hone the big tools, not the small. And like golf, keep it simple.

JUNE 19

---

## The Comeback

The long journey ended with a carcass sprawled out in a chair and wedged between a pair of 20-inch biceps and a pair of man-eating crocodiles. I was beat...and this wasn't exactly what I had in mind.

In December of 1983, I visited Nautilus Sports/Medical Industries® in Deland, Florida to purchase spare parts for my machines in Venezuela. I also sought an update on training ideas and equipment, and - if I was lucky - a glimpse of the eccentric inventor, Arthur Jones.

As I sat in the reception, it was evident I was not alone. To my left groaned a pair of 14-foot crocodiles, each in separate cages, part of a collection that later reached 1,400. To my right paced a man built like a reptile. He sported a beard and moustache, and was dressed in a pair of blue corduroy slacks and loose polo shirt. His size was impressive, but there were plenty of athletic specimens around Nautilus.

Both man and beast impatiently waited for the receptionist.

Suddenly, the man extended his arm toward the counter and out popped a slab of meat from his shirtsleeve. I couldn't help but stare; this was no ordinary arm. I glanced at his face a few times and eventually recognized Boyer Coe, Mr. Universe in the mid-1970's. I had seen him many times in magazines, always clean-cut and in superb condition. Now, at the age of 40, he had officially retired from bodybuilding and was in an untrained state for the first time in his life.

Jones had hired him for an 'experiment' - results were always better using what Jones called "genetic freaks." An out-of-shape Boyer Coe was ripe to produce an optimal training response.

I followed the progress of the 'experiment' through conversations with Dr. Fulton, orthopedic representative for Nautilus, and through Jones' writing. Coe began with one set of 12 exercises three times a week. When he hit a plateau, he trained 'hard' twice a week and 'easy' in the middle session, reducing the number of exercises from 12 to 10. Months later when progress stalled again, he performed eight exercises twice a week. The workout adjustments were made according to strength tests and size measurements. At each plateau, Coe performed *less but harder* exercise, a procedure used by Jones to allow better recovery between sessions.

There were, however, a few unknowns.

Despite his 'announced' retirement from bodybuilding and Jones' advice to stay out of the sport, Coe was secretly using the opportunity for a comeback. To add fuel to the fire, after a few months of training, Jones discovered that Boyer was taking steroids and immediately terminated the arrangement. Coe begged to continue, agreed to stop the steroids and consented to medical testing.

According to Fulton, he slowly lost muscle size from then on, despite the fact that his strength continued to increase. Normally, an increase in size parallels an increase in strength. With gifted individuals, an increase in strength triggers a greater increase in size. The lack of steroids made the difference.

Coe finished the six-month ordeal going through the motions - he did not like what he saw in the mirror. In the end, he was as strong and lean as ever, but did *not* look like a bodybuilder. He looked like a well-conditioned athlete.

To each his own.

## JUNE 20

---

### The Brain Drain

Machines are for this, free weights for that. Use machines like this, barbells like that. Three sets here, one set there. The controversy rages on. And while it is true that some tools provide better resistance than others, it's all from the same pot - with one exception. Contact with free weights appears to stimulate *more* than muscle growth.

Years ago, I watched a half-hour TV show that featured seven-time Mr. Olympia, Lee Haney and a celebrity guest. The topic was low backs, and the guest - a bodybuilder turned physician, Dr. Dumb Dumb.

The first 15 minutes addressed exercise related to low backs *without* equipment. The hosts examined sources of pain, demonstrated exercises to strengthen the midsection and warned of things to avoid. Above all, they stressed and displayed good form - slow movements, proper positioning and good posture.

The segment ended with a promise of more of the same, this time *with* equipment.

It didn't happen. The moment a barbell was introduced, all remnants of gray matter disappeared. Haney threw weights up and down while Dr. Dumb Dumb harped upon the virtues of control. When they switched, the Dr. lived up to his name with form far worse than Haney's, while Lee basked in the wisdom common among bodybuilders - that only chest and biceps count.

The first half was informative, safe and sane; the second half, none of the above, which made it appear that bodybuilders and low backs are better off *without* equipment - the opposite of what research suggests (that low-back muscles can be strengthened *only* by specific exercise on a MedX® machine).

I have likewise struggled with the second half of my show - training clients - but only when the session is an hour. If exercise is as intense as it should be for best results, 30 minutes is enough, and anything more may be counter-productive.

One set of 10-12 exercises for the major muscle groups of the body with little or no rest between is plenty for anyone - from an out-of-shape rehab patient to a professional athlete. Properly performed, few can make it. When trainees are pushed to their limit, the session won't last long.

A trainer must first determine the existing state of the client, then estimate a starting resistance, the amount of rest between exercises, if any, and an appropriate level of intensity. The process is called trial and error, nothing more.

The workout should proceed as follows (from the trainer's perspective):

- Determine an exercise sequence.
- Adjust the seat of the first machine, then set the weight.
- Secure the seat belt (if provided) and scrutinize the first few repetitions to assure good form. Don't 'talk' good form like Dr. Dumb Dumb, demand it.
- Once the form is sound, set the seat and weight of the *next* station, then return to push the trainee through the final repetitions.
- Move the trainee as quickly as possible (in light of his or her condition) from exercise to exercise.
- Repeat until all stations are complete.

Multiple sets, rest between exercises, water breaks and watching someone ride a bike for 30 minutes are some of the common 'tricks' used to stretch a potentially productive session into a dismal, social hour.

# JUNE 21

---

## Impact Force and Exercise

I first learned about the destructive nature of impact when I suffered a concussion in a high-school football practice the year before. But this was different. I was on the giving end and it wasn't pretty.

One cold evening, I decided to visit a friend to work on a music project. The mile run would keep me warm and get me there quickly, but there were puddles to dodge - it had just rained. I kept my head down most of the route, especially in the section of street that was missing lights.

BANG! Something hit my right shoulder and spun me off the sidewalk. By the time I turned around, it was too late. The elderly woman fell back like a board into a large puddle formed by a car rut. As I helped her to her feet, she held her face, blood showing through her gloves. She mumbled something in a foreign language and pointed to a nearby house, where I got my first glimpse of her son - a 6'4", 280-pound Russian man.

"What happen?" he panicked.

"I ran into this lady on the street," I said.

"With car? With car?"

"Not exactly."

Her nose was broken in seven places. The explanation was difficult.

Twenty years ago, I witnessed the effect of impact on something other than a nose during a presentation by MedX® Corporation in Ocala, Florida. A 200-pound man stood on a force plate (a large scale) and jogged lightly. The screen (an oscilloscope) revealed a force of approximately 650 pounds with every foot contact. He then jumped four inches high with both feet and landed softly. The force registered 1,000 pounds - five times his body weight. I didn't quit running that day, but should have.

Unknown to most trainees, impact force is present in many of today's exercises, either inherent in the movement itself, in the execution of the movement, or in the way we are instructed to perform it. In all cases, the result is the same.

The most common impact in gyms is the clang of weights and movement-arms. Yet, the very noise that attracts attention and assists the repetition count, is an open invitation to a clinic...a bargain when compared to the following.

For years, manufacturers of constant-speed 'isokinetic' rehabilitation equipment have instructed clinicians and patients to press *hard* against the resistance pad(s) to initiate dynamic strength tests. The result is increased exposure to impact force inherent in the machine's effort to sustain its speed.

The absurdity of such advice was demonstrated in a TV broadcast of the "latest isokinetic device for low backs" more than 20 years ago. From a standing position, the patient rocked back and forth, repeatedly banging his torso into the machine's front and back restraint pads with such impact that his jowls vibrated. The supervising physician called it "aggressive rehabilitation." Aggressive, yes; rehabilitation, no.

The most incriminating form of impact occurs when coaches promote training methods that increase the risk of injury, such as the common use of "plyometrics" to enhance an athlete's power. MedX inventor Arthur Jones addressed the matter for more than 30 years and concluded, "Anybody dumb enough to use plyometrics will probably get just what they deserve, hurt."

Impact implies high levels of force - and high force, injury - in every language.

## JUNE 22

---

### Dynamic vs. Static Strength

Meaningful strength testing in the field of exercise is doomed without understanding the role of internal muscle friction, and the relation between dynamic and static strength.

Movement creates friction, and when muscle contraction produces movement, it creates friction within the muscle that affects the output of strength. An illustration by Arthur Jones should clarify the point.

"If you were seated at one end of a table...and were holding onto a handle that was attached to a rope that extended to the far edge of the table, passed over the edge, and then supported a 100-pound weight that was hanging from the far end of the rope, how much force would be required from you to cause the weight to rise? Well, if we assume that the rope rubbing against the edge of the table produces 20 pounds of friction, then you would have to exert 120 pounds to lift the weight, 100 for the weight and 20 for the friction. But if you were lowering the weight then only 80 pounds of force would be required, because in that case the friction would help you instead of hurting you."

If a pull-type scale were connected to the rope above the table and another to the rope below the table, the scale below would always read 100 pounds if the speed of movement was constant. The scale above would read 120 when the weight was lifted, and 80 when lowered. Both would read 100 when the rope was *not* in motion.

Unfortunately, the only practical way to measure strength is by output, an output biased by friction when the muscle moves. To eliminate the bias, muscle strength must be measured when the muscle is *not* moving - which is asking a lot in today's science.

"Muscular strength of any kind, dynamic positive, dynamic negative, or static," claims Jones, "is one and the same thing: an output of torque produced by the force of muscular contraction, minus muscular friction if positive, plus muscular friction if negative or without friction if static. But, of course, at least 99.9 percent of the current crop of supposed 'experts' in this field are not even aware that friction exists in muscles and damned sure do not understand its effects... Such supposed experts should be burned at the stake, letting them live is far too dangerous. And no possible amount of punishment would be enough to compensate for the harm they are causing millions of people" (the danger of impact forces encountered during dynamic tests). The problem runs deeper.

"There is an almost universal bias," he adds, "in favor of using a dynamic testing procedure when trying to measure human muscular strength; and the fact that conducting meaningful and accurate strength tests in such a manner is simply impossible has occurred to damn few, if any of the supposed 'experts' in this field. 'Oh,' they usually say, 'we are not interested in static strength, we are interested in dynamic strength.' And, of course, they remain unaware of, or even deny, the fact that there is a direct relationship between static and dynamic strength; having changed one, you have changed the other to exactly the same degree. If you believe otherwise, as many people do, then you are a fool... But not to worry, being a fool has several advantages: it means, for one thing, that you are a member of the majority, and it also keeps you unaware of, and thus not generally disturbed by, the insanity that surrounds you."

The greater decrease in dynamic (vs. static) strength *after* exercise in many studies can be explained as follows: "Dynamic strength has been reduced by an increase in muscular friction resulting from fatigue, but muscular friction has no effect on static strength."

There may be another advantage to being a fool - you might learn from it.

## JUNE 23

---

### The Inaccuracy of Dynamic Muscle Testing

Much of the confusion that plagues the scientific and medical communities concerning the measurement of muscular strength revolves around the fact that strength cannot be measured directly. You cannot insert a strain gauge between the end of a muscle and its tendon. Muscle strength must be measured indirectly, by testing the functional output of force produced by a body part being moved by muscular force.

Unavoidably, this brings joint systems into play and they vary greatly in efficiency. Less than eight percent of the force generated by the front-thigh muscle, for example, is used to move the lower leg in the direction of extension about the knee. In contrast, the output of the muscles that extend the low back is 2-4 times that of the input. Nonetheless, such information, when known, is useless because the relationship between muscular force and functional output changes with movement - in some cases, as much as 1,000% from one end of the range of motion to the other.

When movement is involved (as in dynamic testing), other factors add confusion:

- Internal muscle friction wastes at least 16% of the muscular input in dynamic tests of lifting strength, yet increases the functional output in similar tests of lowering. Unfortunately, a known percentage of friction cannot simply be added to the tested level of lifting strength (or subtracted from that of lowering strength) because friction varies with at least two factors - speed of contraction and level of fatigue. The faster the contraction speed and higher the fatigue, the greater the friction.

- The ability to recruit and involve all of the available muscle fibers varies from one individual to another and from one muscle group to another in the same individual. Fast-twitch muscles recruit quickly but fatigue in the final part of a dynamic test; slow-twitch muscles have better endurance but recruit slowly during the first part. The output suffers at one end (of the tested range of motion) or the other, and a change of movement speed can vary the output by several hundred percent.

- If an 'isokinetic' source of resistance is used during a dynamic test, impact magnifies the level of force produced (when measured as output) by as much as several hundred percent. To add insult to injury, a 'damping' system inherent in isokinetic devices modifies the result. As one study (Sinacore, *Physical Therapy*, 1983) commented, "Note how torque (force) diminishes as damp increases and how the torque curve is shifted to the right (i.e., later in time)." Great information if you like lies.

Arthur Jones, an advocate of *static* muscle testing, concluded that after 20 years of dynamic testing with isokinetic devices, "nothing of any slightest value has been learned. Quite the contrary, such tests have merely added to an already high level of confusion."

Proof? In 1987, the prestigious and peer-reviewed *Spine* magazine reported higher levels of trunk flexion strength during dynamic lifting tests than during static tests - impossible. Static (holding) strength is *at least* 20% greater than lifting strength under *all* conditions (fresh, fatigued, etc.) due to internal muscle friction. *Spine* and other medical journals have also consistently reported higher levels of force at faster movement speeds - another impossibility. Try to bench-press your car quickly. Such test results are records of impact force *added* to the force of muscular contraction.

The data gleaned from muscle testing procedures performed in the majority of today's clinics would lead you to believe that if you jumped off a building, you might go up.

There's only one way to test strength accurately - when a muscle is *not* moving.

JUNE 24

---

### The Dangers of Dynamic Muscle Testing

Startled by a 'tap' on the shoulder in front of my locker, I turned around and saw the high-school Principal 20 feet away signaling me to follow. It was fraternity "Grease Day" and he didn't like fraternities (even if ours was service oriented). My hair was slicked back in a manner "unbecoming a President of the Student's Council." He strapped my knuckles and sent me home.

MedX® inventor Arthur Jones did the same when he lectured to medical doctors on the dangers of dynamic muscle testing. His volunteers, however, required no 'tap.'

"Slowly and gradually push your fist against a brick wall as hard as possible" he said. "Provided enough time is allowed for the muscle to recruit all of its available fibers (normally, a few seconds), you will produce the highest level of force of which you are capable. It will not hurt because you are exposed to the exact level of force you produce."

He hesitated.

"Now...from three inches away slam your fist against the wall as fast as possible."

They hesitated.

"Your hand and wrist will break because of exposure to a higher and more dangerous level of force, even though the force produced by your muscles is *lower* than when you pushed your fist against the wall. Lower because the speed of movement does not afford time to recruit *all* of the muscle fibers." Yet, the impact would produce damaging results.

Jones then demonstrated what occurs during a dynamic muscle test by imposing a known level of torque on a Cybex® isokinetic machine and allowing it to move at a constant speed (by gravity) through a range of 90°. The peak force, measured at 0°, was 100 pounds, exactly what it should be (A, below). The same torque was then imposed upon the machine as it moved at a selected speed of 30° per second. The peak force registered 220 pounds at 7° (B, below) and was then filtered through an electronic lying machine (a "damp") that distorted the force to 76 pounds at 39° (C, below).

| With a Constant Level of Torque (100 pounds) | Peak Force | Angle of Peak Force |
|---|---|---|
| A. What should happen | 100 pounds | 0° |
| B. What did happen | 220 pounds | 7° |
| C. What they said happened (damp) | 76 pounds | 39° |
| D. What happened (with instructions) | 470 pounds | 15° |
| E. What they said happened in D. | 90 pounds | 45° |

"It is obvious to a goat," said Jones, "that an isokinetic machine does not measure torque produced by contracting muscles. It records impact forces produced by the sudden stops and starts of a quickly changing speed of movement (acceleration and deceleration of the movement arm)." High levels of impact only increase the chance of injury.

The situation is worse in practice. The test procedure suggested by Cybex - a sudden movement against the resistance arm - exposes the body to greater impact. In the example above, the same torque (220 pounds at 7°) following manufacturer's instructions rose to 470 pounds measured at 15° (D, above); when "damped," 90 pounds at 45° (E, above).

Dynamic muscle testing with isokinetic machines will tell you as much about your strength as jogging on a scale will about your bodyweight. Yet, the majority of rehab centers in this country use dynamic testing and doctors make decisions every day based upon the useless information it provides. Knuckles on the desk, I say.

Jones will likely spend the next 20 years waiting on a lawsuit from Cybex - and an increased enrollment of goats in medical school.

## JUNE 25

---

### Dynamic Muscle Testing – The Why Not

A static strength test measures the force output of a muscle not in motion. The muscle exerts a maximum effort against a movement arm set at fixed positions (about every 15°) throughout the range of motion. In contrast, a dynamic test measures output as the muscle lifts or lowers. The muscle exerts a force against an arm that moves at a constant speed. Yet, despite a 30-year bias in favor of dynamic testing, it spells nothing but confusion.

Figure 1 shows the results of two dynamic testing procedures: one immediately before a hard exercise; the other, immediately after. Curve A (right side of chart) shows the level of fresh positive (lifting) strength before exercise; Curve B, what remained after exercise. Curve C (left side of chart) shows the level of fresh negative (lowering) strength before exercise; Curve D, what remained after exercise. As can be seen, positive strength dropped significantly following exercise; negative strength, only a bit.

So, how much strength was lost - the 'bit' indicated by comparing negative curves or the large amount implied by comparing positive curves?

Neither. Dynamic test results are rendered worthless by internal muscle friction.

If fresh lifting strength is 100 (units), fresh lowering strength is 140 (40% more, see chart below) and fresh static strength (your real strength, unbiased by friction) is exactly between, at 120. Internal friction in a fresh, slow-moving muscle is about 20. Since friction helps you to lift and hurts you to lower, the strength output is affected as follows:

- Fresh static strength (120) minus friction (20) = positive (lifting) strength (100)
- Fresh static strength (120) plus friction (20) = negative (lowering) strength (140).

With dynamic tests, the output during the lifting phase is always lower than, and the output during the lowering phase is always higher than, the actual strength. The true level of strength can only be determined when friction is removed, that is, by static testing. A static test taken at any point during an exercise will reveal a strength level that falls exactly midway between positive and negative tested levels.

When a muscle is worked to total exhaustion, internal friction triples (from 20 to 60 units) and equals the contraction force of the muscle. The strength output is affected as follows: when lifting strength is 0, exhausted lowering strength is 120 (only 14% lower than its starting level) and exhausted static strength is exactly between, at 60.

- Exhausted static strength (60) minus friction (60) = positive strength (0)
- Exhausted static strength (60) plus friction (60) = negative strength (120).

|  | Positive | Negative | Static |
|---|---|---|---|
| Fresh | 100 | 140 | 120 |
| Exhausted | 0 | 120 | 60 |

Only a comparison of fresh to remaining static strength will show what truly occurs. When worked to total exhaustion, a muscle loses 50% of its strength (from 120 to 60).

Figure 1 demonstrates another error common to dynamic tests. On the left side of the chart (the start of the lowering test, C), positive strength (A) is higher than negative strength, impossible under all conditions. According to Arthur Jones, "The tested level of strength will always be too low during the first few degrees of angular movement at the start of any dynamic test." The muscle doesn't have time to recruit all of its fibers.

Just as cars did not immediately replace horses, static tests will not replace dynamic tests anytime soon. There are too many horses out there, too many people who know how to use them, and far too many of both taking the public for a ride.

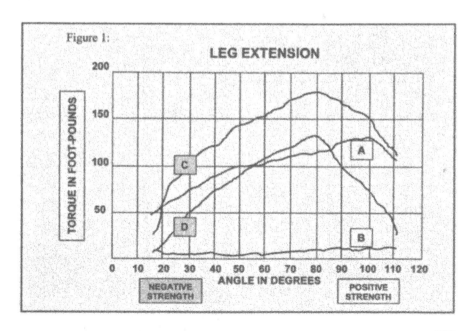

## JUNE 26

---

## The Invincible Man

Phrases like "Timing is everything" and "You finally met your match" make for boring reading, but both were appropriate the afternoon I put on a pair of shorts, socks and shoes and slid out the door for a routine jaunt.

The path was as predetermined as the attitude - to the Country Club and back, seven miles - a piece of cake in my condition.

I was invincible.

Just before the entrance to the club, a set of railroad tracks that paralleled the highway beckoned a challenge I knew well. The distance between the ties banished both leg rhythm and the ability to look up, and forced a run riveted on the task.

I had trained on tracks during cross-country season in a small town where there was little danger. Danville, Virginia was different. The local textile mill used the rail system to deliver goods. A long, loud whistle soon interrupted the riveting.

I scooted down the shallow embankment on my left but stayed close to the tracks. The thrill of tempting fate was on. A second whistle - loud and clear. I held my ground. I'd done it with cars, but I had never shouldered a train.

At once, the sound and rush of air repelled, then drew. I was disoriented, consumed. The blur of freight cars over a right ear that could bear no more gave the impression that I could no longer run a straight line. Was I moving at all?

Thank God, the train was long and always on time.

On more occasions than I care to count, I returned to take it on.

I once belonged to the stubborn and addicted lot of humanity known as 'runners,' at a time when the word 'jogger' was as much of an insult as the word 'belong.'

Cars became an enemy, an obstacle. I flashed a finger when they honked and banged their sides with a flat palm when they cut me off. I later added a spin that shook up more than a few glances in the rear-view mirror. I ran on busy freeways in South America dodging 'locos' that couldn't distinguish red from green.

I endured seven winters of snow, hail and sleet; ran in the sultry heat of San Fernando de Apure, Venezuela (near the equator); ran at night and early morn (only when I had to); and ran sick, in pouring rain. Mom can attest to that.

Three times a week for 15 years, I never missed. Invincible. Not even the Nautilus® inventor's able demonstrations on the 'impact' of running during his exercise seminars would suffice. I was a runner and was not going to stop.

Times have changed. I'm still disciplined and stubborn and tempting fate, but I'm no longer a runner, nor invincible. The impact was too great to sustain. Sure, there are long-time runners still out there, patched up and wounded, enjoying. I would if I could, but a couple of back operations now dictate 'wiser' choices.

It happened exactly as Bernard Darwin once wrote about a golf match in which "a rot set in" (*Green Memories,* 1928). "I always think that that day's play illustrates very well," he said, "the rule of nature which prohibits anybody from holing more than a certain number of good putts in a given time"

I used mine early in life, but have no regrets. There's a time and place for everything - I just haven't figured out when and where for impact.

<br>

## JUNE 27

---

### "The Kid" and His Entourage

"The Kid" had about the same impact as Tyson but his 'entourage' was not up to snuff. In fact, his escort was down to one badly dressed old man - and "The Kid" wasn't far behind in that category.

When Casey Viator entered the room for the pre-judging of the Mr. Teenage America Contest in York, Pennsylvania in 1971, he looked to the casual observer as if he had missed his peak. He was clad in a pair of dress pants and an extra large short-sleeve sport shirt that was 'out' at the waist and covered his upper-arms at the elbow. Casey was short - about 5'8" - and upon first glance looked 'fat' for a bodybuilder. He was anything but. Nonetheless, as bad as "The Kid" may have looked, he was miles ahead of the guy who brought him.

"I noticed a man standing off to the side watching me," said Jim Bryan, a trainer who was there when Viator entered. "He was dressed in a sport coat, I'm not sure if he was wearing a tie. He looked like he hadn't slept in a week. If he was sleeping, it must have been in his car! He had a way of looking straight through you. Very intense! I walked over to him and asked if he was Arthur Jones, and he said, 'Yes.'"

The soon-to-be-famous Nautilus® inventor had warned everybody about Viator. When Casey appeared in posing trunks, Bryan commented, "He had the biggest, most muscular, most powerful looking legs I had ever seen."

Bryan had accompanied a first-time contestant from his gym to the competition and met Jones there. The two went out for coffee during the prejudging and it didn't take Arthur long to light the fireworks.

"We started to talk," said Jim. "Next thing I knew, I was starting to feel like the dumbest SOB that ever picked up a barbell. Arthur would ask me a question, I would answer and he would point out what an idiot I was. I think he even called me an idiot! Several times! ...Boy I felt stupid!"

Arthur always supported his opinions with fact and statistics, that is, he might call you a name, but would then explain 'why?'

Whatever Jones thought or did worked in the eyes of the judges. Viator won every body-part category except "Best Abs," and many thought he should have won that as well.

Before parting, Jones invited Bryan to train at Nautilus headquarters in Lake Helen (Florida) to discover what 'proper' exercise was all about. But Bryan was no dummy.

"I sent two guys from the gym to see Arthur. They trained under him, heaved up just outside the DeLand High School gym door, and fell to the ground for about a half-hour. They came back after resting a few days. One was convinced (of Jones' methods) and showed me what he had learned. The other hated Arthur and never went back!"

Bryan was next to show.

"It took about 30 minutes and I was dead," he said. "Even Arthur's yelling couldn't get the dead man to move. He insulted me, questioned my manhood, and made fun of me. He could get momentary muscular failure, maximum inroad (or whatever you want to call it) like no one else. He wouldn't let you quit! I was dizzy as hell...my wife just stared in horror! I drove back to Arthur's house in my Datsun 2000 and my wife sat in Arthur's lap again. Hell I didn't care, I could barely see or move."

For the sake of historical accuracy, I don't think Arthur owned a tie.

## JUNE 28

---

### The Gym Scene

Perform exercise in a different setting as often as you can. Besides the physiological advantage of using other equipment, the change allows you to showcase your work - after all, no one wants to look like a 'wimp' in front of a new crowd. But be forewarned: It can bring on the unexpected.

Weeks ago, I trained in a facility (Pompano Beach, Florida) owned and operated by a former world-class bodybuilder and witnessed a rebirth of the term *genetic freak* - at least the *freak* part. At each station, one male's strut was prologue to a series of facial gyrations that clearly announced, "Prepare thy loins, world, you're about to witness one of the greatest feats of strength in the history of exercise."

The man possessed two pre-requisites for success on the gym scene - decent genetics and high visibility - and half of another, good form. His slow movements, static contractions and negative repetitions at the end of each set assured that he could do no wrong. Yet, set after set to *near* failure only confirmed what Nautilus® inventor, Arthur Jones believed, that *near* wasn't close enough.

I looked around for things I like to see in a gym: good equipment, cleanliness and concern (on the part of the staff) for good form during exercise.

This place had been newly renovated and had a clean 'feel.' The equipment was well maintained - BodyMaster®, Cybex®, Flex®, Magnum®, Hammer® and one Nautilus machine - but old. And old is old.

The hip abduction machine had thin, non-adjustable pads that applied the resistance to the outside of the upper thigh. It accommodated wide hips and thick legs but was inadequate for the average person. In the starting position, the inner edges of my thighs were 10-12 inches apart *before* I began, which limited the resistance to the last third of the range. Ironically, the neighboring adduction machine had thick pads that reduced its effective range of motion. The pads should have been switched, but no one noticed - or seemed to care.

Five minutes into my 25-minute jaunt on an elliptical cross-trainer, a young lady mounted the abduction machine. There, she performed set after set of exercise and finished a few minutes *after* my effort - 22 minutes of lousy, short-range movement with plenty of rest between. Someone must have told her it was a 'butt' exercise.

I spotted an old friend - a Cybex triceps-extension machine with an adjustable pad for the upper-back. Years ago, I trained on a clone that featured a picture of the pad on the instructional label. The manufacturer had removed the real thing and destroyed any hope of staying in the machine during exercise - all to save a buck.

I failed to spot others. The gym had no pullover (a direct upper-back exercise) and no one performed exercise in what I would call 'good form.' Slow repetitions, pauses in contracted positions, and worse, concern for the same, were nowhere to be found.

The majority of clients were left to fend for themselves and the few who paid *extra* for personal training seemed no better off. The trainers walked about with their clients as if it was, "Tea anyone?"

One staff member commented to my sponsor, "You work hard," but mentioned nothing of her form, easily the best in the gym.

The field of exercise has gone to the dogs.

Maybe the staff doesn't know what good form looks like. Tea anyone?

## JUNE 29

### No Springs Attached

Every so often, I stumble on a set of exercise springs at an antique show that reminds me of what once sat under our Christmas tree when I was 15. Red handles, five springs and an illustrated manual kept me occupied when I had no access to the barbells of the Christmas before. The springs were unlike weights - the more you pulled, the tougher they became - and a step in the right direction.

Springs increased resistance as a muscle approached contraction, which was better than Universal's® attempt at a leg extension machine years later. But it wasn't enough. They ended as they started - in zero - until a recent miraculous comeback in the form of rubber bands.

Rubber bands (in sheets or tubing) first appeared in gyms as a carryover from rehabilitation programs, which should tell you something. Their extensive use in sports-performance and functional training programs should tell you something more. When a muscle is weak, bands may provide an effective initial source of resistance. Yet, beyond convenience, flexibility of use and the fact that they don't rust, bands can't touch the potential loading of springs. Nonetheless, they have become the gold standard in programs designed to enhance athletic ability. How effective are these programs?

According to Ken Mannie, football trainer at Michigan State University, "A common misconception is that fundamental abilities can be trained through various drills or other activities. The thinking is that, with some stronger ability, the athlete will see gains in performance for tasks with this underlying ability. For example, athletes are often given various 'quickening' exercises, with the hope that these exercises will train some fundamental ability to be quick, and allow quicker responses in their particular sports. Coaches often use various balancing drills to increase general balancing ability, eye movement exercises to improve vision, and many others. Such attempts to train fundamental abilities may sound fine, but usually they do not work. Time and money would be better spent practicing the eventual goal skills."

"There are two correct ways to think of these principles," he added (referring to *Motor Learning and Performance: From Principles to Practice*, Richard Schmidt, 1991). "First, there is no general ability to be quick, to balance, or to use vision. Rather, quickness, balance, and vision are each based on many diverse abilities, so there is no single quickness ability, for example, that can be trained. Second, even if there were such general abilities, these are, by definition, genetic and not subject to modification through practice. Therefore, attempts to modify an ability with a non-specific drill are ineffective. A learner may acquire additional skill at the drill (which is, after all, a skill itself), but this learning does not transfer to the main skill of interest."

Nautilus® inventor, Arthur Jones took it a step further by saying the closer the drill mimics the actual skill, the greater the chance of negative transfer. In effect, you could hurt the skill of swinging a 5 ounce golf club more by swinging a 10-ounce club than by swinging a telephone pole - and the strength gain (from 10 ounces) would be negligible.

Jones advocated the separation of strength training and skill training. Identify the muscles used, strengthen them and then plug them into the practice of the skill.

Rubber bands have a place in exercise - rehabilitation, older people, muscle atrophy, to save space and in lieu of no access to other equipment. Their place in the training of elite athletes, however, should remain at the bottom of the nearest trashcan.

Gary Bannister, B.A., B.P.E., M.Ed.

## JUNE 30

---

### Letter to the Editor

I recently read two articles in the December 2002 issue of *Running Times* and was appalled by the nonsense now being passed off as strength training.

*First*, the bias "from machines that control your muscular actions to equipment that you control." Unfortunately, equipment that you control works muscles *indirectly* and, in most cases, muscle failure occurs in the small groups long before the prime movers have been adequately stimulated.

*Second*, the bias toward compound movements over isolated movements ("do not train muscles, train motion patterns"). Compound movements involve more muscle mass - but they fail at their weakest link. Isolated exercise strengthens the large muscles that move you from A to B and decreases the overall chance of injury.

*Third*, the bias toward performing exercises "at 'real world' or faster speeds." There is *no* proof that speed in the gym means speed on the field, while there's plenty to support that slow movement against resistance develops full-range strength without exposure to high forces. Lifting weights builds strength; throwing them produces injury.

*Fourth*, training for endurance is a myth ("The difference lies in the type of strength gained"). Strength and endurance increase *simultaneously and to the same degree*. Performing 2-3 sets of 12-20 repetitions, as advocated, is less efficient and no more effective than one set of 8-15. The fatigue characteristics of a muscle - its genetic fiber-type (*not* subject to change) - should dictate repetition schemes.

*Fifth*, muscles cannot reach their strength and endurance potentials without high levels of intensity. The advice of feeling "good honest effort" in the last few repetitions and stopping before the end of a set is the same as quitting before the finish line to save energy for the next day. In running as in strength training, *no* number of 90% attempts can stimulate the changes triggered by a single, 100% effort.

*Sixth*, the bias toward strengthening core and stabilizer muscles. The abdomen takes care of itself and the low back remains unaffected by traditional exercise (can only be accessed by a MedX® Lumbar machine.) The use of a Swiss ball dictates less resistance, which means fewer results for the large muscles. A man I once trained on a seasonal basis performed six months of exercise on balance cushions only to return in a de-conditioned state with his balance the same - bad.

*Seventh*, specificity of training is a myth. Skill training is specific and demands zero resistance. Strength training is general and demands a maximum load. Exposing sports movements to resistance compromises both. Identify the muscles involved, strengthen them *independent of how they are to be used*, and then apply the new strength to the practice of the skill itself. Anything else is a step in the wrong direction.

The belief in a *special* way to train runners for strength is commercial. Any exposure to resistance satisfies athletes and parents, but the method advocated by your authors is *not* the most productive or the safest, which comes as no surprise - they are certified by a national group that endorses power-lifting for children.

I reference a study by Nautilus® inventor, Arthur Jones (West Point Academy, 1975) in which cadets lowered their 2-mile running times by 88 seconds in six weeks using *proper strength training*. The results would have shocked your authors more than it did Dr. Cooper. The machines did *not* allow feet to touch the floor - a must in your program.

They did, however, (or so we thought) allow heads to get out of the sand.


(**Letter to the Editor** was sent to *Running Times*. As expected, there was no reply)

# JULY

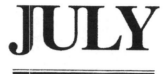

"If race horses were trained as much as most bodybuilders train, you could safely bet your money on an out-of-condition turtle - it would be unlikely that a horse trained in such a fashion could even make it around the track, and certainly not rapidly."

Arthur Jones

## Politics and Physical Preparation

There were advantages to living in South America. First, a North American education was thought superior to that of the homeland. Consequently, most "gringos" were nicknamed "Doctor." Second, North Americans were considered more honest than the average Jose, and their work associated with integrity. Nonetheless, the edge had to be earned on a day-to-day basis.

In 1980, I introduced the Nautilus® system of exercise to Venezuela by learning how to best use the equipment according to research, and by slipping the bulky machines past a corrupt customs system. All the while, I harbored a belief that the process was more than just a business venture.

The effort paid off. Word of mouth turned a trickle of locals into a flood well before completion of the gym's interior. My partner was a man with whom I had worked in the Physical Education Department of Colegio Internacional de Caracas (an American high-school). Pedro Jimenez had represented Venezuela in both Pan-American and Olympic competitions and once held every basketball record in the country.

Our staff of PE majors attracted a clientele that included Venezuelan National male and female water-ski and golf teams, Olympic basketball and volleyball players and a handful of Americans who played in the Venezuelan professional basketball league. We worked with Anna Maria Carrasco (World Champion water-skier, 1988), Carlos Lavado (World Champion motorcycle racer), Cesar Baena (World Cup soccer goalkeeper), Eduardo Fernandez (National swim, cycle and triathlon champion) and Martin Materano (ranked 10th in the world in karate). We even answered the doubts of a karate school (35 black belts) that questioned our slow method of training.

But we weren't as fortunate with others.

In 1983, Venezuela was elected to host the Pan-American Games. Pedro and I approached the President of the *Instituto Nacional de Deportes* with the intent of helping prepare athletes for the competition. At the meeting, more interest was shown in a televised soccer game than in spending money on training programs, much less in a private setting.

We persisted by inviting 20 National basketball team members to our facility one Saturday. They arrived in various shapes and sizes, and after sickness, left a little lighter. Their strength was pitiful compared to our clients. Only a few did anything about it.

Shortly after the Games, rumors of scandal and corruption surfaced, and the day before administrative headquarters was searched for evidence, the building burned down.

The National soccer team fared no better. Every fourth year, Venezuela played Brazil in a home-and-home World Cup qualifier. The Venezuelan players lived all over the country and gathered to practice about a month before the competition. It showed. In one match billed as "the greatest game in the history of Venezuelan soccer," the National team crossed center only four times. Brazil scored on a penalty kick with 10 minutes remaining to win 1-0. It's tough to score on 11 goalkeepers.

The Venezuelans played hard; the system did not.

In 1980, Pedro Jimenez was asked to coach the National basketball team for the Olympic Games in Russia. When he demanded "absolute control of all team members one year in advance," he was laughed out of the building.

If physical preparation is hit and miss, there's no sense doing it at all.


## JULY 2

---

### Bottom of the Seventh

The old warrior stood on the mound, softball in one hand, microphone in the other. "Back when games were real," he announced, "we played a National All-Star Team in a packed stadium. We were up one run with two outs in the bottom of the seventh (last inning) and two strikes on the batter. The opposing coach came out of the dugout, both hands in the air, and called 'Time.' He met the batter halfway to the plate."

"On the last pitch of the game, he likes to pitch behind his back," warned the coach. "I want you to be looking for it."

The batter returned to the box and dug his cleats into the dirt. He was ready.

"I cranked the old windmill and pitched the ball behind my back into my glove."

The catcher's mitt exploded with sound.

"S-t-e-e-e-e-R-i-k-e."

"All hell broke loose. The coach and team stormed the field. Spectators jeered. The batter unleashed on the umpire, his teammates not far behind - and rightly so. What they were upset about was obvious - they thought the pitch was too high. I retreated to the bus and got out of there in a hurry."

The 'Phantom' pitch had worked. It was off to another ballpark.

Such was the legend of Meryl King (alias Eddie Feigner). Few could hit him. Few could see him, which is why his four-man softball team, "The King and His Court," took on all nine-man challenges.

I got my first glimpse of Feigner when I was eight years old (1956) and still remember the size of that arm signing autographs. Like a transplant from a bodybuilder, it was much longer and thicker than the other - the largest arm I'd ever seen. It belonged to a man who could pitch blindfolded from second base, a man who struck out nearly everyone he faced, a man they called "The King" for a reason.

Feigner once retired Willy Mays, Willy McCovey, Maury Wills, Harmon Killebrew, Roberto Clemente and Frank Robinson (in a row), and fanned all-time hits leader Pete Rose twice in the same game. With over 132,070 career strikeouts and more than 8,270 wins, he was the undisputed King of fast-pitch softball for more than 50 years.

His unusual sojourn started on a bet.

In 1946, playing for Kilburg's Grocery in the Green Pea League of the Walla Walla Valley (Washington), Feigner shut out a team from Pendleton (Oregon), 33-0. At a tavern after the game, the Pendleton manager challenged him to a rematch. Feigner replied, "Your team is so pitiful I could lick you with just a catcher, a shortstop and a first baseman. The reason I need four is because you would probably walk us both if I just used my catcher." The next day, Feigner pitched a perfect game en route to a 7-0 victory. As word spread about the four-man team, challenges came fast and furious. They played 250 games in the next four years and expanded their reach nationally, then globally.

They're still going strong.

Thirty-eight years after that first encounter, I revisited the 'arm' in North Lauderdale, Florida. Now in its late sixties, it hadn't slowed any more than my eyesight - I still couldn't see its fastball. For four innings, Feigner worked his magic and then took the microphone. His successor, Rich Hoppe, a former major league baseball player, carried the torch and pitched the last three innings faster than Eddie in his prime.

I wish I could say I noticed the difference, but you can't call what you can't see.

JULY 3

_____

## The Absolute Limit Of Muscular Size

A football inflates the same way a muscle grows - only the width changes. Its ultimate size is dictated by the pliability of the leather, the strength of the seams and the rules of the league. Ultimate muscle size is dictated by genetics, which Nautilus® inventor Arthur Jones made clear. "Some can and some cannot;" he said, "most can meaningfully improve, but not everybody can improve to the same degree." The degree is determined by what he called 'aspect ratio,' the relationship between length and width.

"An aspect ratio of 2-to-1," he said, "would mean that the length of the muscle was twice as great as its width. Which, in turn, would mean that its shape would be long and narrow."

Muscle size and strength go hand in hand. A stronger muscle is a larger muscle; and a larger muscle, a stronger muscle - which led Jones to believe that, apart from practicing the skill of lifting a barbell, bodybuilders and weightlifters should train the same way.

The relationship between size and strength, however, is not direct. That is, a muscle that doubles in strength will not be twice as large, and visa versa. Muscles grow by increasing their width; their length remains the same. As such, the 'aspect ratio' changes, as does something else - the angle of pull.

"Only a part of the muscle that is located on the exact centerline of the muscle," said Jones, "is pulling in exactly the right direction." The other parts pull in a slightly different direction, affecting the efficiency of the output. And the larger the muscle becomes, the greater the change in the angle of pull. "Eventually, a point will be reached," he said, "where the angle of pull of part of the muscle has changed to such a degree that it is no longer functional. Any increase in the width of such a muscle would produce added force of contraction that would be entirely wasted. So there is a limit to just how wide a muscle can be, a limit dictated by aspect ratio."

"The potential cross-section (size) of a muscle," he added, "does not increase in direct proportion (to its length); in fact, the resulting increase in muscular cross-section will be much greater than might be expected. If the muscle's length is twice as great as average, this means that its maximum width is twice as great as average, and that its maximum cross-section is four times as great as average, and that its maximum 'mass' (or overall size) is eight times as great as average. Thus it follows that having muscles that are even slightly longer than average, gives you the potential of greatly increased muscular size."

But note: A muscle twice as large (by cross-section) is not necessarily twice as strong. It may be capable of generating double the force (input), but a large part would be wasted because it is pulling in the wrong direction. Therefore, its output would be less than double its strength.

Nonetheless, a slight increase in strength goes a long way. It leads to a disproportionate, yet favorable increase in muscle size, which is why Jones believed that bodybuilders should make themselves as strong as possible - a thought foreign to the field, both then and now.

Today's trainees believe that muscle size can be increased in many ways - steroids, supplements, training techniques and whatever else - all in the face of the following:

*The only way to increase muscle size within the limits of genetic potential (other than increasing strength) is to get down on your knees and pray for a set of parents more genetically blessed.*

## JULY 4

---

## Build Your Back – Eventually

Chin-ups (or pull-ups) are considered an upper-back exercise. Yet, if a group of untrained individuals performed a hard set of chin-ups, they would experience the majority of muscle soreness in the biceps tendons near the elbow. The reason is simple: Chin-ups work the biceps harder than the upper-back muscles.

The same applies to all pulling exercises: rowing, front and behind-neck pulldowns, and pull-ups in any form. When the small muscles of the upper-arm, forearm and hand can no longer continue due to fatigue, the large upper-back muscles have barely worked, regardless of how much exercise is performed.

Arm strength determines the outcome, and it seems only logical to place the muscles of the arm (biceps, in this case) in their strongest position for the task. To determine that position, try the following: Stand with your right elbow bent at 90° and hand palm-down (as if playing a piano). Pull the back of your hand toward your shoulder and grasp your biceps - soft. Now, rotate your hand to a thumbs-out position and observe what happens. Your biceps becomes hard. The main function of the biceps is not to bend the arm at the elbow but to rotate (supinate) the wrist, as in tightening a screw.

Which means that all pulling exercises should be performed with hands in a supinated position - a shoulder-width, palms-up grip for normal chin-ups and front pulldowns, and a parallel grip (with palms facing each other) for behind-neck pulldowns. Anything else is mechanically inferior.

Despite the obvious, most bodybuilders use a palms-down (thumbs-in) grip for pulling exercises, claiming that it eliminates the biceps and allows the back to perform more work. If this was true, the large back muscles would account for more repetitions, but they don't. Pulling is still limited by the arm muscles, and placing them in a weak position to start results in less work for both biceps and upper-back.

Another misconception relates to grip width. Most trainees are convinced that "wider is better," yet the use of a wide grip during chin-ups reduces the range-of-motion from a possible 135° to less than 90°. And partial range exercise does not produce nearly the results of full-range exercise - the reason Arthur Jones refused to include wide-grip options on his Nautilus® machines.

Weeks ago, I witnessed typical neglect of the 'obvious' when the serenity of my stationary-bike ride was interrupted by the grunting of two bodybuilders doing their interpretation of a "lat" (upper-back) workout.

Besides the use of a wide, weak grip in all of their pulling exercises, both men jerked the resistance during every repetition. The weight was so light in one case that it was easy to throw, and so heavy in another that it had to be thrown to move at all. It didn't matter. The results were the same - pending.

To add insult to injury, they performed too many sets, vacationed between them and ignored the only direct back exercise in the gym, a pullover machine. I clocked them at 45 seconds of bad form, followed by 5½ minutes of rest, times seven.

The 12-minute back, chest and shoulder workout that Jones used with bodybuilders in the early 1970's was nowhere in sight. His combination of pulldowns (one set of 8-12 repetitions) *immediately* followed by a pullover machine and negative chin-ups (quick walk up, 10 seconds down) to fatigue was about as tough as it gets.

With upper-back exercise, you can swim or jet to the 'Promised Land.'

## JULY 5

---

### The Real McCoy

I can't claim many firsts in life, but I can claim a second. After the Brazilian soccer team, I was next to introduce Nautilus® machines to South America (Caracas, Venezuela, 1980). Their arrival created quite a stir.

One of my charter members was a man named Elias Sayegh who owned a fitness equipment business in town. Within weeks of using the machines, he contacted Nautilus Sports/Medical Industries in Lake Helen, Florida requesting to be their official representative in Venezuela, if not in South America. The company showed no interest.

But Elias was persistent.

Four years later, he invited me to a venture in the neighboring town of Valencia - the production of Nautilus clones. When he opened the door to the showcase gym, I couldn't believe my eyes. Someone had secured the blueprints and was making exact copies of the originals. The only visible difference was the color and quality of the finish. "Ciro Sports Machines®" were bright red with black upholstered seats.

One of my instructors was so impressed that he accepted a position in the first Ciro-equipped gym that came to town. Months later, he returned with the scoop. One, he could lift the entire weight stack on all the machines and questioned the composition of the plates. Two, the machines had a lot of friction. In one demonstration of an overhead press, the weights stuck at the top and had to be pulled down. Three, the manufacturer had added details to the equipment that made it 'superior' to the original.

The first opportunity I had to use Ciro machines came during a golf tournament at the Valle Arriba Golf Club in 1988. The club's newly renovated gym and an early tee-off time allowed for a workout after the round.

The machines were unique. The pads were hard, the weights moved roughly up the guide-rods and the change of resistance was, as Hertz® would say, "Not exactly." I gave them the benefit of the doubt until I reached the biceps machine. There, the weight was so difficult in the extended position that I had to lower it twice to start. Yet, it was too easy in the contracted position. I looked for the rotation point of the machine and found it - a foot below the elbow pad.

In adding details, Ciro had destroyed function, and function was the only thing about which Nautilus inventor, Arthur Jones was concerned. It was the equivalent of installing square tires on your car and complaining about its performance.

Jones created the original blueprint for many of today's machines. During the early 1970's, he identified 10 ingredients for a perfect form of exercise and incorporated them into his equipment. His competitors ridiculed his work, then copied it.

In 1994, the gym in which I trained purchased 11 new machines from a prominent manufacturer. The change of resistance through the range of motion on eight of eleven 'felt' wrong and it wasn't because I was used to another 'feel.' They were dead wrong - too hard at one end, too easy at the other. Years later, I helped inaugurate a gym with equipment from five leading manufacturers. One company sent three machines with lousy resistance changes, which surprised the salesman who called months later.

How can someone market a tool that doesn't 'feel' right, unless they don't know what it should feel like? At least Ciro was smart enough to copy the original in the beginning, if not humble enough to remain on that path.

There's a lot of junk out there, even when they claim to have the blueprint.

# JULY 6

---

## Smart Start

The moment Al Jangl stepped off the bus that Sunday evening, his 'hot' weekend in Georgia turned cold. Someone had stolen his heartthrob - a Triumph" motorcycle parked in front of the dorm - the one he roared through Greensboro with at 90 miles per hour.

"No!" he hollered in disbelief as we made our way up the stairs. "Why me?"

"It was taken Saturday night," said Pete "Thighs" Johnson, a semi-pro ball player. "We filed a police report..."

Pete and I burst out before we made it to the room. It was only the beginning.

We spent most of the afternoon hiding the bike in the woods behind the dorm. From there, we backtracked by leaving clues at places that matched Jangl's storied past. It began with a note that read, "Press *Play* on the tape recorder."

The message led to a pair of underwear on a shrub at the foot of the women's dorm. Next - to the back seat of my car, the dance studio, the campus bowling alley (to which we had keys) and finally the anatomy lab where we dressed a skeleton in Jangl's vest, hat, sunglasses and sandals. When he spotted a girl's name etched in a bowling ball chained to its leg, Al hit the floor and laughed until he could barely breathe.

We straggled home at 1AM, unchained the bike, slept some before class and, too tired to disrobe the skeleton the night before, underestimated the reaction of the teacher. If I recall, Jangl failed the course.

Many people in fitness facilities fail to succeed for much the same reason - lack of accurate information, and the fault lies with the guy issuing the clues.

A good exercise orientation is critical. It should be brief, comprehensive, provide a base from which a client can grow - rather than one from which to launch a sales pitch for personal training - and should cover the following:

- Proper equipment selection and set-up, with emphasis on safety and productivity.
- Principles of overload, progression (repetitions, weight), intensity, proper speed of movement and form (and explain 'why,' where appropriate).
- Sequence, time factors (total workout time, between machines, per exercise), frequency, amount (sets, repetitions), warm-up, cool down and the 'when,' 'why' and 'how much' related to stretching and cardiovascular exercise.
- Expected physiological response (muscle soreness, strength/appearance changes).
- Record keeping (excluding inappropriate exercises where necessary).
- Written handouts as reminders of the above.

It should then be repeated to answer questions, review and encourage, so that clients can take it from there. Sure, best results are obtained with one-on-one supervision, but good results can be achieved without paying exorbitant fees if the staff covers the 'floor' the way they should, with *everyday* service.

Unfortunately, good orientations are hard to come by. As new instructors enter a field of expanding myth, they are exposed to, and taught, an increasing number of unsupported theories. Saturated and confused, they seek out 'experts' with the same success the Nautilus® inventor encountered 60 years ago. There were (and are) none, and his work was brushed aside in favor of nonsense passed off as 'superior' or 'necessary.'

When the fruit of the new labor jumps off a building, it will hit the pavement the same way it always has - unless it was taught to go up.

Stick with proper strength training and let the 'old-school' help you find the treasure.

## JULY 7

---

### Coaching Golf at The Other End of the Chain

The prestige of coaching golf at a major university often falls into the hands of former players, successful alumni or established teaching professionals. It's different at a small college.

In 1972, I was hired to coach the men's golf team at Averett College in Danville, Virginia. The 'girls-only' school had just turned co-educational and sought to attract male students with an athletic program. I had played competitive golf in high school, captained the university team and assisted the golf coach during graduate school. My comfort level may have been the exception. Most coaches were chaperones or leftovers from other sports. There was little concern over the win-loss record.

While glancing through an old Averett yearbook one evening, I was surprised by the number of players in the team photo, considering it was a major undertaking to scrounge up four for a match.

On one occasion, I secured a student (I'll call him Tom) who hadn't played in months and who normally shot 120. I reassured him in the van that there were no expectations and a free lunch. Nothing worked. He was fidgety as we entered the club parking lot and a wreck during warm-up. I tried to calm him but his pulse was nearly audible by tee-time. I remained on a distant putting green and glanced away whenever he looked. The last thing he needed was *more* pressure.

The first hole was wide open, a short par four with an elevated tee. Tom hit a glancing blow that turned quickly right and sailed over the fence onto an interstate that, until then, had not been a factor. I kept my head down and putted while his second effort landed safely inside the fence. It would be a long day.

We once played three schools at a course in Virginia upon which a player commented as we drove by, "I hope we don't have to play that dump, Coach." Sure enough we made a U-turn...should have made two.

The first tee was cut into the side of a steep hill. The players gathered below; the coaches above. One competitor "on the tee" set his left hand on the club and glanced up toward the coach standing beside me. Coach gave him the nod. He then placed his right hand on the club and looked up again. A second nod. With that, he took his stance, waggled and glanced a third time. Coach, whose players carried a rulebook in their back pocket, OK'd the 'launch.' It would be another long day.

Long, but fun.

After Tom and the boys teed off, I set out with an athletic director and two basketball coaches. The tee of the par-five third sat in a depression fronted by a stream that begged to be called a ditch, the lip of which protruded about a foot above the fairway some 30 yards away. The left-handed basketball coach addressed his ball amid a courteous silence. Whack. The ball hit the club and split in two - one piece curved low and left; the other, low and right. The whirring sound subsided when both halves simultaneously sucked into the muddy bank.

You could hear a pin drop as the coach pivoted toward us.

"Damn, have you ever seen anything like that?" We couldn't hold it in.

That evening, we laughed all the way home. Tom had blasted a ball from a bunker into a Burger King® parking lot; the others had their own tales of woe.

When fun outweighed score, as it often did, those days were some of the best.

JULY 8

---

### Heads or Tails?

*"Public service is the rent we pay for our room on God's earth"* was the motto that guided our local chapter of North America's oldest international high-school fraternity, Gamma Sigma. I embodied that standard through life, with one regret - I failed to grab the microphone on the final eve of the 1988 National Petroleum Tournament at the Valle Arriba Golf Club in Caracas, Venezuela.

The insult began months earlier on the 15th green of the Lagunita Country Club as I walked toward a 60-foot putt that stopped short of its target. Halfway there, I dodged the coin of a fellow player and glanced downward when he swooped in behind. I couldn't believe my eyes. He scooped up the coin on the ledge of his putter, walked 10 feet closer to the hole and dropped it. I didn't say a word; my playing partners were in a big money game. From then on, I observed his actions closely and saw much the same each time a long putt rolled toward the hole.

The next week I watched the Doctor attempt to cheat on every hole, and finally spoke to a member of the foursome after the round.

"I don't want to cause a problem, but I saw Dr. L. do this...and this...and..."

"Oh, that's nothing," he replied. "You should have seen him last year at the Country Club." For every tale of woe I recalled, he had 10.

I eventually abandoned that group but played with the Doctor on a few occasions. He hadn't changed. I once stooped to mark a ball and noticed a coin rolling across the green. He had tossed it from the front apron - where it settled was his new mark.

The worst was yet to come.

I sat through the Petroleum Tournament's award ceremony and saw the Doctor win his flight with an 81. He had a legitimate - to use the term loosely - 39 on the outward nine but slashed his way home (bunkers, lakes and out-of-bounds) in at least 54 strokes. After the presentation, I went to the scoreboard - hmmm, 42. Doc controlled the pencil.

'Characters' in the field of exercise were not far behind.

I once trained a self-proclaimed bodybuilder who was equally creative, even when I controlled the pencil. Alejandro typically didn't work hard enough to produce best results with his own equipment - barbells - and turned to Nautilus® training. One day, it seemed the ticket to the Promised Land; the next, it was the reason he was smaller.

He thought he knew how to play the game.

Every time he completed 12 repetitions in good form, I increased the weight by 5%. While most gym members were stuck at 11, Alejandro performed a consistent 12 - a count I could not control because of my attention to other clients. One day, however, I set up a machine, walked away and returned in about 30 seconds. He was done.

"How many?" I asked.

"Twelve."

"Twelve? You didn't have time to finish 12 repetitions."

"Um, I'm not really sure. I've got a bit of a headache today."

During his next workout, I set up machines, turned away and counted from behind. He did three repetitions on one, four on another, and reported "12" - another headache.

Don't lull yourself into a sense of security by using heavy weights at the expense of sound physiology to show progress - just because others may be doing the same.

In exercise, as in golf, you'll end up resembling the east end of a horse going west.

# JULY 9

---

## Mickey

To suggest that he looked like a bodybuilder that hadn't shaved his chest, if there are any, might have been enough to start a fight. When you spoke the name Mickey, you were treading on sacred ground.

Mickey was larger than the famous Mouse who lived a few hours down the turnpike, and larger than any bodybuilder Arthur Jones had ever seen. He was also stronger than any bodybuilder he'd seen, and if you really asked, smarter. And last but not least, he was more revered than any bodybuilder Jones had chanced upon.

Arthur took him in like a son.

Mickey was the only African lowland gorilla in the hands of a private collector in the world, and he was lucky. They were good hands. Nautilus® inventor Arthur Jones treated him better than most people are ever treated and, as some have suggested, better than other members of the Jones family.

He purchased the gorilla from the Barnum and Bailey Circus® in 1984 and housed him in a luxurious suite carved within a 60-foot-thick wall of concrete that separated his exotic animal collection from the noise of his jet airplanes.

Mickey was 18 years old at the time and had lived most of his life in a small cage. His new L-shaped enclosure consisted of a space resembling the old environment and a larger rectangular section glassed in on one side so that he was visible to a daily parade of seminar participants. Unfortunately, Mickey wouldn't leave the small space, despite endless attempts to lure him with bananas.

I first saw the magnificent beast shortly after Arthur had finished the runway and protection wall. He was all male - picking his nose with the finger of one hand while wielding a TV remote in the other - except for the fact that he had an affinity for soap operas.

Mickey weighed about 380 pounds, had a 54-inch chest, 33-inch neck, 17-inch forearms and 13-inch wrists. His demeanor was passive other than the occasional barrage of chest pounding or forearm shivers on a nearby wall to demonstrate that he was still king, at least of his immediate domain. In that regard and in refusing to leave a space, Mickey was very much like a bodybuilder (with apologies to Arthur).

Ellington Darden included a profile of Mickey in his book, *Super High-Intensity Bodybuilding*, 1986, to demonstrate the girth of his neck. An adjacent photo had Mickey strapped in a Nautilus pullover machine, his mouth wide open as if suffering the slings and arrows of high-intensity exercise. The stunt was performed with the gorilla sedated, an act that affected him in a negative way for longer than Arthur cared.

Mickey's death was sudden, unrelated to any stunt - an unsuspected heart condition. He died on the spot one afternoon despite efforts by Dr. Fulton and others to save him.

Weeks after the passing, a friend of mine by the name of Jay Valentine visited Ocala for a medical seminar. During the luncheon, he stepped on sacred ground.

"What are you going to do now that Mickey is gone, Mr. Jones, get another gorilla?"

The room went silent. Arthur looked up from his meal and slowly uttered a pledge that few forgot, "**Mickey cannot be replaced**."

When the Nautilus inventor donated $10 million to the University of Florida to establish the Center for Exercise Science, a stuffed Mickey resurfaced at the entrance.

Jones kept him in the deep freeze and, more importantly, kept his word.

# JULY 10

---

## Mr. Nautilus

The sport of bodybuilding never amounted to much - was always bunched with circus pursuits like wrestling and boxing - until 1970. Change was on the horizon.

Nautilus® inventor Arthur Jones had more than a 'commercial interest' in resistance exercise. He wanted to legitimize the sport of bodybuilding by opening its doors and revealing the truth. Those in command thought he 'couldn't see the forest for the trees,' but Jones was a visionary and realist who clearly saw both.

"I used to think that most people were unjustifiably biased against bodybuilders as a class," he said, "but I now realize that the actual state of affairs in bodybuilding circles today is far worse than most people even suspect; which is a cryin' shame, because progressive weight-training could be, and SHOULD be, of very great value to almost everybody, and might be if it were not for the antics and outrages of many of the very people who should be doing everything in their power to promote weight-training."

Jones started from the bottom end of the spectrum. His unique approach to training, novel equipment and open-door policy sought to convert current trainees in the field:

"The very most I can even hope to do is to try to reach a tiny minority of humanity - and even if I can reach them, the most I can then hope to do is to direct their thinking into a logical direction."

He then attacked the upper echelon by putting money on the table. Jones proposed a competition in Los Angeles that offered "a total of $50,000 in cash prizes, as follows: $25,000 for 1st place (the norm was $1,000); $7,000 for 2nd place; $5,000 for 3rd place; $2,000 for 4th place, and $1,000 for 5th place - plus $2,000 for each best body-part winner: best arms, best chest, best back, best legs, and best abdomen."

He devoted the week prior to the event to careful testing "conducted by a group of doctors from a number of universities and research foundations." The tests would determine accurate body-part measurements, drug usage, performance abilities and related physiological factors. Entrants were required "to sign a release permitting free and unrestricted publication of the data," none of which would be made known to the judges until after the award ceremony.

The competition format was designed with three purposes in mind.

First, it was "a sincere attempt to determine and publish the truth so that millions of young bodybuilders would not be led into attempts to duplicate impossible (and false) measurements and performances."

Second, it was a unique opportunity "to bring together a large group of outstanding physical specimens for the purpose of conducting accurate tests for scientific purposes."

And third, Jones hoped it "would attract enough attention outside the actually very narrow field of weight-training to 'change the image' of bodybuilding in the overall public mind." He proposed a one-hour, made-for-TV color documentary on exercise in general, and weight-training in particular, with the contest and testing as the highlight.

Jones assured that "the contest WILL BE HELD and that 'everybody' will be there."

The contest was held but not everybody showed. Twenty-one individuals competed, but not all was lost. Michael Monis (who finished last) recently announced his retirement from drug-free bodybuilding and plans to steer youth down the right path. "Many people think it can't be done (without drugs)," he said, "but it can by dedication and hard work."

Maybe Arthur's input paid off.

Gary Bannister, B.A., B.P.E., M.Ed.

## JULY 11

---

### Exercise Fads

The confusion between exercise and recreation (both of which have value) is more than semantic.

Exercise is a systematic approach to physical and physiological change that addresses the major components of fitness: muscle strength, joint flexibility, heart-lung endurance, body leanness, and injury reduction. Because it involves the use of resistance, its value should be judged by the quality of the resistance and the range of motion over which the resistance has an effect.

Recreation, on the other hand, is instinctive and fun, which leads to the crux of the problem - people continue to call what they *like* to do 'exercise.'

Arthur Jones and, later, Ellington Darden, Ph.D. believed that proper exercise was anything but fun. "Don't try to make exercise fun," said Darden. "Don't try to make recreation exercise. If you do, you grossly compromise the physical benefits of the exercise and the intended amusement of the recreation." (*The Nautilus Book*, 1985)

In the same (book), Darden examined the 'exercise' value of yoga, a popular choice among health-club trainees.

He found, to no one's amazement, that the prime benefit of yoga is flexibility. Some postures (performed the same way as calisthenics) had an effect on the cardiovascular system because of difficulty, sequence and the amount of rest between.

The prime benefit of yoga, however, was not enough.

"Most children and adults do not need increased flexibility," he said. Most women are hyper-flexible and, at the same time, under-muscled which leads to joint instability and ultimately, injury. Adults need muscle strengthening which, when properly performed, increases flexibility.

He wasn't alone with that thought.

Independent studies by Dr. Stanley Plagenhoef of the University of Massachusetts and Dr. Richard Dominguez of Loyola University Medical Center concluded that the importance of flexibility was overrated by sports-medicine professionals:

- If joints are supported by stronger muscles, the chance of trauma is reduced.
- If joints become more flexible without a corresponding increase in muscular strength, the chance of injury is increased.

*Some* activities require extreme flexibility and a supplemental program of stretching. But the average person does not require or necessarily benefit from extreme flexibility. The flexibility provided by proper strength training will suffice to restore a normal range of movement in the joints of most.

Besides the benefits of flexibility, mind control and relaxation, yoga can have an effect on the cardiovascular system. As an overall exercise, however, it is incomplete.

Yoga was popular in the 1970's and has recently fought her way back to the commercial scene - due, in part, to the hard work of sincere and dedicated professionals. But, as Arthur Jones suggested in the field of bodybuilding, "Sincerity is no proof of knowledge - or even good intentions; I have known some very sincere burglars - and if a man runs at you with an axe, you better believe he is sincere."

Darden summed up his thoughts on the contribution of yoga to the major components of fitness, as follows: "Most people would be better off finding something else to do with their exercise time."

## JULY 12

### Full Moon Over Toronto

I was always proud of the fact that my father was born in England, a country famous for the rowdiness of its soccer fans - but now I'm not so sure. Fans of the little-known sport of water-skiing have made soccer look like a pleasantry.

At a recent international competition in England, an off-balance jumper hit the ramp at 70 miles per hour and sailed for the shoreline where the bleachers were dangerously close. He landed hurt, half-in and half-out of the water. A handful of spectators rushed to his aid but, to the surprise of many, picked him up and threw him back in. They wanted to see some "bloody skiing."

The show continued on this side of the pond - in Toronto, Canada - when the British team found themselves well back in the trick-ski event with only a glimmer of hope. The English competitor fastened his foot to the towrope as the boat neared the judges' stand, a series of towers along the shore. It was one mistake and out.

He opened with a flip, a turn and a solid landing, but his next move ended in a premature splash. He was towed to the end of the lake and returned for the hand pass (performing with the towrope in hand), which he initiated with a series of 'normal' tricks. Then he got creative. Holding the rope in one hand, he lowered his bathing suit with the other, and bent over to salute the crowd. Hours of hard training culminated in a pointless (this one wasn't in the book) "full-moon" that exhibited all the features a judge was trained to detect - speed, finesse, agility, balance, poise - and then some.

It's unfair to judge a population by the actions of a handful of lunatics that form a small part of that population. Most people have noble intentions, as do the English, but some simply need to show the world the *other side*.

So it is in the field of exercise, where most enter with noble intentions and try to steer clear of the lunacy around them. It's a losing battle.

The first problem - one that lingers - relates to the fanaticism of body-builders, a fortress that no one has cracked due to the overwhelming commercial bias for nonsense. The second problem - one that continues to grow - is that of trends and myths. Plain Yoga isn't enough. It has to be Yoga for Wimps, Yoga for Menopause, Bikram Yoga and hundreds of offshoots. And the big three - sports-specific, functional and speed training - continue to make an alarming dent in the wrong direction.

Sports-specific training is certain to hurt skill more than help. Its compromise of strength and speed has less positive transfer than the traditional approach. Speed training is a ticket to a clinic or law office and functional training is high-risk calisthenics with about the same benefit as a high-school PE class.

All three provide a poor source of resistance, a limited range of motion and dubious transfer value to other activities.

You can't judge the field of physical training by the actions of a few. When the few, however, become the majority and the sane, the minority - myths emerge. Financial gain and warped physiology play a role in the mix.

The solution? There isn't one, other than to preach the virtues of sanity and hope that physiology will someday salvage proper strength training. Nautilus® inventor Arthur Jones spent a lifetime trying. Few listened.

There are many ways to skin a cat, but the majority of today's proposals deserve little more than a British ski salute.

JULY 13

---

## The Little Guy

I don't have the statistics or the FBI report but the habits of those who exercise in a commercial gym would classify most as 'persons of interest.'

Exercise habits in this country are, at best, pitiful. People come and go, start and stop, intend and fail, and generally feed the coffers of commerce in a way that keeps doors open and space free for the few that show.

Human nature has something to do with it. The body doesn't like exercise - the mind, even less - so trainees take the easy way out. "I'm heavy, I'll hide in the back of the class." "I'm intimidated, I'll stay away from the weights." "I've a headache, I'll do the treadmill and leave." "I'm sore, it must have been the gym." And some can afford to say, "I'll let someone else worry about it and just show up at my appointed time."

Personal training, the VIP service of exercise, brings the promise of more results for those who pay the extravagant fees, and addresses the major problems faced by those who can't afford it, form and intensity. But it rarely delivers.

For that, I have never felt at ease with the plight of the little guy who pays the rent, unsupervised. Sure, the establishment wants him to feel comfortable with his investment, and sure, the last thing they want him to do is break his neck. So, there's an orientation to get him on his feet, an occasional greeting as he enters, and a feeling that he belongs to a community sincerely interested in his progress.

Then reality rears its ugly head. He has to show up regularly, anonymous; repeat a boring routine that includes a station or two he dislikes; and face the same guy in the mirror each day. If he is not willing to shell out half his paycheck, he is ignored. If he asks, he gets an answer; if he asks too often, he gets a sales pitch. No wonder he quits.

Today's gyms provide little 'service' for the majority. Pay extra and get all the service you want - if you can call it that.

Last month I encountered a bump in the road in the form of a pink-slip. Our owner decided to cut costs and four years of employment wasn't enough to stay. Nonetheless, an old gym member called the other day to say 'hello.'

During his workout that day, he approached the reception behind which the new directors hide, asked a question and suggested that the gym wasn't the same. "You guys are never around. People are doing things wrong. When Gary was here, he wandered the floor helping everyone with form, tips, etc..."

The reply was brisk. "Gary lost a lot of money for this company. He gave out too much free information and paid too much attention to females."

It's nice to know you're heterosexual and of some help to somebody (where no one helps anyone). The fact remains that most trainers have very little to say, wouldn't know where to start as far as 'information' is concerned, free or otherwise.

Personal training, as it stands, is a joke, a babysitting gesture that should continue only under the following stipulations:

- No one-hour sessions (30-minute maximum).
- No talking (unless about the workout). Talk after the session.
- Miss once and you're out. A commitment is a commitment.
- Better yet, unless medically necessary, get rid of it.

Personal training means one client doing something right while 100 do everything wrong. The staff should help the little guy and increase the average production of results.

<br>

## JULY 14

---

### Calf Training

I first learned about calf muscles from the family album. Despite the fact that he never lifted weights, my Dad at 18 looked like Tarzan in a pair of swim trunks. He trained in the Welland Canal with a group of world-class distance swimmers who showed up for the annual competition across Lake Ontario from Niagara-on-the-Lake to the Canadian National Exhibition in Toronto. The prominent feature of his physique was calves - I have him to thank.

A second lesson came from the Nautilus® inventor. In the early 1970's, Arthur Jones hosted a bodybuilder who - because of the size of his calves - was about to endorse a machine made by another company. During the conversation, the man revealed that he had an identical twin whose calves were larger, despite the fact that his brother never lifted weights. Years later, Jones met the twin and measured his calves. They were larger, which proved a point: All the training of the zealous brother served only one purpose - to diminish his calves by over-training.

A third lesson evolved from the misfortune of a client who had not trained in years. I warned Mr. H to perform 8-12 repetitions on each exercise and to work 'easy' during his first session. At the time, I was training others and couldn't focus solely on his plight.

"How many?" I asked as I returned.

"First exercise, 34; second, 42."

I summoned enough compassion to warn him about the next, a calf raise: "If any muscle hurts in the morning, it'll be this one. When your calves get hot, quit." By the time I returned, he had completed 54 repetitions...with a smile. Two days later, Mr. H shuffled into the gym with a stride shorter than the distance between his ears and both legs bandaged from ankle to thigh. Following a lengthy medical tale, he acknowledged his error. It was my turn to not listen.

Another calf misfortune occurred years later when three young ladies did listen. From a stationary bike, I witnessed a certified trainer walk three members through their first (and perhaps last) workout on what must have been "National Calf Day." One at a time, they performed three sets of calf raises on one machine, followed by three on a different calf device, and three more on a third.

The result constituted a medical story all its own.

A final lesson came from a surprise paragraph in *The Nautilus Advanced Bodybuilding Book*, 1984. Ellington Darden, long an advocate of one set of 8-12 repetitions, introduced a calf routine consisting of two sets of 50 repetitions, some performed in a normal manner, the remainder in a negative-only fashion. The rationale was to take stubborn calves beyond 'normal' fatigue. Darden recommended that the new approach be performed three times a week for two weeks only, and then repeated every four or five months at most, due to its severity.

Calves are *not* different from other muscles. Their ultimate size and shape is dictated by muscle-belly length, a genetic factor. Daily activity fails to work them through a full range of motion, which is why they can become sore when first exposed to proper exercise. The performance of one set of 8-15 repetitions two or three times a week should produce optimum results. A variety of infrequent, intense activities can stimulate further change, with one caution - overworked calves can lose size and strength on the best of family trees.

JULY 15

### The Power of the Mind

In the early 1970's, without warning, Vic Tanny showed up in Arthur Jones' office at Nautilus® headquarters in Lake Helen, Florida. Apart from training a couple of months in a gym that Vic operated in Santa Monica, California in 1947 (a few years before he opened his famous chain of health clubs), Jones hadn't seen him in 35 years.

"I have never seen anybody who gained as much, or gained as fast, as you did," remembered Vic.

Jones had heard it before. Many people "were surprised and very favorably impressed with my results; but I was never satisfied."

Vic's comments were directed at what Jones called "the arms of a gorilla on the body of a spider monkey." Arthur thought his rate of progress was slow because he failed to understand the cause and effect relationships involved. His search for facts yielded nothing but opinions and he left the gym in frustration. In his words, "Nobody there could teach me anything of value."

It was a blessing. "If some muscles could grow that quickly, why couldn't others?" provided the spark for the creation of the first Nautilus machine.

Jones trained like a light switch for 50 years: either "on" (training hard), or "off" (not training at all). Despite the irregularity, he peaked at 205 pounds in lean muscular condition (at 5'7½") with a cold upper-arm of 17 3/8"; because of the irregularity, he became aware of certain things.

"I learned that all I had to do to produce growth was to decide to start training after a prolonged layoff; that is, if I decided on a Friday to start training again three days later, on the following Monday, then my upper arms would grow at least a full half of an inch in circumference before I did any training at all. The mental decision to start training again triggered the growth. This occurred so many times that I eventually reached a point where I expected it, and it never failed to happen."

Jones wasn't blowing smoke. When Ellington Darden was asked, "Of all the athletes and bodybuilders that trained at Nautilus, who worked the hardest?" he replied, "Arthur Jones." Jones' power of concentration was so great that he could produce a maximum effort and result with an expressionless face. Dr. Michael Fulton trained with Jones during one of his "on" phases and commented, "I've never seen anything like it. His arms grew to an incredible size at an incredible rate."

Darden illustrated the importance of concentration with a 'Pendulum Test' in his book, *Super High-Intensity Bodybuilding* (1986). Try it. With a key attached to one end of a 10-inch string and your forefinger to the other, sit at a table with your elbow propped on the surface and wrist forward. The key should hang a half-inch from the table directly in front of your center. Relax and visualize it moving like a pendulum from left to right and back. Now, will it to move. The key should be swinging.

I've witnessed displays of mind-power first-hand over the years - from magician and hypnotist, Doug Henning to Uri Geller who bent spoons 'with his mind' and to Jack Nicklaus who seemingly 'willed' putts into the hole throughout his career.

As Jones suggested, "The difference between success and failure may be largely, or entirely, your mental attitude. If you are convinced you are going to grow, then you will, but if you are afraid that you will not grow, then you won't."

'Focus' during strength training. Mental attitude has a great deal to do with results.

JULY 16

## Diet and Exercise

A one-time glance at an antique print depicting a swath of hair, thick mustache and set of piercing eyes that belonged to the one and only Albert Einstein triggered two thoughts. One, it probably didn't take a genius to unravel the mysteries of nutrition and exercise back then; and two, *only* a genius could figure it out today.

Nutrition should be simple - balance and amount - but it's not. Bodyweight and fat loss should be simple - input vs. output - but it's not, and the reason is clear: There are too many experts.

The consumer is constantly bombarded by information and products that are countered by future information and products. The result stands.

"Is my excess weight due to a lack of exercise or too much food?"

According to Dr. Megan McGory, a researcher at Tufts University Metabolism Lab, the culprit is food. Physical activity levels, she claims, haven't changed since 1985 but the average consumption has - by 400 calories per day. She blamed the growth on the increased variety of food offered by manufacturers, greater availability, less cost, better taste, larger portions, more restaurant visits and an elevated consumption of soft drinks and snacks.

Yale University psychologist, Kelly Brownell believes that consumers are targets of marketing experts and urges them to take a stand as they did with the tobacco industry. "If so many people can quit smoking," she says, "they can quit anything."

Their suggestions: Become a smarter shopper. Buy a book that indicates the number of calories in food. Put less food on the plate. Seek variety through fruits and vegetables. Curb snacking. Don't eat out as often and get off the couch.

Some view the final suggestion as the key. In a recent study, the obesity rate among children rose from 5% to 9% while the rate of those classified as 'overweight' rose from 15% to 24%. Poor exercise and nutrition habits, low levels of long-term breastfeeding and the pace of life were cited as possible causes.

Today's children are twice as likely to weigh more and have more body fat than children 20 years ago. Since 1985, the number of 'super obese' children (20-30% overweight) between the ages of 6-17 has doubled, while only 32% meet *minimum* standards for cardiovascular fitness, flexibility and strength.

According to the Cooper Institute for Aerobics (Dallas, Texas), 30-35% of school-age children will be at risk for cardiovascular disease and cancer as adults. As it stands, 60% have at least one modifiable risk factor for heart disease - physical activity, obesity, elevated cholesterol or high blood pressure - by the age of 12.

Nearly half of young adults (12-21) are not physically active on a regular basis, 25% don't participate in any vigorous activity, and 15% are completely sedentary. To add insult to injury, only 40% of schools offer daily physical education classes and many no longer *require* participation.

The statistics are confusing. As Nautilus® inventor Arthur Jones called it: "Figures lie and liars figure." The solution to body fat is simple and hasn't changed - input vs. output. The bad news: Addressing the former is quick and short-term; the latter, slow and long-term. The good news: Both have been mapped out - nutrition, by the common sense of Ellington Darden, Ph.D.; exercise, by the genius of Jones.

Start young, add a dash of discipline and keep stirring.

JULY 17

---

## Physical Education

'Porky' was about physical, not education. The typical overweight and over-mature kid found on most playgrounds came from a poor background, but he was likeable - and popular with those he didn't beat up. When we chose sides for teams, Porky was among the first to go. He provided a one-man defense in soccer, a home-run feast in softball and a wonderful ally in snowball fights. When needed, he applied his brawn-over-brain bear hug followed by a bouncing sit on his victim until "Uncle" was heard - not so loud, and not so clear.

Back then, recess and PT (physical training) class provided the same degree of supervision, little. There was no formal teacher - anyone who blew a whistle would do - and only certain days allocated for our shenanigans.

Things changed in high school, where lines of white T-shirts and green shorts were the order of the day. There was only one teacher to blow the whistle, and something I liked about the whole thing. Running in open air was a joy that could lead to success beyond the playing field.

I eventually made it my life, shared that joy with students, teammates, teachers and coaches for eight years, and adopted a philosophy common to the day. Physical education became a series of progressive, skill-oriented sessions (teaching students how to play basketball, golf and soccer, for example) with a sprinkle of rules and courtesies thrown in. Sports and games were a challenge and, above all, meant to be 'fun.' When the activity was directly related to a physical demand or conditioning per se, fitness was improved through participation. The notion of fitness, however, took a back seat to the rest. It was not the major focus.

Perhaps it should have been.

Little did I realize that the 'I-can't-wait-for-recess' feeling in grade school was not shared by others. Most kids dreaded PT (or were not exposed to it in a meaningful way) and dropped all traces of activity the moment they left school.

The first cuts in declining school budgets, not surprisingly, occur in programs such as music, physical education, art and drama. The result is a decline in the fitness level of students and in the probability of their choosing active lifestyles.

The trend has not escaped scrutiny.

"At least 99% of the physical education programs being used in schools today are simply stupid; a total waste of time, at best, and counterproductive or dangerous at worst," declared Nautilus® inventor Arthur Jones in *Ironman* (September, 1995). "Very few people are helped, nobody is helped to a meaningful degree, and quite a few people are hurt...the only results of such programs are the provision of employment for thousands of coaches and the wasting of time of millions of students."

According to Jones, the condition of the participants has not increased in any way, "which certainly does not mean that exercise is 'bad'; but rather that exercise, as it was being applied, was utterly wrong, worse than worthless. The same thing is true today."

Jones was right. Things haven't changed for the better, as statistics suggest.

If exercise continues to command its current respect, the nation could follow the path of Porky, last spotted high atop a commercial pavement-roller wearing the largest orange vest known to man.

I hope he's still around.

## JULY 18

---

### New Kids on the Block

At the age of three, Arthur Jones looked at a globe of Earth and recognized that the continents had drifted apart. It was something he assumed everyone knew until its mention, one day, produced nothing but ridicule. Arthur kept his mouth shut.

One man did not, however, and paid a high price. When Alfred Wegener first suggested the divide in 1912, he was mocked by the scientific community until his death in 1930. Thirty years later, they realized he was right.

It was a typical reaction to something new.

"About 100 years ago," said Jones, "when the first recording of a human voice was played for a large group of leading scientists in England, the chairman of that group denounced it as a fake and walked out of the meeting; he believed it was a fraud based on a ventriloquist. Still refused to believe it even six years later."

The Nautilus® inventor received a similar reception in the field of exercise. Jones first tried to communicate ideas through bodybuilding magazines that he believed were neck-deep in nonsense and had nothing 'new' to say for 30 years. He was right - publishers wanted nothing of truth or logic. Joe Weider's magazines rejected everything he sent. *Strength and Health* and *Scholastic Coach* published one article each. Only *Athletic Journal* and *Ironman* willingly agreed, but at times published them edited. Jones eventually turned to self-publication - but was still not satisfied.

"I have found that meaningful communication is all but impossible when it depends on the published word - primarily, it appears, because there is no feedback from the audience... People usually hear what they want to hear, what they expect to hear, that which agrees with their already established opinions. So, when your statements fly in the face of their opinions, they either fail to understand what you said or reject it out of hand; but in either case, real communication does not occur."

To solve the problem, Jones built an airport at his ranch in Ocala (Florida) to host eye-to-eye lectures. There, he addressed small groups "in an attempt to insert a little common sense in a field where sense of any kind was almost totally lacking."

His efforts were received with the same fervor as that of the continental divide. He resumed publishing 'as is' articles in *Ironman*.

Around that time, I witnessed a similar reaction to something new in the field of politics. In the 1980's, a popular Venezuelan TV host decided to run for President as an independent. Rene Ottolina amassed such a large following with his honest, matter-of-fact style and athletic, good-guy demeanor that the two major parties, then in rule for 20 years, became 'concerned.' One morning, on a trip to the interior, his plane mysteriously failed. It was the end of the problem and served to confirm the belief held by Jones that politics was far worse than exercise.

"I have learned," he said, "that a much better source of bullshit (than that found in bodybuilding magazines) can be found by listening to the statements of politicians, bureaucrats and other supposed 'experts.' There, at least you can be sure that it's pure bullshit, is never confused with anything that is even partially true."

In a current run for governor of California, bodybuilder Arnold Schwarzenegger has intrigued the media with concern over his credentials - he's not a politician. Have no fear. If he makes it, the transition from one level of bullshit to another should be the cause of no concern at all.

JULY 19

### The Knee and Other Nonsense

Nautilus® inventor Arthur Jones once called the knee an 'outrage.' And it is. But it's nothing compared to the advice circulated by many of today's 'certified' trainers - never straighten your knee during resistance exercise.

The knee joint is mechanically inefficient. Approximately 92-94% of the effort of the front-thigh muscle (quadriceps) to straighten the knee is wasted by poor leverage and friction. Only six percent contributes to the actual movement. In other words, a contraction force of 100 units produced by the quadriceps muscle (during leg extensions) results in a lift of six units of weight. Not good, but it numerically whips that of a man who routinely exercises with 650 pounds on a leg extension machine - and some can. The quadriceps requires a contraction force of 7,500 pounds - 3.4 tons.

And that's not the worst of it.

In the starting position (120°), the kneecap is exposed to a compression force 73% higher than the pulling force of the quadriceps. Therefore, if the quadriceps contracts with 100 pounds of force and lifts six pounds of weight, the kneecap is exposed to 173 pounds of compression force. In a 650-pound lift, the quadriceps muscle contracts with 7,500 pounds of force and exposes the kneecap to a force in excess of 13,000 pounds, 5.9 tons. This explains why Jones restricted the range-of-motion on his leg extension machines to 120°, why knee injuries are so common in competitive weightlifting and why it is important to lift weights using a slow speed of movement.

Apparently, word hasn't hit the street.

Most trainees move weights at lightning speeds by creating enough momentum in the first 10-15° of movement - precisely where forces are highest and most dangerous in a leg extension - to allow a muscle a free ride through the remainder of its range. Furthermore, initiating an exercise with a sudden jerk increases the force to which the muscle and joint system is exposed by 3-4 times. Call it what you will, throwing rather than lifting weights is less productive than it could be, and dangerous as you know what. Yet, this borderline insanity is a choice that most have made.

The situation is better in the full-contracted position of a leg extension (the knee-lock position that trainers warn you never to assume - where it feels as if your legs will explode during intense exercise). There, a lift of six pounds of weight still requires a pull of 100 pounds from the quadriceps, but exposes the kneecap to a compression force that equals the pulling force of the muscle, 100 pounds. *It is safer at the top of a leg extension than at the bottom.*

It is also more productive. The muscle demands a larger recruitment of fibers in that position, which increases the possibility of stimulating change.

How about *feel?*

Holding a contracted position during the final repetitions of a leg-extension exercise can make a grown man cry, which scares just about everyone involved. Yet, your strength is so low at the end of a set that you couldn't produce enough force to hurt yourself even if you did jerk the weight - which you shouldn't. Remember, it's not speed of movement that creates injury, but a *sudden change of speed.*

The knee is a mechanical outrage. The next time someone tells you to avoid the most productive and, by far, the safest part of a leg extension - a position of full contraction - walk away. You are talking to a fool.

## JULY 20

---

### Socketing and Other Maladies

There are three diseases in golf: the yips, the shanks (once called socketing) and the blow-by-blow description of 18-holes to an audience who, if given a choice, would rather not listen. The first two come and go at random and have no cure. The third is all too common but has a simple cure.

All three have a close ally in pride - whether viewed a cause, symptom or innocent bystander - and it goes without saying in golf, that pride comes before a fall.

One day I stood on the highest point in the Niagara Peninsula (Lookout Point Golf Club, Fonthill, Ontario) with my Driver in hand. I was 15, it was sunny and I had played the front nine in 41, a good score at the time. But I was lucky in another way, although unaware of it at the time - the shaft of my Driver was nowhere near its face, which was not the case with some other clubs.

It struck exactly as Bernard Darwin described in 1935, "Suddenly, like a thunderbolt out of a blue sky." Every time I hit an iron - on the same grass, under the same blue sky, using the same slow backswing, and the same thoughts that had led to prior success - the ball squirted low at right-angles to its intended line. Shot after shot, I struck the ball on the hosel (where the shaft meets the head), the socket - socket after socket. With 'out-of-bounds' markers bordering the right side of the course, my score quickly tallied to a back-nine 72.

I don't recall how I escaped the grasp of that rot, but just as suddenly, it disappeared, leaving only a memory - and a scar that wasn't as bad as some.

Darwin's 1935 character was pitching balls with a so-called 'socket-proof' club in a garden the day he was struck. His panic multiplied with each errant shot and, with lunch fast approaching, he stayed until he hit 'several' good ones, fearing that "his family would discover that he was raving mad and send for a doctor." Darwin continued, "I recollect that a good while ago this poor man won a certain tournament. In one of the rounds, the enemy had come to such sad grief at the last hole that my friend could not fail to win if he kept topping the ball down the middle of the course. He remarked to an onlooker: 'Thank Heaven, I've got a mashie without a socket,' and by trundling the ball in inglorious safety with this weapon he duly won. If he had known then what he has learned now I doubt whether he would have ever reached the green at all."

Gary Bannister, B.A., B.P.E., M.Ed.

There are three parallel diseases in exercise: too much quantity, not enough quality and too much "well-intentioned" advice, with pride lingering near. The first two have no cure because real education will never penetrate such a commercial fortress, and because it is hard to teach old dogs new tricks. Yet, for those energetic enough to try, I have solutions that may prove as effective as a 'cure' for socketing:

- Enforce a maximum time limit per workout (and per exercise) and a minimum time limit per repetition by using a clock at every station.
- Install pay-per-use equipment. "You want 10 sets? Bring more quarters."

The third disease is all too common but has a simple cure. The next time Mr. Physique embarks on a trail of advice, treat him as we do all golfers who start, "On the first hole...," by taking a sudden and profound interest in your soup.

The other day, an old friend returned - I socketed a pitching wedge from the 13th tee. The ball caromed off a tree, narrowly escaped a trashcan on its descent and confirmed a longstanding belief about the dreaded disease, "Once you've had 'em,' you've got 'em.'"

JULY 21

**Home on the Range**

You can learn a lot about a person on a driving range. I don't know how many times I've seen a golfer, within seconds of dropping his bucket, pull out the driver, perform a couple of jerks in the name of 'warm-up,' and boom, start banging away. As Bernard Darwin put it, "The ball flew straight and high but came down to earth all too soon again." It's not the way to build a golf swing.

Then again, some people aren't there for that. They simply want to see the ball soar with or without basics - grip, posture and ball position. The logical approach is to begin with the short irons and work toward the longer clubs. Once you have a feel for the swing, hit the driver. When you look up, you may like what you see.

The same occurs in gyms where the performance of the first exercise predicts what will follow. When a guy heads to an abdominal station and pumps off 20 repetitions before you can blink, you know you have your hands full.

The abdomen is indirectly involved in every exercise. Working it first detracts from the performance of major muscle groups. Save the 'abs' for the end.

The same applies to forearm exercises, a popular first among golfers and racquet players. Exhausting a small muscle group that will later be involved in exercise for larger muscles spells disaster. Try a chin-up immediately after a hard set of wrist curls, a leg extension after a leg press, a pullover after an abdominal exercise or a chest fly after a bench press. Good luck.

I once owned a gym in Caracas, Venezuela and spent time concocting exercise combinations from the Nautilus® books. Four times, I hosted the company's medical representative who suggested the following non-stop sequence: chin-ups (palms-up grip), arm curls (on a Nautilus Multi-Curl machine) and negative chin-ups. I completed the first, rushed to the second - a few feet away - and back to the third.

At the time, I could perform 10 repetitions of negative chin-ups with 50 pounds strapped around my waist. This time with no weight, I couldn't hang onto the bar to start - a great lesson. Failure in all three exercises occurs in the same muscle group, the forearm and you cannot pre-exhaust a small muscle and expect it to assist a larger muscle (biceps and upper-back) seconds later. The sequence was tough, but lousy.

Fortunately, not all triple-exercise combinations are poor. A pulldown - pullover - negative chin-up is a great upper-back sequence. Although each movement works the same muscles of the back, failure on the first and third exercises occurs in the weaker muscles of the biceps. The 'no-arm' (pullover) exercise in the middle allows the biceps a 'break' before the final onslaught - a break of adequate duration to allow execution of the third exercise.

The combinations: chest press - chest fly - negative dips (parallel bars); and lateral raise - upright row - overhead press are equally effective. Failure occurs in different muscle groups on each exercise but the major muscle is targeted in all three. The 'fresh' smaller groups assist the larger ones to reach a greater level of fatigue.

Unless you are attempting something advanced, work muscles from large to small and avoid combining *more* than three consecutive exercises - as I've seen with a few trainees that should know better.

More than three exercises in a row - properly performed - will have you "come down to earth all too soon again." And when you look up, you may not like what you see.

## JULY 22

---

### Plate-Loaded Machines

According to bodybuilders, plate-loaded exercise machines offer "the best of both worlds." They allow trainees to combine the safety of machines with the joy of lugging barbell plates around the gym.

The modern version of the equipment (notwithstanding crude plate-holding poles attached to pulleys) began with Nautilus® inventor, Arthur Jones. His "Leverage Machines" introduced in the early 1980's were like teeter-totters with a weight on one end and a muscle on the other; between them, a single axis of rotation.

Jones made it clear from the start that the change of resistance on his new machines did not compare with that provided by the 'cams' on his existing line. Both single-joint exercises (leg extensions, curls, biceps, triceps) and compound movements (presses, pulling motions) suffered from too much resistance at one end and too little at the other, or provided a limited range of motion. It was the nature of the beast.

Nevertheless, Arthur's son, Gary "stole" the plans for the new equipment (early in their development) and formed his own company, Hammer Strength®. Arthur countered with a line of machines called "Power Plus," a leverage machine *with* a cam that provided a superior change of resistance, a greater range of motion and the 'feel' of the original Nautilus machines. It was too little, too late. Most bodybuilders had been corralled by Joe Weider to believe that anything that didn't resemble a barbell (or that evolved from Arthur Jones) was trash. In the end, Hammer Strength captured the market using high-profile athletes for promotion, and remained (as had Nautilus 10 years before) the "must have" in gyms.

The Jones family hasn't been the same since.

Around that time, a business associate and I acquired a copy of Nautilus Leverage Machine plans to build a multi-exercise tool in Venezuela. We didn't understand the size of the tubes we cut and welded, but we could copy. The result was a sturdy device that incorporated a pulldown, incline press, leg curl, leg extension and chin/dip station (with steps for performing negative work). Despite the fact that the resistance at each station had a great feel, the project was abandoned.

The exercise field hasn't been the same since.

Hammer Strength quickly became the 'Holy Grail' for those who crossed the line to include machines as part of their training regimen. It was safe to be seen on a Hammer machine, but not on one of the 'others.' It was also safe to say that a derogatory comment about a Hammer machine in a gym would create a conflict. Devotees became defensive in spite of the fact that even a blind man could tell that the change of resistance was too drastic from one end of the movement to the other. It was obvious to everyone but the majority of bodybuilders who, in their embrace of the new equipment, also neglected to find out how to best use it.

None of this is meant to be critical of Hammer Strength or its equipment, but merely to explain the technology. With plate-loaded, single-axis exercise machines, deficiencies in the resistance are found on *at least* one end of the movement.

To date, Arthur Jones has had the last say in the family saga with the introduction of his MedX® plate-loaded "Avenger" series. With a single-axis of rotation (sometimes more), his new machines offer a resistance change that 'feels' as good as a cam.

Bring on the blindfolds.

## JULY 23

### The Reverse Bungee

One blustery day, Mike Sanchez stepped out of an airplane that hadn't stopped flying. The bad news was yet to come.

Mike, a skydiver with 150 jumps under his belt, was among a dozen peers that shuffled toward the open door and the ultimate thrill that day. Out he went in the wind, performing a series of flips and turns before releasing his chute. Life was good.

But things were not down below.

One man's parachute failed to open; his auxiliary, the same - dead. Another had his second chute tangle in the first when it partially opened. Mike swooped in to assist but couldn't get near - dead. Mike crafted a turn for the final descent when a sudden gust of wind collapsed his chute. Down he shot, pulling hard with his arms to brake - near dead.

Mike broke both femurs upon impact and underwent several surgical interventions. Thanks to MedX® orthopedic representative, Dr. Michael Fulton, he walked away with no apparent aftermath.

I've often wondered what it would be like to jump off a bridge with both legs tied to a bungee chord. With my luck, it would be the only time the chord snapped. I've also wondered what it would be like to jump off a bridge with no attachments.

Well, exercise, under the guise of performance, takes it one step beyond. It attaches the bungee to the bottom of the canyon to ensure, like a slingshot, a faster result. As ridiculous as it sounds, I see the same when athletes attach themselves to rubber chords and jump from platforms in so-called 'sports performance' programs.

According to physical therapist, Alvin Ponce de Leon, "It's only for the young."

But while the young may better tolerate impact, it's still no excuse. "Most of the millions of people who are now interested in exercise," commented MedX inventor Arthur Jones in 1993, "are too young to even be aware of the true history of this field, do not know who to believe or what to believe, remain unaware of the many outrages that have occurred during the past 50 years or so in this field, many of which outrages are still occurring. Outrages? You're damned right: isokinetics, plyometrics, power cleans, any sudden movement against resistance, jump squats and a long list of other things that provide no benefits whatsoever and are dangerous as hell."

Add to the naivete of youth - proud parents with the means to pay, a warped notion that athletes require 'special' training, and the endorsement of 'star' athletes - and you have what you have, an explosive and lucrative situation.

In the early 1970's, Jones listened as Gideon Ariel addressed an audience about the high and dangerous levels of impact force associated with jogging. Twenty minutes later, the speaker recommended jump squats as a safe and productive exercise. Jones jumped. "The level of impact force involved in jogging," he said, "is usually about three times as high as the subject's bodyweight, but with jump squats it may be 50 times as high as bodyweight. So, if jogging is dangerous, how in the hell can jump squats be safe?"

According to Jones, you can run faster and jump higher in a safe way, as follows:

- Strengthen the involved muscles by isolated, slow, controlled, intense work.
- Improve the body's muscle/fat ratio (fat creates friction during movement).
- Refine the efficiency of the movement itself by proper skill training.

When athletes leap to their final destination, bungee in place, they may find that their performance *has* improved. Instead of six feet under, they'll be six and a half.

## JULY 24

---

### Figures Lie and Liars Figure

For four summers, I worked in the Ford® Motor Company's glass manufacturing plant in Niagara Falls, Canada, eventually performing almost every job related to the fabrication, packing and shipping of windshields, back and side glass. It wasn't easy.

Students were assigned the least desirable positions, such as loading and unloading furnaces that molded the panes. A few minutes in and a few minutes out, when you removed the asbestos gloves to wipe your brow, there was no sweat. It was as if someone had sprinkled salt on your forehead.

The temperature in the plant was about 95°, and in front of the furnace, double. Workers were encouraged to take salt pills twice a shift - a practice that began during World War II. 'Salt out - salt in' made sense until it was discovered that excess consumption could lead to health problems, including death. Apparently, the daily consumption of salt pills had to be accompanied by the drinking of about half of Lake Erie to balance the system.

The salt dispensers soon disappeared.

And so it is with many things, including exercise - too little creates a need; too much, a danger. As Arthur Jones put it, "Some is good, perhaps essential, but it does not follow that more is better, and it is frequently worse, and too much will kill you."

In the late 1960's, Cybex® (among others) began promoting the idea that positive-only exercise (lifting) was superior to normal or negative-only exercise (lowering), based upon the fact that their equipment was void of negative work. Its removal was somehow an advantage. The premise was noticed by soon-to-be Nautilus® inventor, Jones.

"Once called to my attention," he noted, "it required less than 10 minutes of consideration for me to realize that the negative part of exercise was very important...I still didn't know just how important; but I knew how to find out."

As Jones was investigating the issue, an article was published by Tom Pipes and Jack Wilmore that supposedly 'proved' the superiority of positive-only exercise. It started a landslide. Hundreds of thousands of copies were distributed by Cybex over several years, quoted as 'fact' in scientific books and used in physical therapy schools - all in spite of the fact that it never happened.

"The whole thing was an outright fraud," claimed Jones. "Tom Pipes simply made up the published test results. Which is not surprising, since he has a long history of outright fraud, having called himself a doctor when he had no such degree or training in that direction." Arthur had a three-hour taped conversation to prove it.

The co-author wasn't any better. When cornered, "Wilmore suddenly remembered that he was out of the state during the period when the study was supposedly performed," said Jones, "and thus had no actual knowledge of it."

Because of his work, Wilmore became president of the American College of Sports Medicine and editor of a major scientific journal that refused to publish a low-back study demonstrating significant gains from a brief protocol on Jones' MedX® equipment. Wilmore's letter to Dr. Michael Pollock, who submitted the article, read as follows: "Everybody knows that one exercise each week is worthless; to produce good results you must perform each exercise nine times every week."

Jones promptly added bullshit to his list - too little creates a need; too much, a danger.

Pass the salt, please.

# JULY 25

---

## Crossing the Line

"How you gonna putt?" was the usual reaction from golf professional, Gord McGinnis Sr. "Your body's shaking from your run." Senior knew golf - two of his students won United States and Canadian amateur titles in the same year, Marlene Stewart in 1956 and Cathy Sherk in 1980 - but he didn't know fitness. When I ran to the course or teed off after a workout, there was always that look.

The majority of golf professionals are embedded in theory and reluctant to change. Their stance is rationalized by experience and by the success of players who adhere to or demonstrate at least part of that theory.

Recently, golf was shaken by a rumor surrounding the heir to the Nicklaus throne, Tiger Woods. The message was loud and clear: You can improve golf by improving physical condition. Almost overnight, golf experts began commenting on the role of fitness as it related to performance. At first, they didn't know what to say, but it didn't take long. What Gary Player failed to stimulate in 40 years now inundated the field.

Trainers, experts, therapists, tour trailers, entourages and academies all sought a piece of the pie. But the vote was not overwhelming.

There were those who stepped in one toe at a time, or not at all. Answers to "How much?" "How often?" and "How intense?" provided little comfort. Many tried exercise and gave it up when it failed to meet their expectations or somehow 'changed their swing.' I heard one professional at a golf school for juniors comment to a teen, "You know how it is...you'll get these big muscles that will just get in the way. They won't be flexible or mobile." The worst was yet to come.

Not long ago I watched The Golf Channel® troubleshooter, Dean Reinmuth assist a player with his short game. The instruction was excellent until - in the middle of the show - Reinmuth appeared in a hotel room in front of a mirror.

"What I like to do when I'm on the road is use the desk for more than business," he said as he braced his hands on the edge of its top. He then moved his feet back a step and performed a series of modified push-ups. "What I do is several slow push-ups followed by short, jerky ones," which he demonstrated. "What this does," he said, "is strengthen the muscles of the back, the hands and the forearms to help you hit the ball farther."

Nice try. Push-ups do not work back, forearm or hand muscles; they work chest, front-shoulder and triceps. Second, his full repetitions were less than full and performed too fast. Third, choosing a desk as a prop made the effort easier than the use of the floor. Fourth, why short jerky repetitions?

'Experts' are bad enough, but crossing the line is worse. In Reinmuth's defense, he doesn't claim to know anything about exercise but he is more than eager to relay the latest suggestion of his trainer or some other 'expert.' With the power of TV, he should have been a little more aware of professional responsibility.

The scenario brought to mind a quote from "Rex vs. Haddock" (A.P. Herbert, 1933) in which a man was accused of using blasphemous words during a round of golf.

"It is clear that the game of golf may well be included in that category of intolerable provocations which may legally excuse or mitigate behavior not otherwise excusable, and that under that provocation the reasonable or gentle man may reasonably act like a lunatic or lout respectively and should legally be judged as such."

Dean meant no harm, but he should stick to golf.

## JULY 26

---

### An Accident of Time and Place

Arthur was not impressed with the teacher's explanation and thrust his hand in the air. Calculating the area of a circle by plugging numbers into a formula was not his idea of learning. "Teacher," he said, "I get the same as you every time, but I use the diameter." He had his own formula.

Nautilus® inventor Arthur Jones wasn't joking when he said, "I quit school in the fourth grade, but they kept dragging me back." He thought he knew more than the teachers, and from time to time showed that he did. Fortunately, he chose to apply that brilliance to the field of exercise - only to learn that he was not the first.

In 1996, Dr. Tom DeLorme, medical director of Liberty Mutual® Insurance Company and the "father" of rehabilitative exercise in this country introduced Jones to the work of Dr. Gustaf Zander. As early as 1857, Dr. Zander conceived the idea of practicing "medical gymnastics" and in 1865 began to use a line of machines he designed at "The Medico-Mechanical Institute" in Stockholm, Sweden. By 1894, he had developed 40 different devices; some activated by muscular action, others driven by steam, gas or electric power.

According to Jones, "He (Zander) was clearly aware of, and obviously understood, many of the actual requirements for proper exercise that I introduced in early Nautilus machines." Among those requirements were variable and balanced resistance.

The Zander method used a special apparatus "for exercising each separate group of muscles." The weight was adjustable "from zero to the maximum suitable to each apparatus" and was indicated "with mathematical exactness by means of a scale on the lever. The position of the weighted lever was so arranged that its effect increased or diminished in accordance with the mechanical effect of the contraction of the muscles."

According to the *Monthly Journal of Therapeutics for Injuries by Accident*, 1894, Zander ingeniously varied the resistance "in proportion to the cosine of the angle of incidence of the weighted lever."

Zander's machines also factored in Schwann's law for muscular action that stated, "with increasing contraction, the muscle is able to accomplish less work." In each machine, the resistance diminished during the latter half of the contraction.

Like Jones, Zander viewed his competitors with disdain. Nycander's machines and Gaertner's 'Ergostat' used a frictional resistance that remained constant "whereby," according to Zander, "each movement was too slight in the beginning and required too great an exertion at the end." He found the same with Burlot's and Mager's equipment, devices that "raised weights suspended on ropes running in pulleys." Sach's 'Muscle-Strengthener' had India-rubber straps or tubes that "offered the greatest resistance at the end of the muscular contraction, and thus in the phase of slightest development of muscular force."

Jones marveled at Zander's insight. "Some of his machines, built 140 years ago," he said, "were at least the equal of most of the exercise machines now on the market. If I had been aware of, and had understood, Dr. Zander's much earlier work, I could have avoided many mistakes and saved a lot of time and money."

Jones and Zander had something else in common - they made durable tools. Some of Dr. Zander's machines were still being used in several major hospitals in this country as recently as 40 years ago - 100 years of service.

## JULY 27

---

### Gird Thy Loins

When Arthur Jones first introduced his Nautilus® machines and exercise concepts, he was well aware of the pending reaction from his competitors. There was a lot at stake.

In the early 1970's, Joe Weider had a firm grasp on bodybuilding - equipment, competitions, publications and profit. The new equipment posed a greater threat than that of the Universal® machine (1960's) and its inventor was persistent, intelligent and honest - a combination that spelled trouble.

Weider immediately launched an effort to destroy its validity through his publications, using quotes from prominent bodybuilders under his wing.

- Vince Gironda: "The basic technical concept is erroneous...it is far too costly for what little it can do; and its appearance alone turns many persons away - frightens and confuses them." (as if bodybuilders weren't already confused)
- Frank Zane supposedly said: "Nautilus machines are mainly a gimmick...I actually dislocated my right shoulder." (Eventually, he purchased several machines for training at home, far from the view of peers)
- Ken Waller: "I lost about three-quarters of an inch from my arms!"

- Roger Callard: "Everyone I know who used these machines extensively became smooth." (Smooth is a dietary, not an equipment issue).
- Arnold Schwarzenegger: "I don't feel that the Nautilus machines even come close to training with the standard barbell, dumbbells and pulley equipment. It is my honest opinion that there is no comparison at all." He changed his tune when he visited Nautilus. "Mr. Jones just read me your (Weider's) letter which you wrote to him complaining about the facts he published regarding his new machines and training methods, and I laughed about your complaints because they don't make sense...Visit Mr. Jones and try his machines yourself...I gained four pounds and increased my arm size in the first three days of training, and I am making immediate arrangements to obtain several of his machines for my use in California. If this is not my true opinion, then I will give up all of the titles I have won in the past. I really believe that the new machines are fantastic."

Weider also paid Casey Viator to say that he trained more than what Jones claimed he had ("Casey Comes Clean"). Arthur held his ground - truth has a way of prevailing.

In the November (1976) issue of a Weider publication that featured a photo of Arnold performing curls on a Nautilus Plate-Loaded Biceps machine, a barbell plate had been airbrushed in to make it look like he was curling a barbell. The December issue featured the same photo, with the Nautilus cam airbrushed out. When John Turner showed this to Jones, he "ignited another Pall Mall and turned the page. Arthur doesn't treat paranoia."

Jones dealt with ignorance by using more than 'truth.'

When heckled by a non-believer in the audience at a Duke University seminar, Jones immediately challenged the larger man to "step outside and we will see whose training methods work better." End of challenge.

Weider recently introduced a cheap copy of the Bowflex® to keep his name 'alive' and front his real source of income - supplements. To this day, he remains the antithesis of the Nautilus inventor, adding more water to an already huge flood of lies.

As fellow-Canadian Turner put it, "Arthur Jones is a man so great, Joe Weider would have to stand on his brother's shoulders in order to kiss Arthur's butt."

## JULY 28

---

### While You Were Out...

Every day I return from work, I'm amazed at what happened while I was out. Letters, flyers, E-mail and telephone messages provide a constant reminder that, "If I'm conscious, I'm pre-approved." It's that easy.

There is nothing easy (or conscious), however, about suddenly finding yourself lying flat on the floor during exercise. It happens quickly, without warning or pre-approval.

From the time I started lifting weights, I wondered why biceps exercises were more demanding than triceps; why chin-ups were more exhausting than dips; and why upper-back pulldowns took such a severe toll on the pace of the workout.

I concluded that it had to do with the amount of muscle involved. The upper back was larger than the chest. Chin-ups involved more peripheral work - from shoulders, chest, trapezius, abdomen, forearms and biceps - than dips. And I ruled out intensity because it was consistent from one exercise to another.

I was wrong.

The intensity involved in gripping the bar with the small muscles of the hand and forearm was so great during pulldowns, chin-ups and biceps curls that blood pressure was driven to high and dangerous levels. And recovery was not swift.

When I heard that a bodybuilder in Caracas had lost consciousness while performing biceps curls, my reaction was that he probably passed out from stupidity, his form was so bad. But I guess there was blood in his veins, if not in his head.

Arthur Jones explained the phenomenon in an article, "The Time Factor in Exercise," (*Ironman*, Nov. 1971) with specific reference to standing barbell curls.

"Pause very briefly at the bottom and at the top of each repetition," he advised, "and relax as much as possible under the circumstances; in order to momentarily relieve the forces which will be enormously elevating your blood pressure during a hard muscular contraction. If you don't, you may find yourself 'passing out' in the middle of a hard repetition; one second you will be standing up curling the bar, and the next thing you know you will be stretched out on the floor - possibly having dropped the bar on your leg while you were 'out.' When it happens, it happens so fast that you are not even aware of it - one second you are up, the next second you are down."

He went on. "The human circulatory system is a 'closed hydraulic system' and the mass of applied force is of no importance - only the degree of applied force has any effect insofar as raising the pressure of the system as a whole is concerned. Thus, while it might be expected that a heavy set of squats would be most likely to cause such 'blacking-out' from elevated blood pressure, in fact this almost never happens - because, while the mass of involved muscle is greatest in squats, the degree of contraction seldom if ever is as great as that experienced in a set of heavy curls. 'Amount' of effort is not the responsible factor - instead 'intensity of effort' seems to be the only factor involved."

The pause advocated at the top and bottom of each curling repetition should last only about a half second - "Just enough," said Jones, "to momentarily relieve the blood pressure and restore normal circulation to the brain."

Some biceps machines place a pad against the forearm during exercise to eliminate gripping, but most don't. Perform your machine curls by keeping your hands open during the lowering phase, if not throughout.

The blood pressure 'break' will help keep the lights on.


## JULY 29

---

### Rocket Man

If you thought Vasco de Gama was happy to see land, you missed Cory Pickos. The 11th hole at the Sandalfoot Golf Club in Boca Raton, Florida is a dogleg-right par four with water fronting the green. Cory was used to water, but not this kind. A breeze kicked up as his torso wound for the approach. From 165 yards, he had to get it all.

Suddenly, the same 14 swing flaws that had resulted in such profound and prolonged misery produced one of the most magnificent sights known to man. The ball sailed high and straight, but the breeze held firm as it reached its pinnacle. Tension filled the air, then, SMACK - it struck the middle of the green, 10 feet from the hole. The shout, the neck veins, the fist-pump - you'd have thought Pickos had just won the Open.

I first met Cory in Caracas, Venezuela in the late 1980's when the 35-time world-record-holder in trick skiing was invited to practice with the sport's female champion, Anna Maria Carrasco (who trained in my gym at the time). It was quite a site from the boat. While Anna sought to perfect new combinations, Cory worked on an elusive front flip and a 900-degree turn (2½ times around) off the wake. It was easy to see why they called him 'Rocket Man.'

Champions are born, not made, but there's something to be said about how long it takes to get to the top in trick skiing, and how lonely it must be once there. Cory first broke the world record when he was 13. The record had been broken 35 times since, 34 by Pickos himself. He dominated the sport for 15 years. In the same way, Anna's sister, Maria Victoria Carrasco was undefeated in 44 international competitions from 1972 to 1979, and retired as such. In her final years, with several Russians knocking at the door, Maria made it a point to walk to the dock before the event and stare them down. They were NOT going to win.

Years later, I worked with Cory in Quiet Waters Park (Deerfield Beach, Florida) when a talented Italian teenager showed up to train. At the time, his competition scores ranged from 8,000-8,500 points versus Cory's 11,000-11,500.

"How long will it take him to catch you if he works hard?" I asked.

"About 10-12 years," Pickos replied, adding, "It takes a year to nail a new trick."

In the early 1990's, the sport of water-skiing changed when the US Water-Ski Federation dropped 'trick-skiing' from its pro tour because "it wasn't exciting enough." Cory was forced to take up its replacement, 'wake boarding' to make ends meet. It was a kick in the face for a man who had given so much to the sport.

The other events on tour - slalom and jumping - had more crowd appeal at the time, but they weren't more athletic. When Michael Fulton, MD (US team doctor) performed a battery of strength, cardiovascular and flexibility tests on 18 of the world's top-20 water skiers, Cory emerged as 'the best of the best.'

The last time I saw him was in the US Open at Okeeheelee Park in West Palm Beach. Cory was the last competitor of the day and his peers were closing fast - a glitch on a prior run left his lead in jeopardy. The first part of his final pass was perfect. He set his foot in the strap for the return and took his familiar crouch. Twenty seconds of spins, leaps and jumps later, he landed his last 'trick' at the buzzer.

Once again, the shout, the neck veins, the fist-pump made Tiger Woods look puny.

Cory continues to teach what he knows best - and there was none better - in northern Florida. I hope he enjoys a little golf along the way.

## JULY 30

---

### A Lesson From Experience

"If race horses were trained as much as most bodybuilders train," said Arthur Jones in advocating a universal exercise routine for all, "you could safely bet your money on an out-of-condition turtle - it would be unlikely that a horse trained in such a fashion could even make it around the track, and certainly not rapidly."

The Nautilus® inventor's 'same workout for all' had no obvious appeal to those who considered themselves unique, but it was a dandy.

"The training routine that we are using in DeLand," claimed Jones, "moves so fast that it is almost frightening to watch - but it must move at such a pace in order to produce the results that we are producing. No other type of training will even begin to produce similar results. The entire training program for the legs and lower back consists of only three exercises in most cases - and never more than four exercises in any case. One set of each of three (or four) exercises, a total training time of three or four minutes - performed only twice weekly - a total weekly training time of six or eight minutes. Thirty seconds into this routine, the pulse rate hits a level of 160 to 190 - and will not drop below 130 until the entire workout is completed, a period of approximately 28 minutes for a 'total body' workout covering every major muscular structure, the legs and lower back, the upper back and chest, the shoulders and arms, the abdominals, literally 'everything.'"

The intensity was too high for many - whether they admitted it or not - and the duration, never enough. Jones stuck to his guns.

"The above-mentioned routine is the exact training program that we will use with the Cincinnati Bengals Professional Football Team starting in May of this year (1972). It is the exact program that almost anybody should use, regardless of 'why' they are training. It is the program that almost everybody will eventually use."

Jones continued to pursue the 'exact' program through research using better tools. The process eventually led him to believe otherwise.

"For years, I have been telling people to train in much the same way," he stated in an article entitled *Exercise...1986: The Present State of the Art...Now a Science*, "but I now understand that this advice is wrong...wrong for most people; and I understand why it is wrong for most people. Right for a few, right for me, right for an unknown but probably small percentage of people selected at random, but wrong for most people."

He also changed his tone on intensity. "I have been telling people," he said, "to always continue an exercise to the point that additional movement was impossible...but now I am not so sure; now I realize that at least one other requirement exists...and that it is at least possible that a high intensity of exercise is not even needed."

The 'other' requirement was the effect or immediate consequence of exercise. A large loss in strength led to recovery issues; a small loss failed to stimulate change. The ideal effect (a 20-25% loss) could be obtained by varying the number of repetitions performed.

Jones was aware of this factor before 1986 but, like others, ignored it. "Some people at least have an excuse, since they were not aware of the evidence; but I was, so I have no excuse, I was simply too stupid to pay attention, even when the evidence hit me across the face like a baseball bat, which it did."

In the end, approximately 10% of those tested produced a small effect from exercise; 30%, a great effect. It led Jones to conclude with more certainty that 70-80% of trainees produce best results from strength training by using 8-15 repetitions.


## JULY 31

---

### The Iron Man

Dr. Solleder proudly displayed a copy of her latest article in *Health Education* to a classroom of graduate students. As Dean of the Health Education Division of the University of North Carolina at Greensboro, she encouraged her students to aim high, and most did. Al "Beau" Jangl was no exception.

Jangl first introduced himself as my roommate in the men's dorm in August of 1972. That evening as I was preparing to run, he asked if he could join in, though he hadn't run for months. We set out at a comfortable pace.

Neither of us knew where we were going but were not concerned - runners have good instincts. We cut left at the corner, ran a mile then took another turn. Two miles on, we hit our first sign - **Winston Salem 26 -** not what we had in mind. We doubled back and looked for signs to the college. Nothing.

Desperate, we climbed a high metal fence and found ourselves in a loading zone - boxcars, scrap metal, railway tracks and filth. We scaled the fence on the other side and ran like escapees. Alas, a light - the old convenience store looked like the Taj Mahal.

"Where's the University from here?" I asked.

"University? Well, you gotta go back down this street 'til you get ta..., then..."

"How far is it?"

"About four or five miles, I reckon."

Our misadventure covered thirteen miles and more than two hours. My new roommate never complained. It was only the start of a greater challenge.

Dr. Solleder was Jangl's graduate advisor. She was conservative; he rode motorcycles with 'raked-out' handlebars. Her thoughts were 'old school;' his, radically new. She carried a briefcase; he, chains and a helmet. She lived in a professional shell; he was outgoing, to her, outrageous. She had power; he had none.

His thesis topic didn't help either - Abraham Maslow's "Self-Actualization" applied to classroom teaching - and the hours, nights and weekends he spent typing the thing led to the same end, rejection.

"Ridiculous! Change your topic. I won't have it," she bellowed.

It's tough to console someone who's throwing books around a room. Jangl expanded his ability to cuss and to rev-up an already loud bike.

By year's end, he completed the course work and invited me to his thesis presentation, same topic. During the question/answer phase, he mentioned, "Well, I changed..."

Dr. Solleder rose suddenly from her chair, "You changed **what**?"

If I only had the bike...

No one passed the four-hour written exam - the final frontier - the first time around. We both had to re-write the section we missed. I made it; Jangl didn't. That summer, he saved his caddy money to fly back and try again, but the result was clear. According to his advisor, he was "intellectually incapable of passing the course."

Jangl took his case to the Dean of the University. Nothing. He heaved a few more books, stormed off to teach and applied for a grant from Columbia University to complete his degree. They accepted only eight credits of work. He graduated in 1976.

His radical classroom teaching techniques worked so well that he eventually sent three of his own articles to Dr. Solleder. Yep, Al Jangl, *Health Education*.

Rev-up the bike.

# AUGUST

"Both problems, poor form and lowered intensity, result from a desire to show progress; thus, under the mistaken impression that they are thereby improving at a faster rate, most people quickly start changing the form or intensity of their exercises...and are encouraged that doing so increases the amount of resistance they can handle."

Arthur Jones

---

## Meanwhile...Back in the Playground

Time spent on the monkey bars in the school playground behind the house taught a valuable lesson about chin-ups. First, anything other than a palms-up, thumbs-out grip created nothing but a sudden 'thud' on the final effort, when the lower body swung forward to help. Second, I was right about the first. When it came time to test chin-up prowess, we were instructed to use the 'thumbs-out' grip, with hands close together. Still, there was something discriminatory about the procedure.

While the boys used a strong grip, the girls, who were not expected to perform chin-ups at all, placed their chins over the bar and hung there as long as possible employing a weak, thumbs-in grip. No wonder some used their teeth.

The biceps muscle of the upper arm has two functions: twisting the hand outward and bending the arm. The two, according to Arthur Jones, enhance one other. "Bending the arm increases bending strength - but it also increases twisting strength - and twisting the arm increases twisting strength - and also increases bending strength."

Place your right arm, palm-down, at your side and bend it so that the hand nears the shoulder. Grasp the right biceps with the left hand and notice the lack of firmness. Slowly rotate your right hand to a thumbs-out position and feel the biceps make a stronger contraction. The biceps is barely required to bend the arm, but crucial to twisting it - and twisting enhances the contraction of a bent biceps and its potential output.

Now, take a set of light dumbbells, hold them palms down straight in front of your shoulders, and slowly rotate your hands outward. Then, bring your elbows to your sides and do the same with your arms bent at $90°$. You'll discover more twisting strength when your arms are bent. This time, bending enhances the contraction of a twisted (supinated) biceps and its potential output.

Attempting a chin-up with one arm only will reveal the function of another muscle, the pectorals. Place your left hand over your right chest muscle with your fingers near the armpit. Lift your right arm over your head and pull it down in front. You'll feel your pectoral muscle tighten as the upper arm approaches a position close to and slightly in front of the body. Now, extend the same elbow behind your back and move its hand toward the floor as if to straighten the arm. The pectoral muscle will contract as before. According to Jones, "When the arm is moved into any other position, the pectoral will assist in returning it to that fully contracted position, from any direction."

To get the most out of the biceps, the arm must be bent and twisted to a thumbs-out position. Which means that chin-ups should be performed with a palms-up grip when to the front, or with a parallel grip (palms facing one another) when pulled behind the neck.

Yet, what do I see in gyms? The few who perform chin-ups (because they are difficult) use a reverse (thumbs-in) grip and a wide hand spacing in the mistaken belief that 'wide' provides a better stretch for the muscles of the upper back. Not so. A wide grip decreases the range of motion, providing less contraction and less stretch.

As Jones put it, "The pectoral and latissimus muscles move the upper arms - what happens to the hands and forearms is of no concern to the torso muscles...but if you must involve the arm muscles in torso exercises - as you must in conventional exercises - then at least do so only with the arms in the strongest possible position."

The next time you see someone perform a chin-up with a correct grip, call - I'll fly in with a plaque. Without knowing a thing, we knew more in the playground.


## AUGUST 2

---

### The Ideal Routine – Part 1

According to Arthur Jones, you'd better have a chair and a smile nearby if you ask the 'experts' for an ideal routine - you'll end up with a tearful earful. "If they even think they are right, I am suspicious," he said. "People have opinions and beliefs, they don't think."

With that, he set out in search of a logical, scientific approach to muscle building. What worked? What didn't? Why? His impact was immediate, if not always welcome.

"I tell the truth, and it shocks people. I am against fraud, against deception."

Jones was fully aware that genetics played a role. "People are individuals," he stressed, "and possible variations in individual response to training are literally infinite - so a program that is exactly right for one man will seldom or ever be perfect for another; but while the total number of possible variations is great, the 'range of possible variations' is quite small - and the limits of that range are clearly known."

In an attempt to narrow things down, he discovered that "muscles are best built not by the volume of work but rather by the energy put momentarily into that work." Eventually, his ultimate formula revolved around the words - hard, brief, slow and infrequent.

"Twenty-five years ago (around 1946)," he explained, "I had the distinct impression that the 'exact program' was of greatest importance - but I have long since realized that 'how' you train is of even more importance. Properly performed, even a few basic barbell exercises will produce good results - improperly performed, no amount of exercises or sets will produce equal results." Quality was the key.

Exercise had to be hard enough to stimulate growth without exceeding the system's ability to recover. "It is much easier to do an extra set than it is to perform the last two or three hard repetitions in a properly performed set...The first few repetitions are nothing more nor less than 'preparation.' They exhaust the muscles so that the last few repetitions can make demands that fall inside the momentary existing levels of reserve ability. Without which demands, growth will never occur." One set of 8-12 exercises to failure served the requirements for both stimulation and recovery.

Because it was hard, it had to be brief, and for recovery, infrequent. Jones advocated three weekly workouts of 30-40 minutes in 1970, two (of 15-20 minutes) in 1986 and less by 1996. "I know that one weekly workout is required by most subjects, and that some people do better with a schedule of only one workout every two weeks, and that a few people do best on a schedule of one workout every three weeks."

By then, he had developed the tools and performed the research to support most of his statements.

"Some of my firmly held opinions simply cannot be supported - in some cases I 'know' the facts, but I cannot explain how I know them...How, for example, would you describe a smile to a man born blind? Yet you recognize a smile, and an almost infinite variety of subtle variations in smiles; a friendly smile, a malicious smile, a doubting smile, a sly smile, and many other smiles with distinct meanings - all of these you recognize at once, but do you know how you recognize them? And of more direct importance, should you ignore such knowledge - simply because you can't explain it? I think not." His 'firm opinions' were backed by a high IQ and plenty of thought.

Following a 60-year search, the formula - hard, brief, slow and infrequent - was "so simple, so self-evidently true, that it seems ridiculous to even have to say it."

Yet, it remains as much a mystery to trainees as a smile to the blind.

## AUGUST 3

---

### The Ideal Routine – Part 2

I'm a fool or a liar, or both - that, according to Arthur Jones.

"Anybody who claims to be able to plan an ideal program of exercise for you is either a fool or a liar, and usually is both," said the Nautilus® inventor. "Yet, unfortunately, that seems to be what most people are seeking, somebody who will take them by the hand and lead them to the Promised Land. Most of what I have learned about exercise can be truthfully called 'negative knowledge,' things to be avoided, things that do not work, things that are always foolish, never productive, and sometimes dangerous. 'Positive knowledge,' something that does work, is in short supply, and suffers from the fact that it is not consistent from one person to another; that is, what works for you may not work for me, may even be counterproductive for me."

The process is further complicated by testing tools that are incapable of accurately quantifying what they reportedly measure, which renders most research useless and strands us with the opinions of those who have gone before - a scary proposition. "The simple truth," said Jones, "is that advanced bodybuilders in general have no slightest idea what they are doing - or even why they are doing it."

The result: "Most of the people who are now exercising, for any purpose," he added, "are largely wasting their time and efforts, are producing nothing close to the results that could be produced by much less exercise than they are now performing; a situation that is primarily caused by simple ignorance, a lack of knowledge."

In this era of high-tech computerized exercise, sadly enough, trial and error may be the only way to find out what works, with one suggestion: First consider the ingredients Jones acquired through 'negative knowledge' - less, hard, brief and infrequent exercise.

Now, back to the role of fool, liar, or both...

Find an exercise combination for major muscle groups based on need, not desire, and adopt a simple routine you can use as a measuring stick to test progress. Then, treat each exercise as the *only* one you plan to do. Perform it perfectly, as hard as your current condition allows, and minimize rest between efforts by timing your overall workout. On 'test' days use exactly the same *amount* of rest between exercises (as the week or month before) to get an accurate account of progress.

For those who require the 'Promised Land,' try the following:

| <u>**Machines**</u>   (Option B) | <u>**Conventional Equipment**</u> |
|---|---|
| Leg extension | Leg extension |
| Leg curl | Leg curl |
| Leg press  (Squat on Smith machine) | Leg press (Squat) |
| Chest press  (Pec deck) | Calf raise (with Dumbbell) |
| Lat pulldown  (Pullover) | Chest press (Dips) |
| Shoulder press (Lateral raise) | Lat pulldown (Chin-ups) |
| Biceps curl (Biceps curl) | Seated shoulder press |
| (Triceps extension) | Seated biceps curl |

Remember what Jones often reiterated, "It really doesn't matter why an exercise (or program) works as long as it is clear that it does." And like a computer, it works only if you work - garbage in, garbage out.

The ideal routine is the one you work hardest at, and about which you have no reservations or regrets. It's not necessarily the one you look forward to.

AUGUST 4

_____

### How Not to Make Friends and Influence People

I stood a self-proclaimed bodybuilder before a wall clock with a barbell he insisted he could curl 10 times - the issue was speed. The instructions were clear: "Lift the weight in 10 seconds and lower it in five *without* taking your eye off the clock." I didn't stipulate the number of repetitions because I wanted him to *feel* the resistance through the range of motion. I somehow knew the show wouldn't last - he was thinking 10, I was thinking four.

Bodybuilders generally favor heavy weights and low repetition schemes (6-10). They also love to 'throw' rather than 'lift' weights because it may be the only way to move something heavy. This guy's penchant for speed led me to believe that he had rarely exposed a muscle to resistance for more than a minute at a time. The math was easy - 10 seconds up, five seconds down times 10 repetitions - a 150-second biceps curl was highly unlikely.

The odds were in my favor.

Up he started, slow and sure. Down he lowered, slow and sure. The second attempt was equally noble. The third exposed a twisted lip and reddened face. The fourth barely made it. The fifth did not. He dropped the bar to the floor grasping both biceps. His mouth looked like a patriarch singing "Oh, Canada," without the "Canada." The pain was as obvious as something else - there was little learned.

Despite the fact that he at last *felt* the muscle work through a full range of motion, the next day (and in most cases, shortly thereafter) he was back doing what he did best, the old routine. I had taken him out of his comfort zone.

It is difficult to change old habits, especially amid the social pressure of the gym scene. It results in what I witness every day:

- No one does slow repetitions.
- No one does just one set of exercise, or just 2-3 times a week.
- No one works all the major body parts in a single session.
- No one works to the point of muscle failure, the ultimate way to stimulate change.
- No one dares lower the weight to a level that allows the performance of an exercise in proper form.
- No one risks being seen on a 'machine' when there are free weights available.
- No one combines movements, or moves quickly from one exercise to another (God forbid - headphones might suffer interruption!).
- No one wishes to endure the ridicule of peers by doing something 'off the beaten path.'
- No one listens to someone whose arms are smaller than his.
- And sadly, once they have your money, no one on the staff seems to care.

I apologize for the repeated use of the word, "no one." There are a few people training and teaching in a rational, safe and productive way. Unfortunately, they are not in the majority and certainly not the ones being copied.

The wheel doesn't beg reinvention in gyms.

Swallow your pride, big boy and start wondering what you'd look like if you did something right.

AUGUST 5

———————

## Perception and Injury

Muscles need the surprise of an overload to stimulate change, but they like exposure to surprise applied *their* way.

As a teen, I attended the wedding of a high-school friend in the beautiful lake-district north of Toronto. Following the reception at a remote resort, five of us piled into a Volkswagon® and headed for a cottage owned by one of the parents. To say the least, we were not in good shape.

The 40-minute drive was a mix of laughter and clinging to an elusive line on the road that led to a dark dock in the woods, the island cottage a mile away. The first drunk promptly walked off the end of the winding wood structure, while another strolled directly into the lake with his girlfriend, waist-high in formal attire and singing. The third made it to what I hoped was the right boat to prime the motor. With the wedding party in place (a story in itself), he cranked the cord but the beast was stubborn. He primed, cranked and swore. Finally, during one massive effort, the cord snapped and Charlie flew into the lake. There's nothing like a moonlit row.

I had the same occur on another continent, this time driving down a different elusive line, the middle of the fairway. As I swung a 6-iron through the ball to the final green at La Lagunita Country Club in Venezuela, I felt a sudden loss of resistance. The shaft had snapped sending the clubhead halfway to the hole and my back halfway to the hospital. Of greater importance, the ball found the green.

Back in Canada...exercise physiology professor, Digby Sale once called on a volunteer for a display of strength. On stage was a barbell stacked with heavy plates. A football player braced for the lift and whoosh, up it went with unexpected ease. Most of the plates were fakes.

Injury is not caused by resistance itself, but rather by a sudden change in speed while moving against resistance - and it doesn't matter in which direction. A sudden start can be just as dangerous as a sudden stop.

In the above examples, muscles expected to encounter a certain resistance. When they were suddenly exposed to something different by accident or design, the potential for injury increased significantly.

In a gym setting, muscles expect a 50-pound barbell (or weight of a known level) to have a certain 'feel.' Imagine what would happen if the weight was suddenly and randomly modified by remote control on each repetition of a biceps curl. Fifty pounds on the first repetition, 250 on the second, 95 on the third and zero on the fourth would likely result in smacking yourself on the forehead a few times. Muscles like to know what's coming.

As stupid as that sounds, and is, it mirrors what occurs with the majority of trainees in gyms, with one difference - it's not by accident.

Some do it out of ignorance; others, because everyone else is; and a growing minority, because they pay for, and are taught to engage in, such nonsense. The macho jerk common to most strength training exercises elevates the force to which a muscle is exposed. It makes a 50-pound bar suddenly weigh much more, and then, with resulting momentum, much less. The sensation of dramatic change - easy-to-hard and slow-to-fast - only puts muscles closer to the end of the dock.

If they had their say, muscles would opt for safe, slow and smooth - *their* way.

## AUGUST 6

### The Ungracious Host

One of the most brilliant minds in the field of exercise never looked the role. He anticipated the daily arrival of physicians (to whom he would lecture) by filling a mug with coffee and adopting a familiar stance: feet spread, weight on heels, and shoes splayed outward, curled up at the toes. His footwear was black and old, but clean - except for the coffee stains on one toe, remnants of a right-handed addict.

The stains were patterned around the steady, rhythmic sway of his torso, like an elephant at the zoo. Some drops hit their target; others did not. You'd expect to see a fossil like this sweeping the floor, not selling medical equipment at $60,000 a pop.

Arthur Jones was there for one reason - education - and he promoted his exercise and testing tools with one approach - if you weren't smart enough to buy them, the next guy would. Yet, as superb as his presentation was and as generous as he could be, he often insulted guests along the way... when necessary.

Many times he repelled physicians who had purchased the useless technology of his competitors by calling them idiots, but that wasn't enough. Arthur showed them why they were idiots, stared them down and waited for a reaction.

My first encounter with Jones was indirect, through a receptionist who possessed the social graces he lacked. After attending a lecture on the Lumbar Extension machine, I asked her where I could stay.

"Oh, you don't have a place? Just go to the Holiday Inn® or Howard Johnson's® in town and tell them you're with MedX®. They'll take care of you."

I drove down and mentioned the magic word.

"Welcome to Ocala (Florida)," said the hotel clerk. "Stay as long as you want, eat as much as you'd like and make as many phone calls as you need. Arthur Jones will pick up the tab."

I stayed for a week, thank you.

Despite his desire to educate both the masses and the medical community, Jones excelled with manageable groups - the smaller the better. "The paradox of technocracy," he said in describing the price of fame, "seems to be that survival presupposes the ability to attract crowds - which crowds make survival unacceptable." *Nautilus Training Principles: Bulletin No. 2* (1971).

The feeling surfaced when he felt trapped in his own creation.

Arthur once hosted a gathering of about 500 people (a military or YMCA group) at his home. Toward the middle of the evening, he sauntered to the buffet table - rarely a priority - and plunked a spoonful of beans and a dinner roll on an oversized plate. He then scanned the once-bountiful, now-ravished serving trays and snarled, "Damn, these people were hungry."

On another occasion, he hosted a New Year's party and spared no expense in decorating the premises with dining tents and entertainment areas for the 600 invitees. When he walked out to join the festivities, he immediately sensed the problem.

"Where the hell did all these people come from?" he blurted.

There were more than 1,200 guests wandering around his backyard.

Little did they know that there were not alone. Approximately 1,400 of Arthur's pet crocodiles lurked in their private pens less than 100 yards away.

I'm not certain he would have hesitated to open the floodgates that night.

## AUGUST 7

---

### Where There's a Boot Hill, There's a Way

Whenever I sought the shelter of her arms and the refuge of her silence, I was at once 'King of the Hill,' bounding with energy that no patron could match. The problem was finding her.

"Can you direct me to the nearest cemetery?" I asked.

Once the route was uncovered, I drove through her pearly gates, searched for a shade tree beyond the grasp of humanity and flipped the trunk release. There, I removed the Christmas gift that started it all - the bars, plates and collars - and watched the rear tires sigh in relief. The burden was off.

I was addicted to strength training (at a time it was considered "dumb") and vowed never to miss a workout, which meant lugging its tools around in the trunk of my car any time a session lay in jeopardy.

Why a cemetery?

I felt comfortable there - as we all eventually must - having walked through one to and from high school. And, other than a few pick-up games of basketball in the mausoleum where the floor provided a haunting echo, a cemetery was peaceful, its fresh air disrupted only by an occasional whiff of abandoned flowers. It provided a time and place to feel strong and vibrant - and the motivation to remain as George Borrow described in *The Bruisers of England*, "still above the sod."

It was also practical. Tombstones came in different shapes and sizes, making it easy to acquire the right slab for the task. The toughest find was one that furnished a comfortable width for a bench press. Too wide hampered range of motion; too narrow dug into your back.

Once stationed, I put the one-set theory to task, beginning with squats. Slowly, I lowered my butt until it touched the tip of a stone, and followed with one-legged calf raises from the edge of a plaque that barely broke the surface. Then, it was on to chest flys and presses from the 'elusive' headstone (if found) and one-arm rows from mid-high marble. Seated lateral raises and overhead presses ensued, with arm and wrist work close behind. The non-stop circuit and fear of arrest produced a cardiovascular effect that lasted 30 minutes; then, it was back to the trunk and out the gate.

It wasn't bodybuilding's finest hour - it was her finest half-hour.

The most famous witness to the insanity lay in a plot in Valhalla, New York. Big-band leader, Tommy Dorsey and his glass-encased trombone heard more huffing and puffing that day than during their final performance. For the squeamish, my apparent disrespect for the dead was countered by the fact that I stopped *for one thing only* during a 15-year running career - funeral processions.

The strangest workout occurred between two parked cars in New York City near the end of December when I was forced to park too far from the apartment to lug barbells through snow. So, I popped the trunk, sat on the bumper of the car behind and blended my breath with the adjacent traffic as a jacket, earmuffs and gloves urged the weights skyward in the bitter cold, rep after rep. Only a best effort could generate enough heat to stay warm.

The city wasn't as peaceful as the cemetery - people hustled about too cold to gawk, too busy to appreciate good form - but the two had something in common.

No one batted an eye.

## AUGUST 8

### Star Power

"There's Lee Trevino," I said as I pointed from behind ropes that were set far from the action. It was my wife's first trip to a golf tournament.

"Give me the camera," she said as I dug it out of a pocket. Long before she was aware it was taboo, she ducked under the rope and headed for the practice area. Moments later, she jabbered something in Spanish and asked an adjacent player to take a picture. Later that day, she did the same with Arnold Palmer, Gary Player and Doug Sanders - autographs, pictures - as if there was nothing to it.

Her performance reflected Bernard Darwin's description (from *James Braid*, 1952) of the visit of three-time and current (1879) British Open Champion, Jamie Anderson to Elie, the course where 9-year old Braid caddied.

"To James (Braid) he represented no doubt all that was great and heroic from the far away outside world of St. Andrews, and the boy followed him round with adoring dog-like eyes; followed as near as he could so that he might touch, if not the hem of his garment, at any rate his bag of clubs, hear some of the words of wisdom that fell from the great man's lips and pass them on later to privileged companions."

Hero worship is human nature. The mention of a name in a gathering usually triggers a story from someone. In my case, the word "softball" triggers tales of Eddie Feiner; "golf," stories of Jack Nicklaus, Moe Norman and others; and "exercise," thoughts of Arthur Jones (he barked, I had the dog-like eyes). The knee-jerk response runs deep, sometimes too deep.

I once worked for a man who was adept at attracting celebrity to his gym with his out-going personality. One day it was Jack Nicklaus, the next Jesper Parnevik, then, Jack Welsh, Mike Schmidt and Ivan Lendl. One by one, the stars were passed on to other members of a competent staff, which was apparently not enough to keep customer satisfaction high. He was a tough act to follow.

The next boss would have nothing to do with celebrity, other than his own. He was so obsessed with putting his name on the building, that he replaced a great staff with a cheaper version and slowly sank into the west.

Celebrity may not beef up the bottom line, but it does a resume. I trained a few world champions at the top of their game, but had little or nothing to do with their success. They were champions long before I met them.

'Celebrity' occurs in the gym when we hang our hat on every word of the guy with the biggest arms. In most cases, it matters little what he says or does. Few have any clue as to how they got there (if not by steroids), but they'll be glad to tell you how, which identifies another problem - lack of ropes. More than golfers, genetic freaks are accessible and their information free.

A stock-market 'genius' in our gym once dispensed tips to a captive audience while the market was up, but had about the same to say as a bodybuilding magazine when it went down - nothing. Unfortunately, advice from trainers and peers is much the same. Bold? Condescending? No. Just watch the performance of repetitions in fitness centers. Certified? Big arms? Boo hoo.

One day, I asked a wealthy client the secret of his success.

"Years ago I won the lottery," he replied.

So did every gorilla in the gym.

## AUGUST 9

---

### The Early Arm Routine

When Arthur Jones opened his Nautilus® facility in Lake Helen, Florida (1970), he was still tweaking his approach. After 20 years of training 10 hours per week, he cut his workouts in half and in one week "reached a muscular size and strength level that he had never been able to attain." He was also developing tools that made exercise harder and more productive despite the fact that he believed real progress in the field of exercise "would not be reached by significant improvements in equipment." How you trained was more important than what you used.

Training had to be BRIEF in the extreme. "We will eventually, and rather soon," he said, "reduce the requirement for training to about 1½ hours weekly; and I mean the requirement for an advanced bodybuilder who is training for world-class physique competition - and I also mean that any more training would actually reduce the production of results."

I promoted his brief routines for years, while my audience scoffed at the idea - five minutes of legs; 12 minutes of torso; and seven minutes, 20 seconds of arms.

No one scoffed at the intensity.

The other day I came across the 'old' arm routine (*Nautilus Training Principles; Bulletin No. 2, 1971*) and its long-forgotten sequence:

1. Standing Curl with a barbell - One set of 10 repetitions.
2. Nautilus Triceps Machine (a plate-loaded version) - One set of 12 repetitions.
3. Nautilus Biceps Machine (a plate-loaded version) - One set of 12 repetitions.
4. Wrist Curls with a barbell - One set of 15 repetitions.
5. Reverse Wrist Curls with a barbell - One set of 15 repetitions. Brief **PAUSE**.
6. Nautilus Triceps Machine - One set of 12 repetitions.
7. **RUSH** - Parallel Dips - One set of maximum-possible repetitions.
8. Nautilus Biceps Curls - One set of 12 repetitions.
9. **RUSH** - Front Pulldowns (with a close grip) on a Nautilus Torso-Arm Machine - One set of approximately 10 repetitions.
10. Wrist Curls with a barbell - One set of 15 repetitions.
11. Reverse Wrist Curls with a barbell - One set of 15 repetitions.

The recommendations were to perform the first five exercises in about four minutes with a brief pause between sets, "although little or no harm would result if as much as ten minutes was used." But the RUSH factor from exercise #6 to #7, and #8 to #9 was a MUST to complete as quickly as possible - "and certainly in less than three seconds."

The routine, according to Jones, was "the exact schedule being used by our largest and strongest trainees, some of the strongest men in the world. At times, we do a bit more - but at other times, we do quite a bit less; and when any doubt exists, we always do LESS. And we NEVER do MUCH MORE." He continued, "No *amount* of exercise performed in another fashion will produce equal results...because this actually is HARD exercise - you not only don't need much of such exercise, you literally can't stand much of it."

How effective was it?

"Without single exception up to this point," claimed Jones, "we have been able to add from 3/8 of an inch to ½ inch to the cold measurement of the upper-arms of advanced bodybuilders within a matter of a very few days of proper training."

Try it and I'll guarantee something else. Properly performed, you won't like it.

## AUGUST 10

---

### Thump, Thump, Boom

I had the window down, heard its approach, but never gave it much thought - I-95 is a noisy place. Boom-boom-boom, boom-boom-boom, boom-boom-boom, boom - a car sped by on the left, its front tire thumping from poor balance. A mile ahead, it came to a halt on the side of the road with skid marks leading to its final destination.

Tires are wonderful tools when they're round and cared for. I recently had a set last 72,000 miles by regular rotations and air-pressure checks. It's a different story, however, when they're not cared for...or not round.

One of the major developments in the evolution of the wheel occurred when someone lopped off the sides of a square. Instead of four large jolts per revolution, people were exposed to eight smaller ones, then sixteen, 32 and eventually none as 'round' proved the most efficient and effective way to travel. Whether it was four or 32 bumps, the results were generally the same - negative - and the problem was not limited to the field of transportation.

The craze of 'aerobic' exercise went through a similar series of changes related to impact. From high-to-low-to-no-impact, the experts systematically swept the 'bad' under the table, realizing that the body could only take so much before it looked like the tire on I-95. It didn't take long before other experts flooded the market with 'other' steps in the wrong direction.

In the 1970's, the arrival of Nautilus® machines ushered in an era that preached control of momentum. Machines were safer than free weights, although 'slack' between weight stacks and movement-arms produced a slight impact on muscles. The laws of physics clearly showed that jerking weights with any equipment led to injury and to less work for the muscles as they moved through their range. Few bodybuilders listened, but the average trainee had a handle on safety and productivity.

So why is the field now reverting back to square? Because a bunch of pinheads calling themselves 'performance enhancement professionals' have convinced the world that square is better than round, that four large impacts are better than 32 small ones. Yet, as one trainer commented in reference to the two most popular buzzwords in exercise, plyometrics and periodization, "Two wrongs don't make a right."

Nautilus inventor, Arthur Jones once told a story of an employee named Herbert Prechtel. "I picked him up hitch-hiking," he said. "He knew me from my television show and wanted a job. I didn't really have a need for anyone at the time, but I contacted his parents and he went to work for me. One day I heard a noise upstairs, BUMP, BUMP, BUMP. I went upstairs and asked Herbert what the hell was going on. He was sitting cross-legged on the floor and said he was trying to levitate. I said, 'Herbert, that's impossible. It's against the laws of physics.' He said that he was going to levitate and bet me $10,000 that he would do it. I told him, 'Herbert, you got the takeoffs down but your landings need a little work!' I never did get the $10,000."

The field of exercise has taken a direction that will eventually provide a major jolt to those who follow. Two co-workers recently attended a seminar hosted by a 'pioneer' in sports performance training and were duly impressed with his intelligence.

Intelligence, however, can't change the laws of physics, or, as Arthur put it, "Herbert was one of the most intelligent men I've ever known. He's in an insane asylum now."

He won't be alone.

## AUGUST 11

### The Amazing Journey

On June 1, 1809, Captain Barclay set out on a journey that "attracted notice of the whole kingdom, and raised the highest expectations among the amateurs of pedestrian exploits." He set out to walk "ONE THOUSAND MILES IN ONE THOUSAND SUCCESSIVE HOURS, at the rate of a mile in each and every hour."

It was a daunting task. At the time, the most celebrated walkers in England had tried it, but no one had made it past 30 days (1,000 hours is 41.7 days). This time there was money on the line - 1,000 guineas (then, $5,250) waged by 'a gentleman of celebrity in the sporting world,' Mr. Wedderburn Webster.

The prize forced Captain Barclay into heavy training. A few days before the event, he traveled to Brighton to get some sea, sand and fresh air. As Walter Thom wrote in *Pedestrianism*, "He believed the undertaking would be easily accomplished."

It was at the start. Even with a change of route and accommodations, and amid cries that "the constant exertion, with the short time allowed for sleep, must soon exhaust the strongest frame," the Captain marched on, eventually with "spasmodic affections in his legs." He slept when he could, ate at regular intervals but started losing weight. It mattered little. Bets were in his favor, 2-to-1, and rising.

On the 12th day of July at 3:37 PM, he concluded a final 22-minute mile to the cheers of thousands of spectators. He promptly took a brief bath, went to bed for 17 hours and "seemed as well as before he started" five days later.

Captain Barclay's feat demonstrates a number of things. First, from the beginning of time, there has always been a record to be had and a crackpot to put it to the test.

Second, the repetition of a low-intensity task such as walking 2.5 to 3 miles per hour has little effect on the stimulation of muscle, not enough to sustain its mass. During the ordeal, the Captain lost 32 pounds (from 186 to 154), the majority from his muscle mass (aerobic activity has that effect). His daily regimen of liquids amounted to "a pint of strong ale and two cups of tea" at breakfast and two or three glasses of wine at lunch and supper. If water-weight was lost, and it was, remember: muscle is 72% water; 9%, fat.

Third, leg spasms were a minor issue. The sustained activity taxed his system to the point that a rest of 35-40 minutes per hour proved insufficient for its recovery. Without rest (for limbs, system or both), progress slows or halts.

Many of today's trainees act like the Captain. First, they train as if they are trying to break the record for quantity. Second, they repeat tasks that are easier than they could and should be and, because of the amount of work performed, the intensity falls short of stimulating change. Third, the day-to-day regimen of exercise, combined with a lack of rest for both muscle and system creates a situation where the body does not have enough 'reserve' to fully recover. Sure, the work-rest ratio is about the same as the Captain's walk - one part exercise, two parts rest - but the work is more intense and the system needs a greater repose. Two hours of training followed by 22 hours of rest (that most adhere to) is not enough. The weight of evidence suggests a minimum of 48 hours rest between workouts for best results.

It's a good thing trainers weren't certified in 1809. They would have had the poor Captain walk the first mile normally; the second, backwards; the third, sideways; and the fourth on his hands to spread the fatigue. Would it have made a difference? Nope.

My advice to most trainees: go to Brighton, to the sea, the sand and the fresh air.


## AUGUST 12

---

### Formal Exercise


Charles Herbert Burton believed in the longevity of foolishness and the brevity of youth. He also knew that laughing the night away was not the best preparation for an 8:00 AM cross-country meet, but it was warranted - and miles ahead of the competition.

There was reason to celebrate. It was my 21st birthday, and Charlie and I hadn't seen much of each other since high school.

There was reason to laugh. I stepped off the bus in a Superman outfit, double-breasted Clark Kent suit, fedora and 'new' haircut. I grew a beard for four months and had my hair shaved off just before mounting the bus.

There was reason to run. The meet was scheduled the day after the "Engineer's Ball," a black-tie event of immense proportions. Most of the field would be drunk.

Queen's University in Kingston, Ontario was less than balmy. I played golf there years before in the middle of October. It was just above freezing when we started and much the same after 36 holes. February was worse.

It was cold, damp, and the breeze off Lake Ontario brisk as Charlie headed for a starting line that looked more like a Halloween gala than an athletic event. Had I worn it, the Superman outfit would have gone unnoticed.

Traces of the "Ball" were everywhere - top hats, cumberbuns, striped pants, frilled shirts, jackets, tails, vests and yes, dress shoes. Shouting, drinking, a lone gunshot - the race was on.

Charlie started well amid a sea of flailing limbs but finished 'in the pack' due to a lousy route sign. Nonetheless, the finish was entertaining. Some crossed by diving into the mud-strewn path. Others slid into 'home' with the same end. My introduction to 'formal' exercise was a banner day for the dry-cleaning industry.

I had no room to talk. I spent the rest of the day in a Superman outfit running from phone booth to phone booth downtown and cruising the side-lines of a football game.

And what does this have to do with exercise? Not much, because our shenanigans shouldn't be considered 'exercise' in the first place.

Exercise is movement against resistance, not just movement. Ellington Darden, Ph.D., defined it as "a logical strategy designed around the body's muscular functions, an attempt to stimulate physical improvements in the body" and judged its value by the quality of the resistance and the range of motion. Exercise is hard work, not fun.

Recreation, on the other hand, is instinctive and pursued for personal reasons, mental benefit and for fun, even when it embraces a major physical component.

Properly performed, exercise provides five physiological benefits: strength, flexibility, cardiovascular condition, protection from injury and a reduction in body fat.

Properly performed, recreation and sports provide one or two at best.

Yet, when most are asked about their exercise habits, they respond in the manner of St. Francis of Assisi, "of all his body he made a tongue," and produce a list of recreational activities - swimming, bridge, walking, yoga and racquetball. All are great choices if they are backed up by 'real' exercise - proper strength training that provides the base from which to pursue recreation.

The idiots running around Kingston that day were at least aware that progressive resistance training allowed their instinctive fun to happen in a safe, if not sane, manner.

Charles Herbert Burton and I have lifted weights for years.

## AUGUST 13

---

### "We Now Know..."

I smoked my first cigarette at seven, in grade two, but Dad would have none of it. His backhand saved the day and led me to vow, as a teen, never to smoke - a promise I have kept to this day. No wonder I ignored the advice of a chain smoker on pre-competition warm-up at an exercise seminar. By then, I had coached track-and-field long enough to recognize that this information was hogwash:

*"Keep the fast-twitch athlete in the deep freeze until the gun goes off. Let the slow-twitch competitor run half the race before it starts."*

MedX® inventor Arthur Jones was a master at provoking thought by defending what appeared to be outrageous statements with fact and logic. Years of exercise-equipment design and thousands of isolated muscle tests led him to, one day, spout his pet phrase, *"We now know..."*

It was usually something only Arthur knew, and always on the money.

Jones developed a motorized (isokinetic) leg extension machine that measured muscle fatigue from one repetition to another. It recorded the torque produced during the first repetition (a maximum effort) as 100%, and displayed the remaining repetitions (all maximum efforts) as percentages of the first. Exercise was halted when strength dipped below 75% of its starting level.

One subject's second repetition measured slightly above 89% of his first (a loss of more than 10% strength). His third fell between 82% and 83% (a loss of about 7% from the second repetition); and fourth, 73% (a loss of more than 9% from the third repetition). The total strength loss of 27% from three all-out repetitions represented a typical fast-twitch (fast fatigue) response to exercise.

Another subject's second repetition was 106%; his third, 114%; and fourth, 118% (18% higher than his first). From that point he dropped gradually, but did not dip below 75% until the 11th repetition, a typical slow-twitch (slow fatigue) response.

The fatigue characteristics of a muscle can be determined by first establishing how much you can lift one time. If you can perform more than one repetition with the resistance in trial, test with a heavier weight until you establish a one-repetition maximum. Then, on another occasion, do as many repetitions as you can with 80% of that maximum. A performance of 10-11 repetitions indicates a muscle with an average mix of fibers; 4-5 repetitions, a predominance of fast-twitch fibers; more than 20 repetitions, an abundance of slow-twitch fibers.

For best results from strength training, apply the information as follows:
- If your muscle fatigues at a fast rate, perform 4-7 repetitions of exercise (less than four, the weight is too heavy; more than seven, the weight should be increased).
- If your muscle has an average rate of fatigue, perform 8-12 repetitions.
- If your muscle fatigues at a slow rate, perform 15-20 repetitions.

A muscle's fatigue characteristics cannot be determined by movements that involve more than one joint system. Leg extension, leg curl, hip adduction/abduction, calf raise, pullover, pectoral fly, lateral raise, biceps curl and triceps extension machines (performed in strict form) are valid choices. With free weights, only calf raises, biceps curls, triceps extensions and wrist curls can be considered valid.

Gary Bannister, B.A., B.P.E., M.Ed.

*"We now know..."* that a lengthy warm-up prior to competition will benefit the slow-twitch athlete, but greatly reduce the strength of the fast-twitch.

## AUGUST 14

### Trick or Treat?

There was nothing pretty about what squeezed into the van: an Israeli who looked and played like a bulldozer; two fiery Arabs with curly black beards; a thin-but-game Puerto Rican; a Colombian who had 'game' when he wasn't half-stoned; an African-American basketball diehard who had never played; our last line of defense, a rugged guy named Cam who sported a blonde pony-tail tied at the back; a handful of Americans of varying shapes and sizes with more desire than talent; and a Canadian coach who lacked the glue to hold them together.

The Averett College Men's Soccer Team was off; this time to up-state Virginia.

As we rolled to our destination, English took second stage. 'Cam' became 'Clem' - it was too difficult to pronounce, but not nearly as difficult as the names lanced at two females making obscene gestures from a passing convert-ible.

When things settled, a lone voice piped up from the back of the van. "Hey, Coach, you bring the costumes?"

It was a tribute to the fact that we had just purchased new team uniforms. And to the fact that, other than honest effort, putting this crew on the field was like opening your door at Halloween - you never knew what to expect.

On one occasion, we defeated a Greensboro College team laden with Af-ricans on scholarship. The 1-0 margin was due to a blind leap with closed eyes, a ball that struck the head of a basketball player and nothing but net.

On another occasion we couldn't find the net, but our opponent did, seven times.

It was feast or famine and, in that sense, like many personal experiences in sport where I wore my own share of costumes.

"Nattily dressed in a shocking pink outfit" was the *Hamilton Spectator*'s take on my playoff loss in the 1970 Ontario-Quebec Athletic Association golf championship. Three years later in the second round of the Porter Cup (Lewiston, NY), I selected a dazzling pair of polyester slacks to reach the pinnacle of my golfing career by defeating Ben Crenshaw - 72 to 77. Fifteen years later, I upset European tour-player, Carlos Larraine in the first round of the Venezu-elan Match-Play championship. Yet, on more occasions than I care to recall and to use Dad's expression, "I couldn't hit a cow in the ass with a shovel" while wearing a Superman outfit (and I had one of those).

My preparation was vast and game 'consistent' according to peers, yet I never knew who was going to show up. When the right guy did, the experience was satisfying; when he didn't, it was miserable.

Years of shade for a moment of sunshine, reams of frustration for a line of glory led me to conclude that it was the nature of the beast. The most important thing was the process, the act of knocking on the door.

The gym scene was no different. Strength training kept me in the game but eventually took on a character that revealed the reason I was there - the pro-cess.

Good days were cloaked in measurable progress and, when not, a gallant effort. Bad days were replete with no hint of progress and, too often, a medio-cre attempt. For every good day, there were 10 bad ones - again, the nature of the beast - but I never failed to show.

The next time you open a door that leads to a band of renegades nattily dressed in shocking gym outfits, stick around for the candy.

## AUGUST 15

### The Bull Stops Here

The crowd stood shoulder to shoulder on the fringe of the final green and watched as amateur Jay Sigel stood over a short putt to seal the American victory. He and his partner had breezed through a 22-nation field to win the Simon Bolivar Cup at the Valle Arriba Golf Club in Caracas, Venezuela. The man to my right, my wife's boss, could barely contain himself. When the putt went down, he stormed the green and began shaking hands, slapping backs and snapping photos. God had a different plan.

Manuel was a handsome, worldly gentleman, wealthy, yet down to earth. He walked briskly and kept himself in good shape following a heart attack a few years before. He was a comfortable companion, which made his invitation easy to accept.

"Why don't you join us for dinner this evening?" he asked.

My wife and I followed him by car to an apartment on the way to the Holiday Inn®, where he had rented a room for the weekend. As he grabbed a couple of suits from the closet, Manuel came across an old chest that he simply had to open.

"This is the cape of one of the greatest bullfighters in Spain," he said as he extracted a magnificent red garment from the wooden confines. "He gave it to me in 1969."

One by one he hauled out items, each with a story - a cap, a shirt, a vest, pants, hose, sword, slippers. He carefully wrapped them in the suits and headed for the hotel. Once there, we jumped on the elevator and sat in the room while he showered, dressed and talked...and talked...and talked...about bullfights.

Since I had never seen one, he decided to demonstrate the entire process, starting with the ritual of dress. First this, then that, now the pants, the frilled shirt, the fancy vest and the hat, "not yet." Manuel was stone serious, so much so that my wife high-tailed it downstairs when he entered the bathroom for prayer - a litany of soft and harsh sounds that confirmed her belief the boss had gone "loco."

Five minutes later, the warrior made his exit - tight pants, snug vest, cap and swagger in place. He riveted his eyes on the floor, then the ceiling as he thrust his shoulders back. Ceasing in mid-strut, he offered me the vital role of 'assistant' in the battle - the best offer I'd had since the high-school play. I stuck around to be polite.

My respect for bullfighters rose quickly as the procession moved from the room to the hallway. The cape was heavier than expected; the pace, slow. I silently hung on.

The 'torero' strutted down the empty hallway, tipping his cap to the accolades of a roaring crowd. He signaled for the cape and awaited his adversary. Suddenly, he swished the cloak to the left and pranced away. Then to the right with an elegant spin as a wide-eyed couple squeezed along the wall to their room. The battle continued, back and forth, left and right. Finally, with sweat seeping from his pores, he called for the sword.

Only I sweated more as I relinquished the blade and thought, the first guy out the elevator door was a dead duck. But not so. The matador measured his pace and slayed the beast just beneath the ashtray. The crowd went wild as Manuel paraded for the shower. I bolted downstairs for my wife. Dinner would have to wait.

Nautilus® inventor, Arthur Jones probably missed a few meals because of his battle with the same in the field of exercise. Like Manuel, he must have felt alone in his quest. Perhaps he was lucky enough to have felt something.

Manuel died three days later of a heart condition.

Arthur hasn't done that yet and, from all reports, neither has the bull.

## AUGUST 16

---

### Hoodwinked

The only way to escape poverty in Venezuela was to play the lottery. So, in a moment of weakness and of flirting with that state, I purchased a ticket and won about $500. The system eventually caught up.

"Pst...Epa, Gringo," said the man as he pulled a ticket from his jacket on a busy street. The ticket, he claimed, belonged to a lady unaware that she had won. The prize was mine if I could come up with 20,000 Bolivares (approximately $4,500).

I rushed home for a checkbook, entered the bank with the 'ticket man' and mounted a bus to return to the original scene - pocket full of small bills and head dancing with large. We got off the bus and walked to a corner for the 'exchange.' As I waited for him to retrieve his car, things started to sink in. The good news: I was alive - surely, the man had a gun. The bad news: the money belonged to a business, which didn't please my partner.

A similar situation exists in the field of exercise where new trainees are either left to their own following an orientation or highly influenced by the incompetence of others. According to Nautilus® inventor Arthur Jones, results with both are about the same.

"If the potential productivity of weight training was judged upon a careful comparison of the number of trainees who produce at least some degree of visible results from their training and the numbers that produce NO VISIBLE RESULT," he speculated, "then the only possible logical conclusion would be that weight training is totally without value. Yet the truth of the matter is that progressive weight training is by far the most productive form of exercise ever discovered. And good results can be produced in at least 95 percent of a randomly selected group of subjects - almost without regard for the age of the subjects."

Most people quit before they ever see a result, and Jones thought he knew the reason why: "Primarily - and this is clear from ALL of the evidence - because most subjects train improperly, train in such a fashion that little or nothing in the way of growth stimulation is produced, and usually train so much that growth would be impossible even if growth stimulation is produced."

Consequently, the average production of results from strength training (as in golf) is like the stagecoach wheel that appears to be spinning backwards in the movies. In golf, improved teaching methods and recent advances in technology have kept the Royal and Ancient Keeper-of-the-Gate on his toes. Yet, the score of the average player has not improved. In exercise, the countless new methods of training are, in Shakespeare's words, "Much ado about nothing," Many provide nothing but variety, while others are a step in the wrong direction.

The other day, I entered a gym that featured Free Motion® equipment - a pulley system used to simulate sports movements. The bad news: The machine failed to directly address major muscle groups (the power source in sports) and had the potential to interrupt skill patterns. The good news: It required creativity and a feather duster to use (its use was infrequent). Nonetheless, it will not likely go away without a fight.

"One of the saddest lessons in history is this," said astro-physicist, Carl Sagan. "If we've been bamboozled long enough, we tend to reject any evidence of the bamboozle. We're no longer interested in finding out the truth. The bamboozle has captured us. It is simply too painful to acknowledge - even to ourselves - that we've been so credulous. So the old bamboozles tend to persist as the new bamboozles rise."

## AUGUST 17

### Smoking Gun

The controversy created by the introduction of Nautilus® machines in the early 1970's was the equivalent of a group of bandits riding into town with pistols blazing in a cowboy movie. The intrusion was bold; the town, far from ready.

Nautilus inventor Arthur Jones, one of the few brilliant minds in exercise, didn't shy from conflict. "Recognition has a price," he said. "The price is danger." He wouldn't walk from his bedroom to his bathroom without his "boy's home companion," a Colt® .45 revolver that he kept under the car seat or in his trousers.

He was prepared, but the townsfolk got nasty.

The largest manufacturer of exercise machines at the time, Universal®, reacted as expected: First, they ignored; then, ridiculed, attacked, copied and stole. After a year of ignoring Nautilus, they spread rumors that Jones' innovations were dangerous and unnecessary. Their equipment was perfect, but sales were down.

By 1973, they went on the attack. Jones, now "a member of the Cleveland Mafia," had all of his advertising material stolen at the Mr. America show that year. The next day, it was being distributed (and had been doctored with claims of fraud) by Universal sales manager, Ed Burke at a convention in Atlanta. Nautilus continued to grow.

Universal then hired Gideon Ariel who introduced 'Dynamic Variable Resistance' to their line. The resistance did change, according to Jones, but in a "reverse" manner. He sat tight, collecting sworn statements about rumors until he was ready to make his move.

In an ad titled "Criminal Fraud, or Unbelievable Stupidity" (*Athletic Journal*, Nov. 1974), Jones outlined his accusations. Universal replied with an attack in the same issue. Months later, Arthur began collecting depositions - but one was enough. Burke lied to the extent that his lawyers realized they had no case. Universal settled, but their actions continued - this time in the form of a booklet that savagely attacked Jones.

At a health-club conference in 1975, Jones met Ariel again, in a taxi, on the way to a presentation (by Jones) about computerized equipment. Ariel wanted to get involved. Jones mistakenly signed him to "probably the most detailed contract in history" as 'protection' against stealing credit for his work. Unknown to Jones, Ariel had signed 'exclusive' contracts with other companies and claimed, through phony patent applications, that Jones' ideas were really his, years before. He conspired to take credit for the same with several high-ranking officials of the US Olympic Committee.

Jones eventually cornered him and taped the conversation.

At the 1978 annual meeting of the American College of Sports Medicine, Jones was invited to 'reply' to the introduction of Ariel's computerized machines. Arthur had the proof - and manpower - to bury him on the spot. When Jones took the floor, his entourage stood with him - Jim Flanagan (6'5", 250 pounds), "Foots" Lee (290-pound center for the Tampa Bay Bucs) and Dick Butkus, who, days earlier, had been knocked unconscious in a car accident and had two black eyes, patches of hair missing and enough stitches on his face to keep anyone at bay. The instructions were clear. "Do not raise your voice, and do not raise a hand, except in self-defense; but if we are attacked then I want everybody in that room to end up in the emergency ward of some hospital."

Nobody moved - not even Ariel's 'stooge,' a man Arthur called Dr. Dumb-Dumb.

"Some people need hurting," Jones reiterated. "Or, as a friend of mine says...'I don't care what the problem is, the solution is violence.'" It worked in this town.

## AUGUST 18

### The Lazy Man's Challenge

There are three words in the phrase "Progressive Resistance Exercise," each one a little tougher than the next.

Twenty years ago, "exercise" could well have been synonymous with, "Something difficult to get people to do." In today's society, as solutions to problems become easier and demand for the same rises, the word 'extremely' may need injection between 'something' and 'difficult.'

For those who pass that hurdle, the second word offers more challenge - "resistance." In the past 30 years, the abundance of research and belief that people are dying of 'heart problems' faster than they are of 'strength problems' has produced a bias toward cardiovascular exercise. Yet, injury, mobility and heart-lung ability are all dependent upon muscle strength. Resistance training should be - and may one day become - the focal point of exercise.

For those who cross that barrier, the third word appears the most difficult - "progressive." There is nothing progressive about the training of most people. I once critiqued the card of a lady who repeated the same thing each session. "Oh," she said, "they told me not to increase anything for the first three months." When ignorance is not at fault, human nature kicks in: "I don't want to increase the weight;" "It's hard enough as it is;" or, in the case of the elderly, "I'm not training for the Olympics." When things get tough, people quit.

Only one challenge remains for those who refuse to progress through traditional channels (increase in resistance, number of repetitions, effort expended during exercise or all of the above). Do the same as always (same weight, same reps, same movements and same effort) with one minor change - spend less time between exercises.

If trainees took their current routine and reduced rest between efforts, their results would increase significantly, as follows:

- Increased cardiovascular ability (or less time spent performing the same).
- Increased overall strength (despite fewer repetitions on your last exercises).
- Increased metabolic conditioning (the ability to sustain a high level of intensity).
- Increased energy.

- Increased efficiency (less time in the gym).

If you think not, try the following: Perform one exercise and relax. In seconds, you'll feel your heart rate respond to the signal. Though your muscle takes the brunt of the load, your system takes a smaller hit. Now, perform a second exercise with a different muscle and check the aftermath. The shock will be about the same for the new muscle, but the system takes another hit. A third and fourth exercise will produce an accumulative systemic response, and a higher level of training. Without checking your complexion in the mirror, or allowing your system a chance to settle, continue until you have completed the workout...if you can.

Your system may fail to meet the demand.

A few words of caution: GRADUALLY reduce the time spent between exercises to a minimum. At first, the metabolic system cannot make the necessary chemical changes rapidly enough. But ultimately, like all systems, it will adapt to handle the same workout at a faster pace.

The question remains: "Can you?"

## AUGUST 19

---

### Heat Loss

Don't be fooled by sweating - and you might if you follow your instincts. Most people judge the value of their physical endeavors by how much they sweat, which has led to a number of misconceptions in the field of exercise.

The first time I performed negative work, I sweated like never before and attributed it to the new format. I was wrong. The recommended weights were too light, allowed too many repetitions. The prolonged workout produced more sweat.

Muscle contraction during exercise results in the production of heat. Because many bodily functions are more efficient at higher temperatures, the body resets its thermostat and allows its core temperature to rise and stabilize. To handle the increased temperature, the body activates heat-dissipation mechanisms, the most important of which is increased circulation in the area of the skin where the vaporization of sweat occurs.

The amount one sweats depends upon a number of factors:

- Genetics - some people sweat a lot, others don't. Regardless of your tendency, when you start a program of exercise your body becomes more efficient at dealing with heat dissipation, and you will sweat more than you normally do.

- Amount of exercise performed - the work-rate and duration directly affect muscle and core temperatures. The longer an exercise, the more likely your core temperature will be affected. During marathon running, deep-muscle temperatures can reach 109°F and body-core temperatures, 106°F, while skin temperatures may be in the mid-80's (if environmental temperature is low).
- Environmental temperature - exercise in heat creates a greater need for cooling.
- Relative humidity - heat loss requires atmospheric conditions that result in evaporation, where humidity is low enough to accept water vapor from the skin. Dripping sweat has little cooling effect, which is why most people are attracted to indoor workouts in Florida, especially during summer months. I once worked at the mouth of a large furnace at the Ford® glass manufacturing facility in Niagara Falls. In very hot, but dry, conditions, the evaporation rate was so high that only salt remained on your forehead when you wiped your brow.
- The amount of fluids available to escape - the more you drink during exercise, the more you sweat.
- The size of the trainee - large men have more difficulty dispelling heat and cannot sustain hard work for long periods of time.

The implications are clear. If sweating is more related to the amount of work than to its intensity, it may explain the preference of cardiovascular training over strength training, of long workouts over short. Heat loss meant something else to Arthur Jones. It rationalized the lax training practices of bodybuilders he observed over the years.

"Maximum-possible power production," he said, "simultaneously and unavoidably produces a maximum-possible heat rise. And since the body's efficient operating range is narrow insofar as internal temperature is concerned, this means that a large man will not be able to sustain actually hard work as long as a smaller man can - everything else being equal...and this, I think, is another reason why most advanced bodybuilders fall into a habit of working at a lower intensity of effort and at a slower pace, with more frequent and longer rest periods between sets - which, in turn, reduces their production of results."

...as if bodybuilders needed another excuse for their irrational behavior.

## AUGUST 20

---

### The Dynamate

In 1973, I couldn't stuff a Nautilus® machine in a suitcase or dorm room, so I bought the next best thing. "The future of exercise" fit anywhere.

The device was a two-foot long, one-inch-square tube with a nylon rope exiting from the groove of a small wheel at both ends. The rope had sturdy plastic handles and a metal clasp to adjust its length. The instructions had long disappeared but photos of all 15 exercises were visible on the outer package.

The 30th anniversary of the Nautilus Dynamate® was on.

On first glance, the device wasn't anything to rave about (although it was as smooth as silk), but there was something to be said about its technology.

The Dynamate was a home version of what Nautilus inventor Arthur Jones called 'infimetric' (sometimes 'infitonic') exercise. It represented the application of full-range resistance to a muscle *without* the use of a weight stack, yet with all the advantages of a barbell, Nautilus machine or other conventional exercise. And more.

An 'infimetric' device was safer, and easier to enter and exit. No weight stack meant low friction and better control of forces. The movement compelled trainees to focus on the lowering phase of exercise and made, in Jones' words, "'cheating' almost impossible" by demanding good posture. It also allowed movement to positions normally inaccessible (because both limbs were never in the contracted position at the same time).

The concept was bold - the Dynamate provided no resistance at all. "You will be the source of your own resistance," said Jones, "providing resistance for the concentric (lifting) exercise of one limb by the eccentric (lowering) work of the bilateral limb."

A leg-, shoulder- or chest-press helps illustrate. As one limb is straightened (performs positive work), the other resists by bending, as it must, to perform and provide negative work. Because negative strength is always greater than positive strength, "the positive working limb cannot force the negative working limb to do anything. Instead, the negative working limb must permit movement of the positive working limb. The result is that you are literally provided with an infinite source of resistance, as much as you can handle while working at a 100% level of intensity and more...or as little as you want...or anything in between." (*The Future of Exercise - An Opinion*, 1978)

The bilateral, self-generated resistance, like traditional exercise, allowed for a high level of intensity, yet exposed muscles to low force. It was productive and safe, and addressed things that annoyed its inventor.

"Both problems, poor form and lowered intensity, result from a desire to show progress; thus, under the mistaken impression that they are thereby improving at a faster rate, most people quickly start changing the form or intensity of their exercises...and are encouraged that doing so increases the amount of resistance they can handle."

Jones built several 'infimetric' prototype machines but never hooked them to a computer to record intensity, progression, speed-of-movement and duration. He was at odds with the testing protocols and concerned that, "without weights, it will be hard to convince many people that exercise is being provided."

Hardly. Ten properly performed repetitions were about all anyone could stand.

There are people currently attempting to do what Jones opted not to pursue. If, or when, they are successful, it might indeed be "the future of exercise."

Until then, I have the Dynamate on standby.

## AUGUST 21

### Play It Again, Sam

I don't recall where I first met him, but it was probably the first tee or the 19th hole. Sam was overbearing in both.

On the highest tee in the Niagara Peninsula, the Sicilian was hard to miss. He arrived in plain, long pants slightly bowed at the knee and a multi-colored shirt whose opening - about four buttons deep - exposed a thick gold chain perched on a tanned, barrel chest. The hair on his head was a thinner gray than that on his chest, and always whipped by the breeze. His protruding nose was put into perspective by an ever-present cigar, above which was a twinkle; below which, a grin.

Sam triggered his golf swing with a pair of trademark left-arm practice swings. He then set his feet, wiggled his hips, attached the other hand, stiffened his resolve and whacked it down the middle. Neither the cigar nor the two-handicap wavered.

At the 19th hole it was much the same, with only the volume amplified. Laughter, beer, peanuts and stories flew as Sam topped whatever was on the table, his voice easily piercing the general buzz. The laughter ceased only when the cigar blocked its exit. He was loved by some, but not by others.

Sam owned a kitchen-cabinet business that was a front for what he really did - bookmaking. When I was still a teen, he was charged with a crime, lied in court and sent to prison for less time than he figured. He had a blind daughter.

A year later, I stood on that same high tee to share his return. Once again, the familiar shirt, hair, chain, cigar and pre-shot routine produced a familiar result. His ball sailed down the middle.

"Oooh...hooh," he hollered, "like swingin' a pick axe." The laughter never stopped.

Sam was proud of his son. It was always "Joey this" and "Joey that" - and why not. At 6'3", 210 pounds, 15 year-old Joey could hit a golf ball to places that would make any Dad proud. Sam also showed an interest in my brother and me. He called Al 'Wristy,' in reference to his swing; and me 'Whizzle,' in reference to who knows what. We loved him dearly.

People make mistakes and learn. As someone said, "We learn, when we learn, only from experience; and then only from our mistakes; our successes merely serve to reinforce our superstitions."

Many people would do things differently if given a second chance. Nautilus® inventor Arthur Jones would be no exception.

"If I could do it all over again," he said, "just what part of my life would I change?

Damned near all of it. But in order to do that, I would have required the knowledge that I now have at the start of my life; which, of course, was impossible.

Almost nothing that I ever did turned out, after the fact, to have much in common with my expectations or hopes. Sometimes things turn out to be better than you expected in advance, but most things turn out to be worse than you expected.

So is it even possible to ever be satisfied with anything?

Briefly, perhaps. Which may make you feel good for a while, but which will usually cause you to reduce your efforts."

Would Sam have changed much, or entertained a second chance? Or would he have agreed with Jones on reincarnation: "I hope not. Once around is enough?"

Of one thing I'm certain: Once around was never enough for that laugh.

Gary Bannister, B.A., B.P.E., M.Ed.

# AUGUST 22

---

## Going Up?

In 1977, I purchased a low-mileage 1962 Ford® Galaxie 500 from its sole-owner, an elderly gent in Caracas, and had it checked by a mechanic who operated a fleet of buses at the local high school. When I got 'thumbs up' from Senor Wency, I cruised town for four years and only once had to be towed - after an accident that was my fault.

I pulled out of a hotel driveway onto a major road and was hit from the side by a vehicle moving approximately 30 miles an hour. The other car was crushed in the nose; the Galaxie moved about a foot. The lesson - that heavy objects don't move easily - provided the only explanation I can find for what I witnessed in a gym on a recent trip to Canada.

Welland, Ontario, famous for the canal joining the Great Lakes of Erie and Ontario, was once a bustling center for the steel industry, remnants of which dot its altered skyline. The new canal now bypasses the city leaving only rowing crews to ruffle the surface of its otherwise vacant waterways. The downtown area was abandoned 30 years ago when a not-so-large shopping center opened on the outskirts of town.

"Bulldoze the whole damn thing and make it a park," was one suggestion but it would have meant losing a landmark - a gym. And Welland could ill afford that.

The gym occupied the old two-story building of Switson Industries, a small machine-part manufacturer in what was once the heart of the industrial zone. The entrance was a shade below street level and covered by a black awning that read, "Galaxy 2000."

The layout was replete with nooks and crannies connected by a creaky, single-file wood staircase. The bottom floor housed a modest reception and office; the second, just steps above, a free-weight section that could only be described as "museum quality." With the exception of a few Cybex® machines, nothing had seen a lick of paint in a while, and for good reason - many stations were dysfunctional. I stepped over bars, attachments, cobwebs and safety hazards to peer at a few unfamiliar Canadian names: Global®, Dotmar®, Atlantis®, Ironco®. What paint remained - a dull and fitting black - blended with the rust that spelled in capital letters, LACK OF USE.

The high metal roof and gray cinder-block walls were interrupted by an occasional mirror and a pair of elevated windows that provided more light than expected. At one end of the room sat a rack of dumbbells, among them the kind used by circus strongmen at the turn of the 19th century - two large balls joined by a handle, awaiting the arrival of Louis Cyr. At the other end was the only drinking fountain in the place, a garden-hose lever that dispersed a warm, tasty liquid.

The trek to the third floor hinted of civilization. Halfway up was an aerobic room, locked except during infrequent scheduled times; across from it, the men's locker room, a pleasant surprise. Further up was the main fitness chamber with a complete line of Cybex machines - some old, some new - an array of cardiovascular equipment, a ladies room, three TV's and several portable industrial fans. The best was yet to come.

In the corner, near the stretching area was a fenced-off platform that partially concealed a gaping hole in the floor. Above it, attached to the ceiling was a hoist, a remnant of the old steel days and the only way equipment could ascend.

So, what appeared a step up in Galaxies - from the 500 to the 2000 - was not. But the charm of the latter provoked a return. My only regret was not wearing a belt strong enough to have tried the elevator. Going up?

## AUGUST 23

---

### The Mystery of Muscle Soreness

Those who live overseas huddle around anything that reminds them of home. When the first McDonald's® came to Caracas, I rushed in for a taste. When I opened a Nautilus® facility there, the reaction was the same - nearly every 'gringo' in town jumped at the opportunity to exercise 'home-style.' It kept the doors open.

In the early 1980's, an American businessman showed up with shoulders that filled the doorway as thoroughly as any athlete. Sonny Litz played backup quarterback for Roger Staubach at Navy in the mid-1960's.

His only backup now, however, was the one against the wall. He had let himself go and needed an aggressive program of exercise - a perfect fit. Sonny worked hard and set a goal of 'acing' the leg machines, using the entire weight stack. He had the legs, the drive and the form to do it. It was just a matter of time.

Six months later, Sonny reached his goal, a gym first. You'd have thought he won the Super Bowl the day he completed 12 repetitions with 250 pounds on each of the Leg Extension, Leg Curl and Adduction/Abduction machines. He left a few plates behind on the Hip and Back and Leg Press.

Weeks later, he hobbled into the gym in pain. A weekend, parent-child softball game at the local school left him disabled, muscle sore. We discussed how muscles, regardless of their strength level, could get sore playing a game as seemingly passive as softball. He improved by the time he walked out.

There are many ways to create muscle soreness:

- The trauma of accident or impact.
- Resuming exercise after a period of inactivity.
- Exercising with a heavier resistance; or a normal resistance, a prolonged time.
- Performing exercise or using muscles in a different way.

Yet, none of the above is a sure thing, nor is the site of soreness.

According to Nautilus inventor, Arthur Jones, "Muscles do not have the types of nerves required to produce pain, and thus it is not the working part of a muscle that becomes painful following some hard exercises. And please take note of the fact that I said 'some' hard exercises; because, in fact, some hard exercises do not produce so-called muscular soreness. And secondarily, while a first hard workout may produce later soreness, following hard workouts tend to reduce or even remove this soreness."

The mystery is further enhanced by the following:

Take a dumbbell that you can curl for 10-12 repetitions with one hand. Lift the weight with the right hand, and lower it with the left. Up with the right, transfer it to the left to lower, and then back to the right to lift. The right hand performs all of the 'positive' work; the left hand, all of the 'negative' work.

Continue until the right arm can no longer lift the weight and stop with both. At that point, failure will occur in the right arm only; the left could continue for many more reps.

The right arm will 'feel' exhausted; the left will not. Yet, the left arm will get sore, or sorer than the right. Negative work produces more muscle pain than positive work.

Says Jones, "Just what muscular soreness is caused by we do not know, nor do we know what it really is." But we know how to produce it, know when we have and know what provides relief - heat, stretching and exercise.

The mystery remains an open door.

## AUGUST 24

---

### Bassackwards

I once came across a strange putter - the toe of its blade faced toward you, instead of away. I never tried it long enough to find out if it worked, which was typical. Its function was overshadowed by its looks and both spelled eventual doom for the club with the funny name, 'Bassackward.'

Many concepts in the field of exercise are equally 'strange' - that less exercise produces more results, that the hardest repetition is the safest, that slow repetitions improve the speed of muscle contraction - and like the putter, strange spells doom.

In 1975, the Cincinnati Bengals sent a newly signed lineman to a research study conducted at the US Military Academy in West Point. With an $80,000 signing bonus and a lucrative contract on the line, the 300-pound man had 12 days to get strong enough to pass a physical test, part of which involved the performance of at least one chin-up. The director of the study, Arthur Jones, applied one of his 'strange' concepts to the challenge - that progressive lowering can improve lifting strength.

When first tested, the lineman could not pull himself up, so a tall stool was used to raise his chin over the bar to start. "When the stool was removed," said Jones, "he dropped like a stone." The man couldn't lift or lower.

The crew got him to the top of the movement again, supported his butt just enough to help him lower in control and repeated the same on each attempt. He trained every other day using one set of 7-8 repetitions, eventually without help.

"Twelve days later," said Jones, "he returned to spring-training camp and was tested, and was then able to chin himself 4¾ times, pulling himself up all of the way and then back down slowly under his own power."

With less on the line (but of equal importance), I did the same with world-champion water-skier, Anna Maria Carrasco. When first tested, Anna performed 1½ chin-ups. Following months of 8-10 'negative' repetitions twice a week, she ultimately performed 13 chin-ups, slow and controlled - and left many male biceps drooling.

Lowering weight in a progressive manner can increase lifting strength, and why not? It's the same muscle, just a different direction. Strength is general, but the application of strength is specific. A strong biceps muscle will help an athlete in any sport that requires biceps input, regardless of the way in which the muscle is used, including the plane in which it moves.

If negative work is so effective - and it is - why is it rarely used?

For starters, when it was introduced, bodybuilders overused it and proclaimed it didn't work. Second, negative work requires heavy weights and spotters, although it can be performed safely alone on some equipment. A chin-up or dip bar with steps in front is effective, as is a two-limbs-up-one-limb-down technique on machines with single movement-arms. The same format can be used with biceps and triceps by exhausting one arm first and then the other. Third, lowering weights is the hardest way to train and, as such, appeals to few. It takes a huge toll on the recovery system if continued to failure (when lowering control is lost). As Jones put it, "Some is very good, but more may be a disaster."

Knowing that, don't be surprised to see sports performance gurus (who train 'specific' movements against resistance yet fail to realize that 'specific' evaporates the moment resistance is applied) train golfers to swing backwards for 'power.'

AUGUST 25

---

### Abdominal Exercise

If infomercials are any indication, the single most important facet of training for any purpose is abdominal exercise. A flat, defined stomach is revered by teens, models and bodybuilders. Abdominal strength is the pillar of functional training, yoga and Pilates, and is thought to play a major role in the prevention of low-back pain.

Enter the cast - Ab Slide®, Ab Dolly®, Ab Rocker® and Ab Cruncher® - and the claims that take you from fat to firm "in just minutes a day." One man reportedly lost 50 pounds of weight and 13 inches from his waist in six months, and "it didn't even feel like exercise." One device claimed to "aerobically burn fat in one easy fat-burning circular motion." But the fact remains: Results are tied to the nutritional guidelines enclosed, not to the equipment. How much you shovel in is more important than how you expend it, and abdominal exercise is one of the least efficient ways to burn calories.

One set of 15-20 repetitions of abdominal exercise (properly performed to fatigue) consumes approximately five calories (4 sets X 5 calories X 30 days = 600 calories per month). Since a pound of fat has 3,500 calories, it would take 5 months and 25 days to burn off that pound, if other factors remain the same. But they don't.

Caloric expenditure increases before (in anticipation of) and after (in recovery from) exercise, and elevates when muscle is added to the body (by 50-100 calories/day/pound), which helps reduce the time factor, but not by much. Reducing body fat by performing daily abdominal exercise is a slow process.

Nautilus® inventor Arthur Jones took a different approach: "If you train the rest of the body properly, the abdominal area will take care of itself." It nearly did.

In 1971, 19-year-old Casey Viator, a trainee of Jones, won every category in the Mr. America contest *except* best abdomen, despite Jones' claim that Viator's abdomen was "on a par with any man living or dead." Casey had performed "no direct work for that area of his body in more than a year."

In 1982, I visited the Nautilus complex in Lake Helen, Florida to purchase 13 exercise machines, including the new abdominal tool. The salesman, a former NFL player, echoed Jones: "You don't need it. I'll put you on the machine at the end of a workout done my way with a weight that, fresh, you could perform 20 repetitions. If you get two, I'll give you $100. That's how hard you'll work your stomach before you get there."

I was in great shape at the time but didn't relish the idea of leaving breakfast on a carpet to discover *his* way.

Jones rattled the establishment again in 1986 when he declared: "The strength of the abdomen has *nothing* to do with low-back pain." His research showed that the lumbar muscles were, by far, the weak link in the chain of mid-section support.

Once upon a time, I performed abdominal exercise three times a week on a Nautilus machine. After two back operations and two additional crises, I heeded Jones' advice and stopped altogether. Eighteen years and no abdominal exercise later, I enjoy a pain-free lifestyle. I strengthened my back.

The fact that your largest fat deposits settle in the abdomen has no bearing on exercise requirements. You can't lose fat locally and probably don't have the genetic potential to ever see a 'six-pack.' So, save yourself three easy payments and treat your abdomen as you would any other muscle. More exercise will *not* produce better results...

...unless you call within the next 30 minutes.

## AUGUST 26

---

### Isokinetic Resistance

"Any test performed with a Cybex® machine, or any other so-called 'isokinetic' tool, is worse than worthless and is frequently dangerous," declared Arthur Jones who held nothing back in justifying an opinion that flew in the face of 'wisdom.' Like spitting on the Pope, the Nautilus® and MedX® inventor became the lone critic of isokinetic technology.

In the late 1960's, fitness equipment manufacturers began bashing negative work, the lowering part of exercise. Jones examined the available tools - a handful of scrap - and concluded, "The only real advantage provided by isokinetic resistance is the fact that it does not require a heavy and expensive stack of weights. This 'advantage,' of course, is purchased at the price of almost total destruction of the function."

And more: "It results in greatly elevated blood pressure and the involved forces are far higher than either necessary or desirable."

That was only the beginning.

When isokinetic technology hooked up with the computer age, Cybex jumped in and sold thousands of units to rehab clinics and research labs around the country.

Jones decided to build his own version to control the level of force to which subjects were exposed. "Increase the force, even slightly," he said, "and you increase the danger. Reduce the force and you increase the safety." In the end, "the best isokinetic machine ever produced" (that of Jones) did not behave.

The force levels during dynamic tests were higher than that produced by static tests on his old tools. He then tweaked an old prototype and developed a 'work-capacity test' that reduced the force of a static test by 50% - to a level less than 10% of that encountered on his isokinetic machine. "If reducing the levels of force something on the order of ninety percent doesn't increase the safety," he said, "then I have somehow misjudged the cause and effect relationship involved in injuries of any kind."

At the same time, he reduced the velocity of the weight stack on his own tools by 87.5% to control the high forces associated with momentum.

Jones' prototypes - forerunners of MedX medical machines - were more accurate in delivering a desired force throughout a range of motion during exercise. A force of 75 foot-pounds used by a first-time subject working to fatigue, for example, produced a variation in force from the desired level of less than 1% (due to machine friction). In contrast, an isokinetic resistance of 75 foot-pounds, with an experienced subject and sub-maximal effort, varied more than 20% from the desired value.

In addition, the inability to move smoothly in the new tool resulted in force variations "from a low of 2% of the desired level to a high of 257% of the desired level."

"We are not biased against isokinetic forms of resistance," said Jones, "quite the contrary, we spent years of careful work and millions of dollars in research in attempts to produce the best isokinetic machine that could be produced, without regard for cost or other consideration; and we did...and have a very clear understanding of both the problems and the limitations that are simply unavoidable with such machines."

"We wanted to, we tried to, and we failed," he concluded, "and everybody else that tried failed as well, and always will fail." Yet, the majority of clinics in this country continue to embrace such nonsense.

If nothing else, when you get hurt, you're in the right place...or are you?


## AUGUST 27

---

### Man is Capable – Part 1

Man is capable of performing incredible feats when he puts his mind to it, but at some point, something tempers the accomplishment with, "for a man his age."

Father Time has a way of telling us to hang up the cleats, as stubborn as some may be. Gordie Howe played NHL hockey for six decades, although his performance was less than stellar on the curtain call. Nicklaus won the Masters at the age of 46 when no one but Jack believed he could. Sam Snead finished third in the PGA Championship at the age of 63. George Foreman fashioned a 'comeback' well after his skills had eroded. Some for the money, most for pride - they simply couldn't let it go.

Athletes generally fade from the scene when they feel they can no longer compete. The average retirement age for swimmers and gymnasts is young. It stretches beyond 50 in golf, although most seniors are no longer 'threats' on the PGA Tour. In sports like basketball, soccer, hockey and football, barring injury, the age falls between 35-45.

But there are exceptions.

Gary Bannister, B.A., B.P.E., M.Ed.

A major sports magazine recently ranked the 10 greatest pitchers of all time. The most interesting thing about the list was the name at the bottom - it belonged to a man who did not play baseball.

Meryl King (alias Eddie Feigner) traveled the country with an entourage of softball players known as "The King and his Court." His four-man team of pitcher, catcher, first baseman and fielder took on 9-man squads at a rate of 2-3 games a day from 1946 to the present, and were rarely defeated. Few batters could see the ball, let alone hit it...and then age crept in.

In 1973, Feigner signed a two-year contract to play the winner of the National Softball Championship. Besides the publicity generated and the interest stirred among fans, the game promised to be a beauty. It was not. Feigner was blanked in the neighborhood of 15-0, the most embarrassing performance of his career. The score bothered him less than the taunting, the rumors that he was 'over the hill' and 'didn't have it anymore.'

Eddie wasn't convinced.

When the next year rolled around and much to his delight, the same team won the National Championship. But all was not well. To add insult to injury, they sent him a check in the amount of half the contract, opting to play in an event that would generate more revenue. Feigner ripped it up and returned it with the message, "I'll be there. You better damn well be."

The game was on.

All season Feigner worked his circus-like schedule around that game, reducing the number of exhibitions two weeks prior. The day before the match, he didn't pitch at all - a first. An hour before the game, he performed a 15-minute warm-up in the parking lot of a motel adjacent to the stadium.

When he entered the ballpark, he went through his normal routine, 6-8 pitches. The first batter hit big and more than a few sensed what they had the year before. But Eddie wasn't convinced. In what his catcher called "the most amazing performance he had ever seen," Feigner fanned the next 20 batters in a row - at the age of 57.

The list of 'best pitchers ever' should have been reversed. Eddie Feigner dominated his sport more than anybody on that list could ever have hoped to dominate baseball...and for a lot longer.

AUGUST 28

## Man is Capable - Part 2

Man is capable of performing incredible feats when he puts his mind to it, but not all are positive, especially when money is involved.

Eighty years ago, there were few ways to make a living in the field of exercise. The gyms that existed were small and dumpy. If they attracted enough members for a profit, there was no room to house them. And the sale of equipment was no better: Once a client purchased a barbell, it was over, forcing the leaders in the field to pursue more creative avenues such as publishing and mail-order courses, the most famous of which was the 'dynamic tension' program of Charles Atlas. That was only the beginning.

The real boom in exercise occurred with the introduction of alternatives to barbells in the late 1960's. Exercise machines brightened the horizon in the eyes of the public, but those running the show hadn't changed. Everyone jumped on board...and some took it a little too far.

A man named Alvin Roy began opening, promoting and closing 'new' gyms in New Orleans. He sold as many long-term memberships as he could, packed things up on a weekend and repeated the process - once doing it twice within a 2-3 year span using the *same* location.

Similar things happened all over the country and the potential good brought about by machines was negated by the poor reputation of clubs. Lousy exercise information was one thing, but when the doors didn't open to get that information, it was another - perhaps a blessing. But it was no blessing for the industry. Laws that passed in Ontario, for example, required consumers to pay no more than 1/12th of an annual gym membership up-front. Many turned away from exercise.

Somewhere in the process, Alvin Roy became the NFL's first strength coach and nearly went to jail for dispensing steroids. That was the good news. According to Nautilus® inventor Arthur Jones, "Later he was almost solely responsible for one of the worst outrages ever associated with the field of exercise." Roy convinced both coaches and players of the supposed benefits of 'explosive' training.

In the early 1970's, Roy visited Nautilus headquarters in Lake Helen, Florida, where Jones first heard of his training ideas. "I initially assumed that he was simply stupid," said Jones, "that he really believed what he was telling people." But Arthur was wrong. On a visit to the spring-training camp of an NFL team, he found Roy doing everything but 'explosive' training in an effort not to hurt anyone, and nothing that would otherwise produce worthwhile results.

As Jones got to know him, Roy finally admitted that he was "well aware of the dangers from explosive exercises but still promoted them as gospel because 'that was what coaches wanted to hear.'" Sounds like bodybuilding magazines.

Several years ago, I assisted a high-school baseball team with their strength training. One day, I entered the office of the athletic director/football coach who was studying videotapes about power-lifting techniques. It was not my place to interject, but I sure left mumbling.

The incident reinforced the statement that Jones made in one of his final articles in *Ironman*, "Bullshit is rather easy to establish, but once accepted, it is almost impossible to eradicate."

Thanks, Mr. Roy and Mr. Atlas, who has recently emerged as a dot com.

## AUGUST 29

### Explode!

A friend of Nautilus® inventor Arthur Jones once commented, "Kenneth Cooper (the originator of aerobics) will probably go down in history as the man who destroyed America's knees, rather than the man who saved America's hearts." Jones added, "Yet many of the people who eventually became aware of that danger (the high impact of running) are still telling people to move suddenly during weightlifting exercises."

We share gym space with a "sports performance" group that trains athletes to run faster and jump higher, the FAST program. To say the least, they use their equipment, and sometimes ours, in a unique way.

Last week, a FAST instructor trained a high-school athlete on our plate-loaded chest press. Once the youth was set, the instructor hollered emphatically, "Now, Explode. EXPLODE!" Arthur would have shot him on the spot.

It was reminiscent of the suicide bombers who literally explode at the push of a button and always produce the same result - death and destruction. While exercise rarely leads to death, it *can* lead to destruction - especially pushing that button.

Injury is the only *direct* result of exercise. Increases in strength, flexibility and cardiovascular capacity; and decreases in body fat and injury probability are all *indirect* results. Exercise stimulates change; the body makes the change at its leisure.

But not so with injury; it is sudden and occurs when a muscle or joint system is exposed to a force that temporarily exceeds the integrity of the structure. Unfortunately, the only way to determine the integrity of a joint or muscle is to expose it to a progressive force until it breaks - not a practical way to deal with limbs.

The determination of muscle strength by a one-repetition lift generally produces a force less than the 'break' point. During such an effort, the body allows only 30% of the muscle to get involved as a protective measure. When it allows a full contraction as in an emergency, bones break. Logically, the 'break' point must lie somewhere between a maximum contraction (100%) and a maximum effort (30%).

To avoid injury, there are two choices: strengthen the structure, or keep the force to which it is exposed as low as possible. Both are best accomplished by slow movements.

An average trainee who can lift 100 pounds once, can lift 80 pounds approximately 10 times. During the first repetition with 80, an application of only 81 pounds of force to the resistance will initiate movement - a force well below the 'break' point, and a low level of intensity. Assuming an average strength loss of 2% per repetition, the trainee is left with 98 pounds of strength for the second rep, another 81-pound effort. After 10 reps, only 80 pounds of strength remain to lift 80 pounds of weight. Despite the intensity at that juncture, the trainee has exposed the muscle to a force slightly above 80 pounds throughout - a safe level from start to finish, **if the movement is slow.**

On the other hand, if the weight is jerked during the first repetition, the force to which the muscle is exposed can spike to 2-3 times that of the resistance. Eighty pounds can suddenly become 240 - a level of force that, in light of unknown structural integrity, Jones calls "dangerous as hell," **if the movement is explosive.**

The other day, a FAST instructor complained that area coaches were "old school" and reluctant to commit to the program. Ignorance pays: "Old school" was at least school. "Explode?" The concept hopefully will. "Faster athletes?" If there are any left.

Good thing there's a dumpster out back.

## AUGUST 30

---

### Removing the Weak Link

Two days before the competition, Casey stepped to the plate. He performed one set of leg presses with 750 pounds (20 repetitions), one set of leg extensions with 225 pounds (20 repetitions) and one set of full squats (to the floor) with 502 pounds (13 repetitions). Said his trainer, "Each set of every exercise was carried to the point of absolute failure - and there was no rest at all between sets."

According to witnesses, the brutal sequence was followed by two sets of leg curls and three of calf raises - the leg portion of the workout completed in about nine minutes.

Two days later, Casey Viator won the Mr. America contest (did anyone have a chance after that?). His trainer was Nautilus® inventor, Arthur Jones.

The three-exercise leg sequence was one of Jones' favorites because it attempted to eliminate the weak link found in all compound movements. When more than one muscle or joint structure is involved in an exercise, the small, weak muscles fail before growth stimulation is provided for the stronger ones. In the case of squats, failure occurs when the low-back muscles can no longer continue, "...long before," according to Jones, "the much larger and far stronger frontal thigh muscles have been worked as hard as they should be for the production of best-possible results."

The solution was to "pre-exhaust" the thigh muscles immediately *before* performing squats. The leg-press-extension-squat sequence assured that failure during the squat would occur in the larger front-thigh muscles. Because of its difficulty, Jones recommended little weight for the squat portion, less than half of what was normally used (approximately 135 pounds for a squat of 300 pounds or more). He also reminded egos that stimulation was related to intensity - and intensity to the muscle's *momentary* ability. It only mattered how it *felt*.

Jones applied the pre-exhaustion principle to his Nautilus 'double' machines, which featured two exercises from the same seat. The targeted muscle was first worked to exhaustion with an isolated exercise and then forced to further fatigue with the help of a fresh muscle in a compound movement. The combinations included: a leg extension followed by a leg press; a pullover, front pulldown; a chest fly, chest press; a lateral raise, shoulder press; and a behind-the-neck (upper-back) movement followed by a behind-the-neck pulldown. The machines allowed quick access from one movement to the other.

The instructions - to move "INSTANTLY from one set of an exercise to the next, with no rest at all, not so much as two seconds of rest." The reason, according to Jones, was physiological: "Resting as much as five seconds between sets will reduce the production of results by as much as fifty percent."

The following combinations of three exercises (an isolated movement sandwiched between two compound ones) were later proven effective: pulldown, pullover, negative chin-ups; regular chin-ups, pullover, pulldown; chest press, chest fly, negative dips; and regular dips, chest fly, chest press. Try them, but be forewarned:

- Prepare all stations in advance so that no rest is permitted between. Rest after.
- Use less weight on the second (isolated) movement, and much less on the third.
- Perform one combination per workout (3x/wk.) to start; and two (3x/wk.) or three (2x/wk.) per workout for advanced training. Recovery from hard exercise takes time. If growth stalls, reduce the AMOUNT of exercise performed.

More exercise might remove more than the weak link...as in "Casket anyone?"


## AUGUST 31

---

### Too Good to be True

While touring a potential client through the gym last week, I mentioned that most of the machines (MedX®) were made by the original Nautilus® inventor, Arthur Jones.

"Oh, yeah," he blurted, "I saw him in the early 1970's. He was *quite* a promoter (implying all hype and no substance)." I saved my dissertation for more deserving ears.

Like most things in the field of exercise, the Nautilus system of training introduced in 1970 sounded 'too good to be true.' Twenty minutes, three times a week, one set of 12 exercises appeared an *easy* way to optimize strength and fitness. The public went for it in a big way...until they discovered it was anything but easy.

The machines provided a faster voyage from A to B, but Jones was more focused on the philosophy: "Nautilus is first and foremost," he said, "a concept applicable to any worthwhile exercise tool." In *Nautilus Training Principles:*

*Bulletin #2* (1971), he sought "to point intelligent trainees in the direction of logical training." Most bodybuilders, he thought, performed too much exercise and nothing hard enough; and those who took up his challenge didn't last long enough to stimulate a change, or stay long enough to get a result. Jones didn't stop there.

His *Ironman* magazine articles were so hard-hitting that the editor's wife objected.

"I don't approve of you calling our readers fools."

"I didn't call ALL of your readers fools - just some of them; but in any case, I didn't make any of your readers fools, God did that - I just pointed it out. But should I lie to them? Should I encourage them in outright foolishness? Or tell them the truth?"

"Well, you're still calling them fools."

"Some of your readers are fools, and calling them fools won't change them, or help them, it will only serve to infuriate them; but a lot of your readers aren't fools, they're intelligent people - you have to take a stand, support the truth and let the chips fall where they may. If that outrages a few fools, then so be it..."

It outraged more than a few. "Weider published a long series of articles," said Jones, "that were nothing short of attacks upon both me and my products; which was not surprising, since...he invented everything from sex to money to fire, the wheel, the airplane and damned near anything else you can name, so he naturally objected when any credit was given to anybody else. I have followed Joe's career from the start, and if he ever invented or discovered anything it has escaped my attention." (*Ironman*: Mar., 1994)

Jones took a similar stance in the *National Strength Coaches Association Journal* (Vol.1, #4). "We realized from the beginning that what we wrote and what we built would be reviewed by: those who are biased for and believe everything; those who are biased against and believe nothing (too many years invested in their own beliefs); and those who are capable of logically assimilating information and formulating sound conclusions. This third group has been our major source of support through the years."

The marketing of his MedX medical tools proved an equal challenge. Like bodybuilders, doctors were unaware of the shortcomings of their equipment (isokinetic machines) and its proper use. It led him to conclude that things had only gotten worse. "In 1938, a few people were exposed to a trickle of bullshit, but in 1996 millions of people are exposed to a flood of bullshit." (*Ironman*: Jan., 1997)

In seeking the support of intelligent, open-minded people, he learned that there weren't many around.

# SEPTEMBER

"Over the years, I have steadily reduced the level of my presentations to the point that they are now somewhere between a kindergarten level and a second grade of grammar school level, and they are still far over the heads of most of my audiences."

Arthur Jones

## Cheating

There are 23 ways to cheat during a bench press and the guy in the red shirt managed to combine all of them into one magnificent effort. He wasn't alone. The gorilla at his side was busy writing his own script - clear proof of what Nautilus® inventor Arthur Jones said about the learning process: "There is no education like self education."

No trainer would dare teach 'cheating' during an orientation or push new trainees to exhaustion, where cheating generally surfaces. The focus should be on good form, strict movements and the safe and proper use of equipment, not on seeing how hard one works.

If so, from where did 'cheating' emerge? Who taught these wonderful techniques? You might be surprised. It was the body itself.

Throughout the orientation, it screamed blue murder, "What are you demanding now? And how long will it last?" It never appreciated the first intrusion, nor the second or third; but it got used to it - and got by - in its own rebellious way.

I once watched a lady whose form during exercise was poor. She lingered at each station for too many sets but made up for it by working harder than most - that is, until she hit the leg extension. Where she averaged 10-12 repetitions on most exercises, she performed no more than six consecutive reps before surrendering to pain. The resistance was low compared to other machines, which allowed her to move it at a faster speed. Her facial expression told the story - her muscles wanted out.

You might like exercise, but your body doesn't; and when forced to perform, it initiates its own damage control. The 'tricks' it tries, conscious or otherwise, include:

- Lifting weights slightly faster than normal throughout the workout.
- Lifting slightly faster during the first repetitions to ensure reaching a quota.
- Setting a quota (and settling for it, once there).
- Lowering at a speed that doesn't allow you to feel the resistance.

- Insisting on the same weight and settling for the same number of repetitions.
- Failing to complete the range of motion (at both ends).
- Pausing in a contracted position without squeezing the muscle.
- Lingering near a locked-out position during compound press movements.
- Not holding the weight in a static position once movement has ceased.
- Jerking the resistance to create momentum on the final repetitions.
- Not hustling to the next exercise (water, conversation, waiting for a machine).
- Taking a break of 1-2 minutes between strength and cardiovascular exercise.
- Not 'cheating' toward the end of a set to effect one more repetition.

Certainly, no one has to be goody two-shoes or blessed by the Pope in a place where 'cheating' is required to produce best results. But in the case of exercise, it had better be quantified and timed.

According to Jones, cheating should occur only *after* momentary muscle failure, when movement is no longer possible in strict form. And how much? "The absolute minimum amount required," he said, "to make the last two or three repetitions possible, not to make them easy. Properly performed, the cheated repetitions should be brutally hard."

'Brutally hard' explains why so many of us choose to cheat in a way that makes exercise infinitely easy.

## SEPTEMBER 2

### Advice to the Elderly

Age takes its toll on strength, flexibility and overall physical condition, but it doesn't change the laws of physics - and shouldn't change the goals of a fitness program.

The five potential benefits of exercise - improved strength, cardiovascular condition, flexibility, body composition and protection from injury - should be central to every well-designed program, regardless of the age of the participant. Older trainees simply have medical conditions to sidestep.

The potential for strength gain does not vary with age. An old man can increase his strength at the same rate and to the same degree (percentage increase) as a young man, though his ultimate level will be less. Therefore, progression should follow normal guidelines (8-15 repetitions with a 5% increase in weight at 15), respecting the comfort zone of the trainee with medical concerns. If weights seem heavy or create problems, a higher repetition scheme (12-20) or equipment that allows for smaller increments in resistance can be used.

In any case, exercise should focus on major muscle groups - hips, thighs, hamstrings, calves, chest, shoulders, back, biceps, triceps - with exercise for smaller muscles addressed as required. Full-range strength is best obtained on machines with variable resistance, as neither barbells nor functional training provides full-range exercise for the prime movers.

The need for flexibility increases with age. Short walking strides and golf swings are signs of a limited range of motion. Relaxing muscles (a) during stretching movements or (b) as you lower a weight to a position of full-extension during strength training (where the weight stack almost touches, or to where a stretch is felt) can increase that range. Machines are superior to free-weight exercises for flexibility because they provide resistance in full extension, and therefore the pull to facilitate a stretch.

Cardiovascular condition can be achieved by moving quickly from one exercise to another, but care must be taken with the elderly to ease into the process. Unless contraindicated, start by performing two or three consecutive exercises, followed by a rest of a few minutes. Gradually reduce the overall workout time to keep the heart rate in its training zone. If it is too difficult, include a 15-20 minute cardiovascular exercise after strength training, on a device that features *no* impact.

Protection from injury is a product of structural integrity vs. applied force, and a by-product of proper training. The strength of the structure is greatest when the muscles surrounding a joint are as strong as they can be through as great a range as possible - a condition made possible only by the performance of isolated exercise. Once the parts are strong, the nervous system can coordinate them by skill training. If injury is involved, the coordination can be assisted by a physical therapist.

The loss of body fat for old and young is best achieved by adding muscle to the body through progressive resistance exercise.

The current trend of using elastic bands, balance cushions and Swiss balls for the elderly has shifted the focus away from the very exercise (and equipment) that should form the core of all training - at any age.

Everything has its value on the exercise continuum. But, if exercise is judged by the quality of the resistance and quantity of the range of motion, most things now offered senior citizens should be at the back of the closet, instead of at the front entrance.

## SEPTEMBER 3

### Sources of Information

As kids, my brother and I often relied on a source of information we could trust - Mom and Dad. We didn't know about their 'education' and didn't care. They had - as we ultimately learned - the best form of education, experience.

The Nautilus® inventor discovered the same in his search for the secrets of strength training. As a kid, he wrote letters to sources he assumed were trustworthy - 'experts' in the field - and was surprised when they responded. He was more surprised by the cordial reception he got when he knocked on their doors; after all, he had nothing to offer them. But Arthur Jones was most surprised by the impression they left - the 'experts' knew nothing about exercise.

For the next 40 years, he sought alternate sources with much the same result, eventually ranking them from best to worst as follows:

- Experience. Like most, Jones learned by trial and error. Unlike most, he determined what worked and what didn't without the veil of growth drugs, exotic diets and extreme habits that clouded the cause-and-effect relationships. Jones kept precise records, used a strict style of performance and exhibited general superiority from the shoulders up. He not only discovered what worked for him, but what worked for others by performing more research than all of his competitors combined - with tools that *accurately* measured results. And he was honest. During major research at West Point in 1975, he appointed a man from the PE staff to secure individuals that had no affiliation with either Jones or West Point to perform the pre- and post-study testing. He did not want to be accused of having 'influenced' the results.

- Bodybuilding magazines. Jones deplored literature that fed a stream of nonsense and lies to hungry souls. "Yet, as ridiculous as they usually are," he said, "you can learn a lot more of value by reading current bodybuilding magazines than you can by reading everything published by the scientific community."

- Typical Gypsy fortune-tellers.
- The scientific community. The majority of past research employed worthless tools. "Yet, the scientists are the supposed 'experts' the media, the medical community and the government go to for advice on the subject of exercise; they would learn a lot more of value if they sought the advice of a typical Gypsy fortune-teller, because in that case they would not get their heads stuffed with a lot of pure bullshit based upon utterly meaningless research performed by a group of near idiots."
- The medical community. Jones believed doctors knew nothing about exercise due to lack of education. As the host of daily seminars, he asked them two questions: "When did you graduate?" and, if it was 10 years ago or more, "How much of what you learned in medical school do you still *believe*?" The average response was 10-20%, which meant they no longer believed 80-90% of what they learned. And they didn't learn much about exercise in the first place, which reflects in their performance. "Consult a doctor before initiating a program of exercise?" Not yet.

"Perhaps the most important bit of advice that I can offer you," concluded Jones, "is to point out the fact that you should be very cautious about just whom you go to for advice."

For most trainees, his experience, tempered by your trial and error, would provide a great start.


SEPTEMBER 4

_____

### Pilates

Joseph Pilates had a tough start in life. He was ill and too frail to play outdoors with kids his age, so he decided to shape his own destiny. He turned to exercise.

By the time he moved to England in 1912 (at age 32), he was a gymnast, pugilist, self-defense instructor and circus performer. From his morning warm-up sessions with a group of acrobats, he developed a system of exercise that focused on the abdomen.

During World War I, Joseph worked in an 'enemy alien' (POW) hospital where he rigged a series of springs to the beds of wounded soldiers and had them perform exercise to prevent atrophy and speed recovery. His creation was the precursor to a spring-based device called "The Cadillac."

In 1926, he moved to New York City and established an exercise facility next to a dance studio, marketing his ideas to boxers and other athletes. His methods were quickly embraced by the dance community.

Pilates was ahead of his time and made valuable contributions to exercise from his study of human movement. He would have been proud of the legacy carried on by his students and of the recent surge in popularity among dancers, athletes and the public.

The success of Pilates parallels that of the Nautilus® system introduced by Arthur Jones in 1970. Both men believed in the value of resistance exercise, in fewer repetitions, and in building tools to convey their message. There, the similarity ends.

A recent Pilates ad - "Imagine an exercise program that you look forward to, that engages you, and that leaves you refreshed and alert with a feeling of physical and mental well-being" - was not what Jones had in mind. If you didn't finish in a near-dead heap on the floor, Arthur would 'question' your commitment.

The Pilates method of conditioning, according to its disciples, improves flexibility and total-body strength without bulking up, by strengthening and stretching at the same time. The result - "long, lean muscles."

Let's set the record straight.

Pilates machines, if they have anything in common with the original, are basic pulley stations that use the weight of the body or its parts as resistance, which is why muscles don't bulk up. From a strength perspective, the quality of the resistance and its effective range of influence are limited. In addition, the machines work within the limits of pulleys instead of the limitations of human muscle, and classes amount to little more than a Total Gym® session for those who have misplaced the instructions.

The claimed 'advantage' of simultaneous stretching and strengthening is no different to that of a barbell, properly used. And the claim of building long, lean muscles? Try again. God handled that already, and neither you nor Joe had any say in the matter.

Pilates enhances flexibility, increases strength and stimulates a cardiovascular change if no rest is allowed between movements. Its contribution to body leanness and injury prevention is compromised by its inability to stimulate maximum strength changes.

Jones shared one other trait with Pilates.

One of Joseph's students, Bob Seed, a hockey player turned 'enthusiast,' was one of only two people to open a studio while Pilates was still alive. He set up across town and attracted some of Joe's clients by opening earlier in the morning. One day, Joe visited Seed with a gun and told him to get out of town, which he did.

Arthur would have enjoyed that.

## SEPTEMBER 5

### Preparation

The country of Colombia was full of surprises - some good, some bad and some neither. I was rarely prepared.

I first arrived with a group of high-school teachers from Caracas who had to be flown out of the country a minimum of 24 hours for immigration purposes, Bogota the haven of choice. There, the hotel was grand, the climate brisk and the time right for a run. I changed into my gear, heeded the 'no-jewelry' warning and shot out the door.

The venue was exhilarating - scenery, temperature, country - and the pace brisk to start, but it soon faded. I caught my breath and accelerated again only to fall into the same trap. In the end, the run was lousy.

Bogota was 8,000 feet above sea level; Caracas, 3,000, and it takes approximately one week of training to adjust to every 3,000 feet of altitude. I was not ill, just ill prepared.

Yet, what worked against one activity, helped in another. A doctor invited me to play golf at The Country Club, where the ball sailed so far it was hard to select the right club. After nine holes, we stopped for lunch, then resumed. I cruised along until my ball found the lake at the 13th. When I reached into my bag for another, it was empty - two dozen new balls gone. It made lunch expensive but club selection easy.

On another occasion, my wife and I drove from Caracas through the Colombian border-town of Cucuta to the mountain village of Pamplona, where we dodged cargo-laden mules on top of the world. When we finally pulled into the hotel parking lot in our personal battering ram - a 1962 Ford® Galaxy 500, we lucked out. The rooms were as nice as a Holiday Inn®, the best in town.

We cleaned up and went downstairs to dine in a room overlooking the valley, and to embrace the hallmark of Colombian restaurants, service. As we scanned the menu, I watched a lady struggle to cut a roll a few tables over. The waiter arrived in a tuxedo one size too large in the jacket and two too small in the pants. Between, he sported a twisted bow-tie. That was the good news - the food was the bad.

I needed a chainsaw to cut the role, an axe for the meat, and a hard floor upon which to bounce the Jello®. The food was far from the exquisite dinners in Cali, where the staff did everything but kiss our shoes between bites. When the bill arrived, I was unprepared. It was dirt cheap.

I was equally unprepared when I heard Nautilus® inventor, Arthur Jones advocate training every day, a statement that ran contrary to his philosophy of brief, infrequent exercise. Jones was as full of surprises as Colombia - some good, some bad - but he was prepared. The good related to his introduction of new equipment, something the others could copy. The bad related to the errors he made along the way, errors that others continue to make. Arthur Jones freely admitted his mistakes but learned from them, which is more than could be said of his competitors.

He rationalized his statement in two ways: daily workouts during the first week only help rid of muscle soreness common at the start of training; and, intensity (a requirement for best results from exercise) was hard work. It had to be learned, and learning takes time. He advocated a break-in period of a few weeks for novice trainees and to those initiating a program of negative work.

Jones' machines and philosophy represented years of trial and error. When he said something, there was no crooked bow-tie behind it.

## SEPTEMBER 6

### A Farm Boy's Negative Dream

Arthur Jones did not discover negative work, although you would have thought so by the way he was attacked. He first believed it had value, performed research to confirm his premise (1972), and then created practical ways to use it - at least on a few exercises.

Negative work was in use long before Jones arrived. In the early 1950's, Tennessee strongman Bob Peoples (in Arthur's words), "used a negative-only style of exercise; he rigged up a tractor to lift a very heavy weight that he could not lift, and then trained in a negative-only fashion by lowering this heavy weight back down to the bottom position."

Instead of a tractor, Jones used 'people-power' to lift the weight in his studies and arrived at the same conclusion - negative-only exercise was, by far, the most productive way to train. But it was neither practical nor, in some cases, safe.

The reason you can lower a heavier weight than you can lift is due to a factor that was 'discovered' by Jones - internal muscle friction.

The same friction that works against you as you lift works with you as you lower. It allows you to continue an exercise long after exhaustion, but introduces the possibility of excess fatigue and poor recovery. As Jones put it, "Exercise with no resulting fatigue is largely worthless, but too much fatigue from exercise is counterproductive, may cause losses in strength rather than gains."

He broke it down into numbers for a better understanding (see chart below).

"If positive strength of a fresh muscle is 100, then negative strength will be 140 (40% higher) and static strength will be 120 (the true level of strength); but when a fresh muscle has been worked to the point that its remaining level of (positive) strength is zero, then remaining negative strength will be 120 (nearly as high as it was when fresh), while true strength, static strength, will be 60, having been reduced from its fresh level by 50%. Reaching that level of fatigue while performing only positive exercise is all but impossible, would require a very high number of sets of the exercise, far too many sets; but reaching that level of fatigue from negative-only exercise is relatively easy."

| | Positive Strength | Negative Strength | Static Strength |
|---|---|---|---|
| A. Under FRESH Conditions | 100 | 140 | 120 |
| B. With Total Positive Failure | 0 | 120 | 60 |
| C. With Total Negative Failure | 0 | 0 | 0 |

Under normal conditions, muscle failure during a lift (B) does not reduce positive strength to zero. An average muscle loses approximately 2% of its strength per repetition - at 10 reps, the resulting loss would be approximately 20%. A 100% loss in positive strength would require, as Jones suggests, the performance of an excessive amount of exercise and weeks to recover, if not an ambulance. And guess what? Your negative strength would still be high.

When positive strength is reduced by 100%, the resulting fatigue is the same as that encountered when negative strength is reduced by only 18% (from 140 to 120).

Jones suggests the following for negative-only exercise: on select exercises, one set of eight repetitions (lowering in 8-10 seconds per rep) until the descent can no longer be controlled - with no rest between. How often? "We have a man on our staff who loses strength if he exercises once a week, neither gains or loses if he exercises once every two weeks and gains only when he exercises once every three weeks."

How do you know when you've had too much? When the tractor bursts through the gym doors - which, for far too many, would be nothing more than a good start.

## SEPTEMBER 7

### The World's Most Aerobic Exercise

The best source, if not the entire definition, of aerobic exercise is thrown into confusion each year the "World Aerobics Championship" crowns a victor based upon three minutes of intense cheerleading. But not to worry.

If old physiology texts are valid, and they probably aren't far off, the highest aerobic capacities ever measured (and the highest year after year among athletes) belong to cross-country skiers - not swimmers, runners, rowers, wrestlers or cheerleaders. End of discussion, but not end of story.

The world's most aerobic demonstration of exercise occurred on a device that was not originally designed for aerobic work. The Nautilus® Duo Squat Machine, introduced in 1982, was a leg press with independent movement-arms that featured three performance styles: alternating legs (one leg at a time); both legs at once; and 'akinetic' (one leg pushed while the other provided resistance).

The 'akinetic' method was by far the most difficult and so aerobic that the machine's inventor, Arthur Jones, called it "...not 'one of the best sources'...THE BEST POSSIBLE SOURCE OF CARDIOVASCULAR BENEFITS. And probably the safest." The machine allowed exercise with any resistance at any speed through any range of motion without the production of kinetic energy (weight stack acceleration), impact, or the sacrifice of negative work. The stage was set.

Dr. Michael Fulton, orthopedic representative for Nautilus at the time and team physician for a USFL franchise, invited one of his young football players to participate in the experiment. The choice was good. According to Fulton, this kid was "more likely to walk through a wall than fold in a challenge." The object was to raise his heart rate as high as possible, and sustain it as long as possible. The machine, set in the akinetic mode with 150 pounds, required the subject to produce a force equal to, or in excess of, 150 pounds with his leg muscles to remain in that mode.

It was tough - the most anyone had lasted was five minutes.

The kid's pulse soared to 200 beats per minute after 90 seconds of exercise. At five minutes, agony was apparent on his face. He plowed on. At eight, the staff murmured to one another in disbelief. Their encouragement drowned his grunts. Ten minutes. Sweat was heavy. His pulse held the line. At 15, he was still going. No one had touched the weight stack. Eighteen minutes. The effort was taking its toll. At 20, he abandoned ship, leaving a spent carcass at the base of the machine. His heart rate - 200+ beats per minute for 18½ minutes - was possibly the highest sustained rate in the history of exercise.

The experiment left no doubt and only one message: Don't try this at home.

The subject revealed that willpower alone allowed him to elude the pain at eight minutes, but that something nice happened at 12 - his legs went numb. At 20 minutes, searing pain "deep in the bones" forced him to quit out of fear.

Nonetheless, the effort was superhuman. The kid couldn't walk for days.

Upon hearing the tale, a hardened, veteran instructor (in my gym) decided to try it with the same weight. He lasted a miserable 45 seconds.

The Duo Squat Machine provided all of the advantages of full-range exercise for the muscles of the hips and legs without any of the dangers of traditional squats. It also provided a level of cardiovascular condition second to none.

The only problem: too few would walk through a wall to get there.

## SEPTEMBER 8

### If Henry Only Knew

Al and I took turns at what became a three-day paid vacation in Niagara Falls. While one slowly painted the pump, the other, coveralls stripped to the waist, basked in the sun on a raft tied to the dock. It was Ford® Motor Company's annual two-week shutdown, a time for maintenance, cleaning and painting - for some.

A veteran of sly, Al O'Brien volunteered to paint the machines in the pumphouse by the river. Once instructions and foreman were gone, he picked the best spot from which to 'vigil' the situation without being caught - all on time-and-a-half.

Twice daily, the foreman waddled down the path from the plant to view the progress, and twice daily, Al reminded him of the difficulty of the task.

"How we coming along, boys?" asked Big Jack in a gruff voice.

"Doing pretty well," replied Al. "You know how tough it is to paint under the machine in those corners, Jack."

"M-M-M," he grumbled, "Keep working at it, boys. We need you to finish things in the plant. Only got a few days left."

The charade continued until Al ran out of every line but his tan line.

The final day left a host of uncompleted tasks. With Jack in panic, Al and I took on a task that, if done like the last, might have taken eight days. We promised to paint the cone-shaped roof on a service shed in the final hours.

"Get to it, boys," said Jack, with what voice and hope remained.

Al and I first gathered everything on the roof and took turns dumping gallons of paint from the pinnacle. As it ran down, the other brushed as if he was possessed. We got the job done in a couple of hours.

When the plant re-opened, things weren't much different. The midnight shift met 80% of their quota by employing a frenzied pace the first four hours and then dogged it to finish just as the day crew arrived. They could have doubled production.

The parallels to exercise are numerous.

When left to their own, most people will do the absolute minimum to maintain their status quo. On command, their bodies will do what it is told but cease when quotas are reached. If it strives for 10 repetitions, it will likely stop at 10 and reward itself with a drink of water for a job well done. If it gets only nine, it has overestimated its strength and done itself a favor. That is, it probably tried the final, impossible repetition because it assumed it would get there. Exercise should stop only when the resistance stops in the face of a full effort.

The body must be taken beyond its comfort zone, pushed and tricked into submission before it will re-evaluate its current needs. If there is no challenge, it will fall asleep - which is where proper supervision comes in.

My brother, another Al, once took a nap in a crate in the shipping department on the midnight shift and was not warned (again, improper supervision) that it was time to leave. When he punched out 30 minutes late, the day shift HOOTED him out of the building.

The same with exercise - by the time most people learn anything of value in strength training, it's too late.

Two men who revolutionized their industries, Arthur Jones (Nautilus®) and Henry Ford, realized the value of proper supervision. Had Henry pushed us at the right moment, Al and I would have made headlines. The river was adjacent to the Falls.

SEPTEMBER 9

---

## Either You Know, or You Don't

Put a tie on a donkey, give him a gun and badge, place him in a third-world airport, and cross your fingers. Customs agents at Simon Bolivar International Airport in Maiquetia, Venezuela could be sieves or concrete walls depending on the time of day, the number of bags they had to check, and the amount of money in their pockets.

It was already too late. The plane had arrived.

We scanned the confusion from an external corridor for signs of our guest - a thinning shock of blond hair, blue jeans and cowboy boots - and stood helpless as the goods neared their fate.

Suddenly, the customs agent flung both arms in the air as if to say, "What's this?" Our guest was speechless. The man in uniform signaled again with an amplified gesture. The 'gringo' knew no Spanish and retorted by throwing his arms in the air as if performing a military press. The agent didn't know a barbell from a bag of peanuts, but understood sign language. The barbell got through and Michael Fulton, orthopedic representative of MedX® Corporation, learned the basics of communication in South America.

Fulton's mentor, Arthur Jones spent a lifetime creating what he called "a thinking man's barbell" by first identifying 10 ingredients of "a perfect form of exercise," and incorporating them into his new Nautilus® machines. He was so far ahead of his competitors that they literally waited for him to make something to copy. Like our agent, they didn't know a barbell from a bag of peanuts.

Jones later turned his focus to medical equipment and bluntly proclaimed that the leading technology (represented by isokinetic machines) was inaccurate and dangerous. He spent the next 20 years criticizing the leader in that field, Cybex®, for selling tools that, according to him, "their vice-president admitted were fraudulent."

I attended a series of medical seminars hosted by Jones in the late 1980's in which he hammered isokinetic technology in general, and Cybex in particular. On one occasion, a guest piped up, "Those are strong accusations, Arthur. Aren't you afraid they'll sue?"

"I hope they will. It'll take about two minutes in court to show that one and one is two, not eight as they suggest." Jones could clearly illustrate the fallacy of isokinetic equipment, but was wrong on one issue. It took about three minutes.

On another occasion, he halted in the middle of a verbal assault and said, "I will give them (Cybex) one thing, at least they're consistent. Everything they make is worthless."

He wasn't far off.

The pad that supports your back on today's Cybex leg extension machine is fixed at 90° to the seat bottom (instead of leaned back), an error that could have been avoided 30 years ago by copying the original. They're still wandering - and not alone.

The other day a new two-pronged management team decided to reconfigure our gym. As they did so, Fiddle Dumb criticized the MedX machines with particular reference to a "bad" seated leg curl.

"How is it 'bad?'" I asked.

"Obvious, they put the restraint pad on the lower leg instead of the top of the knee."

"Have you heard of action-reaction?" I injected. "When the lower leg moves toward the butt, the pad on the shin prevents the knee from moving forward. Properly secured, the knee remains in line with the axis of rotation and *does not move up.*"

Peanuts anyone?


## SEPTEMBER 10

---

### Banana George

As 35-time world-record holder, Cory Pickos ran his students through their morning paces at the World Ski Center® in Tradewinds Park (Deerfield Beach, Florida), the antique horn of a yellow Cadillac® signaled its arrival.

Out stepped an old man dressed in yellow from head to toe - socks, shoes, pants, shirt, hat, watch and a pair of stripped sunglasses. He waved as he shuffled from the driver's seat to the trunk from where - after a moment's delay - he began carting bunches of bananas to the dock.

"Banana George" Blair was doing his thing, bananas first.

The sprightly man exchanged pleasantries with Cory and then introduced himself to the students, as if it was necessary. George was on 'break' from a hectic schedule in Orlando and had stopped by to check out the new school.

"Do you want to ski?" asked Cory.

"Naw, don't feel like it. My day off."

"C'mon, George," urged the students. It didn't take much. He headed for the car.

With the help of his boat driver, George pried himself into a skin-tight yellow wet-suit, not an easy task for a man in his late seventies. As he suited up, a throng of youthful eyes (kids from the campground) stared from the bank. No skis, no hair, maybe no brains - what was this old guy up to?

George grabbed the rope and walked to the far end of the dock, 30 feet from the water's edge. The rope slowly tightened as the boat steadied.

"Hit it."

George ran to the end of the wooden structure and threw himself feet first into the water, landing on his back. As he grazed the surface, a rooster-tail wiped out all signs of life. Not to fear. Like the Lochness monster, the banana man mysteriously emerged from the swirl and initiated a repertoire of moves that would have left the best of Scottish eyebrows up, and jaws down.

The barefoot skier was legendary. His introduction to the sport at the age of 56 led to daily performances at Cypress Gardens® and television features that included ads based on products for health and vitality.

Rightly so. George was in phenomenal physical condition - and he wasn't alone.

During the 1980's, I worked with a number of professional water skiers through my association with Michael Sanchez Vegas, Venezuelan National Water-Ski Coach. Mike first brought the reigning World Trick-Ski Champion and record holder (overall World Champion in 1988), Anna Maria Carrasco, to my gym for conditioning and rehabilitation in 1980. Her sister, Maria Victoria, was undefeated World Trick-Ski Champion from 1972-79. Mike was a devotee of the Nautilus® system of preparation and lured Cory to train with Anna for several months in Caracas (during which time he surpassed his own world record).

I was left with the utmost respect for the sport. The physical demands of skiing were evident in the low body-fat levels among its competitors. Even spectators - from former skiers to the youngest of viewers - displayed lean, tanned physiques, with not a cigarette in sight. And more. Research has shown that competitive water-skiing is the only sport that meaningfully strengthens the muscles that extend the lumbar spine.

My advice? Eat bananas and ski.

## SEPTEMBER 11

---

### Of Sense and Senses

Four of us sat down after the "Grand Opening." We had worked the gym through its pre-construction and construction phases, a nine-month grind - hundreds of tours, thousands of calls and reams of referrals.

"Who was the guy that came in Monday asking about a family membership?" I asked, lucky to remember my own name.

"John ...ah...Conklin...795-0864."

Mike was his own Yellow Book®, associating telephone numbers with a birthday or life event. Some flashed to his head in the standard form; others arrived in Braille, and many as both.

Mike Chastain was blind, yet could walk through a space he had just been shown without bumping into anything and, of course, without a cane. He could overhear conversations from remote corners of the gym and commit voices to memory. His other senses had heightened to extraordinary levels.

We often fail to appreciate things until we no longer have them...as was the case with my vision one day playing golf.

The Junko (pronounced "Hoonko") Golf Club was truly a sight to see. Glued to a hillside 4,000 feet above sea level and 90 minutes from downtown Caracas (Venezuela), the course was one of unspoiled beauty - undulating, scenic and tree-lined. From one vista, four fairways cascaded down the mountainside with golf-course green scattered everywhere. A Jeep® took players to the next tee at three junctures, while the rugged terrain planted seeds of uncertainty every step of the way. I held my own for 11 holes...little did I know.

As I stepped onto the 12th tee, the wispy clouds that had passed by throughout the day suddenly lingered. The reason why I was alone became clear - a heavy fog rolled in at 2PM every day. I had no warning or map.

I lined myself up where the tee-markers aimed (always a mistake) and saw only the faint outline of trees as I set to swing. It was hit, listen and hope. Sometimes the feel of the swing triggered a clue that the ball sailed right or left, but it was mainly ears that told the tale - and they were not up to the task. I lost eight balls coming home and ruined what was otherwise a perfect day.

On the other side of the coin, I have had perfect days ruined by sight - the sight of 'bad form' in gyms. First off, most people perform exercise in a way that would lead the sane to wonder if they've done anything right and the insane to form habits that might take a lifetime to correct. Second, there's an

412

over-emphasis on watching weights move up and down, a reminder that the ability to see only dulls the other senses, while the inability heightens them.

Mike Chastain listens to the cadence of the machine's friction and keeps a hand on the movement arm when he trains clients. It provides feedback about speed, range of motion and intensity. He trains himself the same way - by feel - and it shows.

Close your eyes during exercise and learn. What muscle is working? How does it feel? How relaxed are non-working body parts? Can the muscle feel the resistance at this speed? Is it moving through a full range of motion? What is muscle failure like? What's your threshold for pain?

Use sight *between* exercises and your strength training will likely improve.

## SEPTEMBER 12

### Use Your Head, Fred

The value of exercise, movement against resistance, is determined by the quality of resistance and the quantity of movement. Movement without resistance has little value; and resistance without movement, as in a static contraction, has its value tied to the angle of effort.

*Only full-range movement and an appropriate resistance throughout that range* deliver the best of both worlds.

Perform a standing biceps curl with a barbell and focus on 'how it feels' - easy at the top and bottom, hard in the middle. The 'hardest' position, when forearms are parallel to the floor, suffers from poor leverage and the full effect of gravity.

The same applies to a sit up. Lie on your back with your legs bent and pull your torso toward your knees. The exercise feels 'hardest' at the start - when your torso has barely cleared the floor - because leverage is poor and gravity high. From there, the movement becomes progressively easier to the point that when your torso is perpendicular to the floor, there is no resistance.

Sit-ups (and abdominal curls) would be more effective if they started 'below' the floor so that your torso could 'finish' parallel to the floor - in a full-contracted position against the greatest possible resistance.

The other day, I saw a trainee perform sit-ups on a decline bench that allowed him to start 'below' the floor. Despite the proper tool, the young man lowered his torso less than halfway down (from vertical) and then swung it up to a position beyond vertical, where gravity was actually helping an excess of useless reps.

"You can perform a hundred sets of a hundred repetitions in the curl and press with a pair of five pound dumbbells - a total of 10,000 repetitions - and you can do so daily for the rest of your life," said Nautilus® inventor Arthur Jones, "and you will NEVER produce much in the way of worthwhile results."

Another popular exercise, a chin-up, is difficult because you must pull your body (not part of it) straight up against gravity. Your arms rotate at the shoulder and elbow creating poor leverage about halfway up. Although it 'feels' hardest in that position, muscle failure could occur anywhere because of the involvement of the small muscles of the hands and forearms - which makes grip position essential.

Yet, what do we see? The same as Jones saw 30 years ago:

"Do you really believe that 'wide-grip' chins stretch your lats (upper back) more than narrower-grip chins?" he asked. "If so - wrong again; such a wide hand spacing literally makes much in the way of stretching impossible (limits the range of motion)."

"And why do you turn your palms forward," he added, "while performing behind-neck pulldowns? Since such a hand positioning reduces the strength of the upper arms to the lowest possible level - and thus reduces the degree of producible results from this exercise by at least 70%. Since the arms are already too weak to provide much work for the much stronger torso muscles involved in this movement - and since you are limited insofar as torso muscle development is concerned by the strength of the arms (or the lack-of-strength of the arms). And yet you make a bad situation far worse by putting the arms in an even-weaker position than necessary."

If a large amount of exercise raises a flag about quality, the performance of an exercise a certain way by the majority of trainees should raise another.

Use your head. Solutions to what we once perfected in grade school are rather simple.

SEPTEMBER 13

---

### Fill and Fodder

I once rejected an offer to work as an assistant golf professional at the Homestead in Hot Springs, Virginia in the early 1970's. But the dreams of strutting down TV's garden path to victory were shattered by something more grandiose - what some called 'lack of competitive drive' and what I called 'genetic inability.' The earth-moving decision may have been a blessing.

In the end, the field of exercise came to the rescue and made what appeared to be a step backward, a leap forward. It also provided the opportunity for a TV debut.

A man who promoted health and fitness on a morning talk show (and who had joined my gym in Caracas in 1980) asked me to introduce the Nautilus® system of training to a nationwide audience.

What should have been a pleasure turned into much less.

The opportunity quickly morphed into 10 minutes of self-glorification - the host determined to show the world *everything* he knew. We had an expression for it in high school, "I've got some friends I haven't even used yet."

It was my first and last experience with makeup, and reminded me of some trainers I'd met who were quick to reveal everything *they* knew about exercise, which took about the same time - 10 minutes.

I recently reviewed the workout chart of a new client who was seated 'in the clouds' on a biceps machine despite an orientation with a co-worker the week before. On machines with multiple settings, only one had been marked, the least important at that. Several settings had been ignored completely, along with the sound advice that should have accompanied the initial session. Day One: Two sets of a slew of lower-body exercises; Day Two: Two sets of a slew of upper-body exercises; Day Three: A whole-body workout. I hadn't read that book yet.

To add injury to insult, my helping hand was interrupted by the frequent thump of a weight stack in an adjacent 'sports performance' program. The name of the equipment in use, Pro Implosion®, was never more appropriate: 'Pro' - for professional (I suppose); 'Implosion' - a cross between impact and explosion (both negatives); and 'Imp' - an elf or gnome. All pointed to the introduction of bad form and danger to a new generation by a group of so-called 'educated' instructors who should have their collective heads examined. The task of de-warping that scene was so beyond human effort that I was tempted to call upon an 'old' friend.

During my college days, a girlfriend put together a Superman outfit - complete with Clark Kent suit, fedora and portable phone booth - so that I could save damsels in distress at football games. It worked - saved a dozen or so - which is more than can be said of the success of our TV host.

He inundated the media with plans to open an athletic club/Nautilus gym high atop the wealthy hills of La Lagunita, 30 minutes from downtown Caracas. Years later, only the ravaged remnants of a single tennis court remain.

Pretending to be someone can be fun, but it doesn't work in exercise. If you can't deal with basics and a measure of common sense, you're no better off than Lois Lane at the end of a Superman episode, when she asked, "Clark, how come you're never around when Superman's around?"

Some people just never get it.


# SEPTEMBER 14

---

## If I Was King

Chronic low-back pain was not considered life threatening until I came along.

In 1981, a neurosurgeon instructed me to lie in bed for a month and get up only to go to the bathroom, all to avoid a second surgery. I stupidly obeyed, lost 15 pounds and could barely stand. One day, while swaying above the toilet, I fell back and cracked my head on a marble floor - out cold. At least my back felt better than something.

Bed rest in 1981? "It has been proven beyond any shadow of a lingering doubt," said Arthur Jones, "that total immobilization of a joint in the human body unavoidably produces changes in the muscles, the tendons, the ligaments and the bones that are very difficult, and frequently impossible, to repair." I should have known better.

Ninety percent of back pain is acute - it comes and goes at random - which makes it difficult to establish a cause-and-effect relationship. Did pills, rest, traction, ice or a combination make the pain subside? Maybe none. In a study funded by the Dutch government, all traditional treatments for back pain were deemed useless.

Fortunately, cause-and-effect is more readily discernable with chronic pain. In 1986, Jones identified three muscular causes of back pain and believed that the treatment least used - exercise - was the only one capable of producing tissue change.

In 1994, the government saw it differently. With the health-care cost for chronic spine pain at $300 million dollars per day, they leaped into action, as described by Jones. "A committee of supposed 'experts' that was recently formed for the stated purpose of determining just what treatment is of actual value in cases of chronic spinal pain consists of a lot of people who generally know little or nothing about the actual cause and effect situation... Somebody once said that a camel is a racehorse designed by a committee."

It wasn't as if exercise was the new kid on the block.

Fifty years before, in 1944, the Surgeon General ordered a military doctor named Tom DeLorme to evaluate and discharge the wounded from service. He began, instead, to rehabilitate them with exercise and wrote the first scientific article on the subject.

DeLorme later became chairman of Liberty Mutual® Insurance Company and was guest speaker at a spinal conference hosted by Jones in 1993. "In the overall field of medicine," he said, "less than a dollar's worth of benefit is produced by every hundred dollars of expense." In the case of spinal care as practiced by his company, "the benefit is less than one cent for each hundred dollars spent. The program is utterly worthless."

The main problem is fraud. I once worked for a woman who kept busy beneath a cloud of smoke in a 'smoke-free' office filing claims for an empty rehab center. By the time the Feds caught up, Jan Fedderman had taken Medicare for a 1.5 million-dollar ride. She was last rumored to be hiding in Maryland under an assumed name.

If I was king, I'd do the following:

1. Eliminate the legal system. As Jones put it, "If Clinton's wife is really serious about straightening out the current mess in the health care system, the first thing she should do is kill all the lawyers."
2. Eliminate worker's compensation fraud - false back, neck and knee claims can be quickly detected by MedX® equipment.
3. Reject *all* claims related to the use of isokinetic tools (both testing and exercise).
4. If the above puts people out of business, I'd force them to hide in Maryland.
5. Go to Maryland and hunt them down.


SEPTEMBER 15

---


### The Best Form of Training

At six feet, seven inches, Tom Laputka barely squeezed through the door of the 30 year-old metal building behind the Deland High School in 1972. Inside, the lighting was so dim that the pro football player could barely see across the room, but the stench was familiar - hot, damp, smelly air - what you'd expect in a locker room. The space was filled with wall-to-wall Nautilus® machines and, on workout days, with football players, bodybuilders and weightlifters who had accepted the challenge of the man orchestrating the show, Arthur Jones.

Training sessions involved the use of negative-only exercise - no lifting, just lowering - and subjects worked in small groups of four by necessity. "I needed two strong men to pull the movement arm to the contracted position," claimed Tom, "and another one, sometimes two, to stand on the weight stack while I slowly lowered the movement arm." The assistants quickly lifted the resistance then carefully passed it to him to limit recovery between repetitions. They jumped on and off weight stacks and shouted encouragement while Arthur cracked the whip. The place was "alive with muscle-building excitement."

The work was heavy. After three months, Laputka reached the following strength levels: Hip and Back machine - 700 pounds (one leg at a time); Leg Extension - 500 pounds; Leg Curl - 350 pounds; Pullover - 700 pounds; Dip - 463 pounds (bodyweight plus 200 pounds around his hips); Torso Arm (pulldowns) - 350 pounds; and Triceps Extension/Biceps Curl - 150 pounds. It paid.

Tom reported to football camp with more size, strength, endurance and speed than ever before. "That year," he said, "I played the best football of my career."

The most productive method of training looked dangerous, but Jones knew otherwise: It was the safest way to train.

Growth stimulation occurs when muscles work near maximum levels of momentary ability. Injury occurs when a force exceeds the breaking strength of the muscle/joint system. Work intensity has to be high for best results, but the force to which the system is exposed has to be low for safety. Negative-only work provides both.

EMG studies show that muscle input (intensity) is greater during negative work than during positive work; while logic demonstrates that force involvement is at its lowest. Place a 100-pound barbell on a scale; it produces a downward force of 100 pounds. Apply an upward force of 50 pounds to the bar without moving it and the scale will read 50. Apply an upward force of 100 pounds without moving the bar and the scale will read zero. A force of more than 100 pounds is required to create movement (lift).

On the other hand, if a 100-pound barbell begins in a lifted position, a force of less than 100 pounds is required to lower it. Why? A 100-pound force would stop its descent, while more than 100 would make it rise. When lowering is neither stopped nor reversed, the force is as low - and the exercise as safe - as it can be.

Tom Laputka met one drawback with negative-only work: "It was easy to overtrain." He hit a plateau after four weeks and reduced his training from three days a week to two. Four weeks later (for the same reason), he reduced his frequency to three sessions every two weeks. On both occasions, his strength increased immediately.

The best form of training takes a toll on systemic recovery and should not be used frequently - once a week to start, once every two weeks to advance.

## SEPTEMBER 16

### Negative-Only Training

In the fall of 1972, Arthur Jones wrote about the benefits of *lowering* (vs. lifting) weights in an article that was read by an American physiologist who attended the Olympic Games that year in Germany. At the games, Dr. Paavo Komi, a physiology professor at the University of Jyvaskyla, addressed the Olympic Scientific Congress on his use of negative-only training with Scandinavian weightlifters (one gold medal, two bronze). The American telephoned Jones when he returned to the US and was surprised to find that the Nautilus® inventor's research was far beyond that of Dr. Komi.

In 1972-73, Jones conducted several six-month studies that involved football players, bodybuilders, athletes from other sports, and non-athletes. All subjects were restricted to lowering weights (not lifting) and performed one set of 10 exercises (8-12 repetitions) three times per week. Each set lasted approximately two minutes and featured a 10-second lowering cadence per repetition, with no rest between exercises. Workouts lasted 18-20 minutes, never more than 30.

The starting weight for each exercise was set at 40% more than what could be lifted in good form for 8-12 repetitions. Subjects were instructed not to stop the downward movement of the weight during the first repetitions (even if they could) and to try to stop the weight when it became impossible during the final repetitions (even if they couldn't). The exercise ended when the lowering phase occurred in 2-3 seconds, despite a full effort from the subject.

The results were spectacular.

One defensive lineman from the Buffalo Bills added 20 pounds of muscle, cut 2/10ths of a second off his already fast 40-yard dash, added 5½ inches to his vertical jump and doubled the strength of his hip, thigh, chest, upper-back and neck muscles.

A professional football player from Canada, who began with 275 pounds on a pullover machine, performed several repetitions with 675 pounds two months later.

A young bodybuilder completed 32 repetitions with 400 pounds in the leg press to start, and later performed 45 repetitions with 840 pounds under the same test conditions (quit at 45 due to muscle pain rather than failure).

Every subject produced a result superior to what had been produced by traditional exercise. The advantages of 'negative-only' training were clear:

- The pressure of force pulling against the subject in a position of extension (at the end of lowering) stretched muscles to improve flexibility.
- The stretch also activated a 'pre-stretch,' the neurological stimulus required for high-intensity muscular contraction.
- The pressure of force pulling against the subject in a position of flexion (at the start of lowering) provided resistance in contraction - a prerequisite for full-range exercise.
- A maximum resistance applied to the muscle through a full range of motion using a slow speed of movement eliminated poor form. It's easy to *throw* a weight up or 'cheat' during the lifting phase, but impossible to throw it down.

Negative-only training exposed muscles to a maximum overload, facilitated a high level of intensity, provided full-range exercise, increased flexibility and ensured good form in the process.

So, the next time someone says, "Lowering is more important than lifting," listen.

Better yet, apply.

## SEPTEMBER 17

### Negative-Accentuated Training

Would you buy a car with no doors?

When you first heard that it was "more important to lower than lift a weight," you probably nodded your head and smiled - with reason. First, the concept was most likely left unexplained. Second, it *felt* easier to lower a weight than lift it. Third, the information could not be used in any practical way, other than trying to lower weights at a slower pace. Fourth, it took an entourage of assistants to perform negative work; and fifth, with strong trainees, the process became dangerous for the helpers.

The car had no doors.

Nautilus® inventor Arthur Jones was aware of these shortcomings and created a practical way to lower weights that he called "negative-accentuated training." It required less resistance than negative-only work, no outside help and could be performed on any machine that had a single (connected) movement arm.

A leg extension provides a good example of his solution:

- Select a weight that represents 70% of what you would use for 'normal' exercise. That is, if you use 100 pounds for 10 repetitions in your routine, select 70 pounds.
- Lift the weight with both legs in a slow fashion.
- Pause in the contracted position for a full second and slowly transfer the weight to the right leg only. Pause again.
- Slowly lower the right leg (in approximately 8 seconds).
- Lift the weight to the top position again with both legs. Pause. Transfer the weight to the left leg. Pause again, then slowly lower the left leg (in 8 seconds).
- Lift with two; lower with one. Lift with two; lower with the other. Repeat until you can no longer lift the weight to the contracted position with both legs.

A proper set of negative-accentuated exercise consists of 8-12 lifting movements and 4-6 lowering movements with each leg. If the weight is correct, you should reach momentary muscle failure at approximately 12 repetitions. When you can perform more than 12, increase the weight by 5%.

My first experience with negative-accentuated exercise followed eight months of hard training on Nautilus machines in Caracas, Venezuela, and left two impressions. One was the frustration of reaching fatigue. The use of 70% of the normal weight permitted too many lifting repetitions (my form in those days was, and still is, impeccable) which increased the total workout time, something I didn't need. At the same time, it stimulated the 'sweat' glands, something I did need. The second impression appeared two days later - I could barely move.

I continued once a week for three months and increased my starting weights by approximately 20-25%. I could now pause and lower the weight I once lifted with two limbs, in control, one limb at a time and the increase in negative strength reflected in 'normal' workouts. Some recommendations:

- Select 80% of your normal weight (provided you can maintain good form).

- Train once a week using 'negative-accentuated' exercise (the final workout of each week) to allow better recovery.
- Try it with the following machines: leg extension, leg curl, leg press, calf raise, pullover, chest press, overhead press, biceps curl and triceps extension.

Negative-accentuated is harder than traditional training - but the doors are wide open.

# SEPTEMBER 18

---

## By the Rules

"Dear Sir,

In playing the 15th hole on Saturday afternoon, I discovered my ball in an unplayable lie, and after dropping it over my shoulder in accordance with rule 22 I was astonished to find that it was nowhere to be seen. Having searched diligently for some time, I then took another ball from my pocket, which I also dropped, but it disappeared as well. In this manner I lost five more. Later I discovered that the balls had fallen into the mouth of my golf-bag, which was slung across my shoulder. Kindly inform me how many strokes I played."
(from *Letters to the Secretary of a Golf Club*, George C. Nash, 1934)

Some people play by the rules; some don't.

I entered a profession with no rules, the field of exercise; in a country with fewer, Venezuela; and was left to adopt my own based on the principles outlined by a man in the process of establishing his, Arthur Jones. It was a great choice.

"Fifty years ago," said Jones, "most of the commonly accepted theories in this field were wrong; today almost all of these same myths are still widely accepted, and in the meantime, hundreds of other superstitions have taken root. So we are now stuck with most of the old myths and a lot of new ones."

It shows.

"Look around at the people in the gym," he continued. "Do they all produce equally good results? Of course not; in fact, most of them produce very poor results, regardless of what they try. Which should tell you that what they are doing is wrong - wrong at least for them, although it might work very well for somebody else."

According to Jones, the first step in solving a problem is recognizing that a problem exists; the second, discovering its nature and magnitude; and the third, finding the means to solve it. "It helps if you clearly understand," he said in reference to the final step, "that there is no place to go for help, that nobody out there can provide you with the required answer; and the fact that something that apparently worked for them does not mean that it will work for you."

The study of exercise physiology was supposed to solve all that, but merely added to the confusion. Why? The majority of research over the past 30 years was conducted with lousy tools - which raises a question about 'certification.' Where do trainers get their information? And why do they have such opposing philosophies? The field needs education, not 'certification' from a pile of garbage.

No one has all the answers, but enough information exists to provide a set of rules based on valid research with appropriate modifications for genetic differences. For those who don't like rules, it beats renting incompetence. In the early 1970's, Jones worked with bodybuilders who modified his concepts to suit their taste - and then claimed they didn't work. Those who followed instructions got more than they expected.

An international group is currently in the process of establishing exercise centers that replace myth and political correctness with common sense, logic and 'certification' based on the training principles and research of Arthur Jones. Brainwashing? Hardly. Did Jones need a 'formal' education to do what he did? Hardly. I call it a great start.

I've had a few regrets in this field - once allowed my beliefs to 'bend' in a sports performance program, and supervised a myriad of oddities from other trainers - but I won't drop the ball anymore.

## SEPTEMBER 19

### Akinetic Exercise

If not for the creativity of bodybuilders, equipment manufacturers and guys like Juan, progressive resistance exercise would be nothing but boring.

I first introduced Juan (I can't recall his last name) to the Nautilus® system of exercise in Caracas, Venezuela in the early 1980's. He was 6'3", 200 pounds, a hard worker, but restless. The Nautilus system allowed one set of 12 exercises three times a week; Juan, among others, wanted more. So, I spent my waking hours pushing clients to the point that they could barely complete the circuit and later introduced advanced techniques that were both brutal and effective.

They had my attention; I had theirs.

One day I showed Juan a method of performing what Nautilus inventor Arthur Jones called 'akinetic' exercise on the Multi Biceps and Multi Triceps machines. Both tools featured an optional restraining mechanism (stop) between the top of the weight stack and the frame of the machine. Once in place, the device halted the movement arm about halfway up. From there, the pull (and bending) of one arm was resisted by the effort (and straightening) of the other. The object was to prevent the weight from dropping (or the restraint stop from losing contact with the frame) during exercise, a phenomenon visible from any seat position. The trainee could vary the resistance on the arm that lifted by varying the pull of the arm that lowered.

The exercise was called 'infimetric' when the selector pin was removed from the weight stack and 'akinetic' when the weight stack was engaged. The object of akinetic exercise was to exert a force equal to or greater than the selected weight (usually a medium resistance) as both arms moved through a complete range of motion. Properly performed, the weight remained suspended at the same height throughout the exercise. With akinetic exercise, you were instantly aware of an effort less than that of the weight stack, but seldom aware of the magnitude of any effort beyond.

As such, progress was difficult to measure.

For that reason, I advised Juan to use it sporadically. He thought akinetics was the greatest thing since sliced bread and used it on both machines every workout. Six months later, I had him perform arm curls and extensions with the weight he used prior to the new toy. As expected, he lost 2-3 repetitions per machine.

I like to measure things, but it's difficult with akinetic exercise. The theory of pushing with an unknown effort (and, as strength increases, with a higher unknown effort to progress) has its problems. The effort could be high today and low tomorrow, and leave trainees guessing as to whether they are making progress, which leads to another point. People love to see weights go up and down. There's no excitement watching a suspended weight or no weight stack at all, which is the problem with resistance equipment based on air and water pressure.

If you encounter 'akinetic' exercise (with Nautilus or MedX®), try the following:

1. Select a weight and support it as long as you can (time the effort).
2. If you support the weight for less than 60 seconds, it's too heavy.
3. If you support the weight for more than 90 seconds, increase it by 5%.
4. Maintain exercise duration between 60-90 seconds to progress.

5.  Use akinetic exercise as a technique immediately after a muscle fails (to take it beyond normal fatigue).

## SEPTEMBER 20

---

### The Snake Charmer

I wonder what Joe Weider was thinking when he witnessed the new rival to his empire calmly descend the stairs with a rattlesnake larger than the height of a man in his bare hands? Perhaps he found comfort in the thought, "What's a snake charmer going to know about exercise?" or "If he's that eccentric, I might be able to use it against him."

Whatever his thoughts, he got his money's worth.

That day, famous equipment inventor Arthur Jones decided to videotape a brief program about one of his not-so-brief rattlesnakes at the world's largest television studio in the Nautilus® complex (Lake Helen, Florida). He set up a camera with a telephoto lens at the far end of a 100-foot corridor to capture the stage - two chairs separated by a two-foot-high platform. Jones would place the reptile on the platform between the chairs while he and a guest discussed rattlesnakes.

A small group of 20 employees and visitors (including Weider) gathered around the set as Arthur made his way to the serpentarium on the second floor. He soon appeared carrying a huge snake down a flight of 20 stairs using his bare hands and a long stick that was curved at one end. He moved his way through the parting crowd and carefully placed the snake on the platform between the chairs.

The female guest, who had experience with wild animals, took her seat beside Arthur and the snake. The show was on - but the snake had its own agenda.

It began to rattle with growing intensity, forcing onlookers to make eye contact with one another and edge away from the stage. The cameraman was caught between the instructions of an irate Jones (who was rattled about the camera focus) and those of the director in the video booth on his headset. The rattle grew louder.

The snake suddenly left the platform, plunked itself onto the floor and slithered toward an open door. The audience scattered as Jones tried to keep it in the room by pulling its tail. In the midst of the confusion, as only he could, Arthur decided to measure it, instructing someone to hold the end of a tape measure on the floor near the end of the tail. Someone boldly stepped forward and put his foot on the end of the tape.

"The brave tape person," according to Joseph Mullen (present in the audience), "was told directly and in what can be best described as 'barracks language,' 'I said to hold the (BLEEP) tape; I did not say to step on it!' One must be precise when around Arthur Jones."

They finally measured the snake and Jones picked it up again at arms length.

By now, someone wanted to take a picture. Arthur walked into an adjacent studio and mounted a stage that stood about four feet above the floor. He held the snake at head height and let its body stretch below the level of the stage (Arthur was 5'8"). Once pictures were taken, the snake was returned to its cage.

The death-defying stunt, all in a day's work at Nautilus, left a few in shock and awe.

"The ease Arthur displayed when handling the snake," said Joe Mullen, "had a lasting effect on me. It was one of those, 'If he can do it, I can too' feelings."

Somehow, I don't think the other Joe felt the same.

Arthur Jones didn't think much of Weider's integrity - even before he arrived - and claimed that he (Joe) "knew nothing about exercise."

Weider was probably more intimidated by Arthur than the snake. Nonetheless, he returned to California to focus on his own snake oil - nutritional supplements.


## SEPTEMBER 21

---

### Stress and The Mind

The ground shook when I heard my name - I could barely breathe, let alone find a chunk of ground in which to stick a piece of wood. The first-tee jitters of the Ontario Junior Championship at the Aurora Highlands Golf Club were unlike anything I'd faced. I don't recall 'if' or 'how' the ball advanced.

Years later, the same occurred in the Porter Cup at the Niagara Falls C.C. in Lewiston, N.Y., but the toll was greater. I experienced all three stages of Selye's theory of stress - alarm reaction, resistance and exhaustion - and lost 10 pounds in four days. In contrast, competitor Bill Rogers strutted around as if he owned the place in shooting 66 - and may have gained a pound with a sandwich at the turn. The difference was attitude.

According to Hans Selye, in *The Stress of Life*, "Stress is the common denominator of all adaptive reactions in the body." He believed that the source of stress was non-specific, that is, could be anything, but that the body's reaction to stress was always specific, usually manifesting itself as something negative.

Months ago, a job search left me drained, depressed and deflated. So, I focused on the positive: Time off allowed me to write, play golf and not work - attitude.

Nautilus® inventor, Arthur Jones once developed a throat problem flying to and from South America. It surfaced the moment he came home, and ceased the moment he left (the opposite of my experience - every time the plane landed in Venezuela, I asked, "Why am I still here?"). When Jones identified the cause-and-effect relationship and 'stress' as the culprit, his problem vanished. On another occasion, he connected a high level of emotional stress to what he called "the worst case of piles in recorded medical history." By addressing the cause, the condition disappeared.

Jones believed that the mind had a great influence on the body, but made it clear he was not endorsing psychiatry. "Far from it," he said, "I have yet to meet a psychiatrist who was on the right side of the bars, have wondered for years whether it is cause or effect; that is, does the study of psychiatry attract lunatics or produce them?"

He also realized that stress could reflect in positive ways. Whenever he decided to resume training after a layoff, the mere thought triggered a growth response. "On one occasion," he claimed, "my arm size increased by a full half inch within a couple of days after I decided to resume training, but before any training was done." It was the alarm-reaction stage at work, the body preparing for stress.

In retrospect, much of what Jones hypothesized about exercise was a reflection of the General Adaptation Syndrome (G.A.S.) theory of Hans Selye:

- Jones believed that results from strength training were directly related to the intensity of exercise. Selye: "The alarm-response of the body is directly proportionate to the intensity of the aggression."
- Jones believed that the stimulation provided by overload produced a direct inroad into the muscle's local energy stores and an indirect inroad into the system's recovery ability. Selye: that the limited stores of local adaptation energy during the body's resistance to stress are replenished by the deeper energy stores of the system.

427

- Jones believed that muscle growth ceased or reversed if the system was not allowed time to properly recover between workouts. Selye: if the deeper stores (of energy) are used up, exhaustion or death follows - neither, a good result.

Stress can be productive; but too much, never so. And the mind can only do so much.


## SEPTEMBER 22

### The Science of Exercise – An Opinion

According to Nautilus® inventor Arthur Jones, the event that triggered an explosion in scientific research in this country was the launch of the first Earth satellite in 1957. The problem was, the Sputnik was Russian.

The United States government was thrown into panic by the realization that they were, for the first time, behind. In response, they allocated billions of dollars to research projects of any kind, which created the first problem. "Most of the researchers," said Jones, "had not the slightest interest in worthwhile results; were, instead, interested only in getting their hands on easy money." When the research was complete, they concluded that 'more' was needed, the equivalent of, "Send more money for more waste."

The second problem developed over time - the rush and requirement to get things published in scientific peer-reviewed journals, a system that prevented the publication of anything new, true or important - and produced nothing but regurgitation. "If it is really 'new,'" said Jones, "then it will fly directly in the face of the opinions of the supposed experts, will put the lie to their statements, will prove just how stupid they really are."

Scientists were not about to prove that, certainly not in the field of exercise.

The event that finally merged science and exercise occurred almost 30 years later, in 1986, with the introduction of tools that could accurately measure muscle function, tools made by none other than Arthur Jones. He criticized the scientific community and its process, believing that private-funded research, despite its pitfalls, had more value due to a greater concern for cost, efficiency and practical results. And he criticized the supposed scientific discoveries in exercise. "Just how can you evaluate the results (of tests) if you cannot measure them?"

To prevent what should have launched an explosion of interest and valid research from the quagmire of publication and review, Jones initiated his own campaign to educate the masses with truly 'new' discoveries. He lectured daily at his home in Ocala and twice monthly at the University of Florida in Gainesville to doctors, therapists, exercise physiologists, trainers and other 'experts.' What he learned was no surprise.

"Over the years, I have steadily reduced the level of my presentations to the point that they are now somewhere between a kindergarten level and a second grade of grammar school level, and they are still far over the heads of most of my audiences." And his audiences were far from stupid. They simply knew nothing about exercise, and most of what they believed was wrong, a reflection, perhaps, of too many scientific journals.

"In general," said Jones sadly, "they not only do not understand the actually quite simple laws of physics but are not even aware of them." To clarify his point he noted that muscle function was affected by gravity, internal muscle friction and stored energy. Yet, "apart from the research conducted or funded by me, nobody else on the planet has ever considered any of these factors while trying to conduct research in the field of exercise."

And worse, approximately 30 years of garbage was published and taught "to hundreds of thousands of poor fools who have been misled into believing that they are being educated; when instead they are being brainwashed into believing things that are untrue at best and dangerous at worst." The picture wasn't pretty.

The value of exercise, he concluded, will never be realized "until the subject is widely and clearly understood and applied, and there is not the slightest indication at the moment that such an understanding will be reached anywhere in the near future."

## SEPTEMBER 23

---

### The Ritual

I stood on the porch of the clubhouse of the Sedgefield Country Club, home of the Greater Greensboro Open (1972), and watched a car roll up. Much to my surprise, out popped the man I most admired in golf, the only competitor bold enough to lift weights at a time it was considered taboo, Gary Player. He lingered at my side, waiting the arrival of his wife. I couldn't have written a better script.

Gary Bannister, B.A., B.P.E., M.Ed.

The awkward greeting quickly vanished when the conversation turned to exercise. As a graduate student at the University of North Carolina, I had keys to the gym and invited him to train while he was there. Mr. Player respectfully declined, claiming that he didn't lift weights during the competitive season but that he would likely jog the golf course later that evening.

I was disappointed, yet relieved - the 'gym' wasn't much of a gym.

It slept in the basement of a building that housed the Rosenthal Gymnasium, an ancient basketball court. Its path led down a long corridor, through a pair of double doors, down a few more steps and into a hallway that played host to two rooms. One, directly in front, had its own swinging doors and floor covered with gymnastic mats. The other, the doors to the left, housed the University's sanctuary of strength training - a small, ill-equipped room that required a map to find and a key to open.

Therein, lay its beauty.

Three days a week, roommate Al Jangl and I descended the frail stairs to the empty room for our training ritual, often more ritual than training.

Jangl was a good athlete - soccer, skiing, basketball, track, tennis, gymnastics and golf - with a great sense of humor. Our workout time was sacred, an outlet graduate students needed to release pent-up energy. We co-operated fully.

On most occasions together, but sometimes alone, we'd change in the locker room and head down the corridor. The moment the first set of double doors shielded us from humanity, we broke into a primal frenzy of stomps, struts, grunts and groans. It was five minutes of King Kong vs. Godzilla dislodging equipment, throwing dumbbells and generally assuming the role of idiots. Once the place was in shambles, we'd laugh like hell and begin the workout. It was a great warm-up and not unlike the antics practiced by some of today's trainees - *during* their workouts.

Little by little, we refined the process and made it a point to be over-courteous with fellow classmates and teachers in the hallway on our way in.

"Good morning, Dr. McKinney."

"Nice to see you, Dr. Lawther. Hope you're having a wonderful day."

The Eddie Haskells of UNC-G somehow found the contrast sweet.

One day, while training alone, I left the door unlocked at the top of the stairs - Jangl was on his way. Finally, the sound of his arrival signaled promise that this performance would be the finest the gym had seen. Godzilla kicked the door of the adjacent room ajar, as he so often had, and found himself face-to-face with a dozen half-naked girls taking body measurements for a self-improvement class.

"Oops. Sorry."

It was much the same as the response he got at graduation time.

Mr. Player would have been proud of our dedication and discipline. But he would not have embraced the gym, even if he had survived the warm-up.

## SEPTEMBER 24

### To and From California

It was not a reception you'd expect from a five-star hotel. First through the doors strode a stunning brunette in her early twenties, dressed to the hilt, a 10-star woman from head to toe. Terri was followed by a man who admittedly wouldn't change his underwear unless she made him, her husband, an old man with only a few strands of hair. Arthur averaged minus 2½ stars - 10+ from the neck up (not counting aesthetics) and minus 15 from the neck down (counting only aesthetics).

The third was a middle-aged orthopedic surgeon who looked more like a surfer than a doctor - blue jeans, blonde hair and colorful shirt. The fourth member of the entourage was a British man with a bushwhacker outfit that placed him somewhere between an overdressed bounty hunter and a low-end safari director.

At least someone was on the 'alert.' The bellhop quickly and politely steered the motley crew away from the reception where a dignified group had gathered, and hustled them into the elevator, up to the penthouse. Arthur Jones had a standing reservation at the Beverly Wilshire Hotel in Beverly Hills.

It wasn't always that way.

In 1970, Jones borrowed $2,500 dollars from his sister, rented a trailer and hauled a metal structure to the Mr. America contest in Culver City, California, where his reception was much the same. The structure looked like a spaceship: 15 feet long, six feet wide and eight feet high with four seats (representing four exercises), one behind the other.

His ideas were equally out-of-this-world. His rhetoric was powerful, unique (to many, unintelligible) and reflected what Ellington Darden called, "the power of logic."

Despite claims to the contrary, Jones had nothing to sell. The pre-cursor to the Nautilus® machine and its system of exercise was a hobby that soon became a lucrative venture.

Decades later, Jones returned to California to pursue another hobby. He stripped down a Boeing® 707 (purchased from American Airlines®), flew it from his home (Ocala, Florida) to a reptile farm that had declared bankruptcy, and returned with "23,000 pounds of crocodilians" to add to his growing collection of animals.

Around that time, he returned on a more serious note - to establish a medical exercise research center in conjunction with the University of California in San Diego. It would serve as a rehabilitation venue for chronic spine problems, collect data on related research, and certify MedX® technicians, as it had at the University of Florida.

Jones left his mark wherever he traveled, much like that of Canadian golfer, Moe Norman. While both may have worn the same pair of underwear for years, there were fundamental differences. Arthur didn't sleep in a bunker, break the course record the next day and hide in a toilet stall when it came time to speak. He may have slept in a motel that resembled a bunker at times, but he welcomed speaking engagements - though his reception often resembled that of the Beverly.

Moe Norman, the genius of golf, was recently awarded $5,000 per month from Titleist® for using their golf balls throughout his career. Arthur Jones, the genius of exercise, will get his due long after oxygen has abandoned his airways.

A few days ago, I looked up the Beverly Wilshire Hotel and read a 'who's who' list of those who have stayed at "The Hotel of the Stars."

There was no mention of Arthur Jones.


SEPTEMBER 25

---

### Chipping and Other Efforts

It pays to listen. Years ago, I caught the tail end of a golf program that featured veteran Phil Rogers' chipping system - a numerical formula that matched the distance to the pin you wanted the ball to land with an appropriate club. The combination, properly executed, would leave you "dead," so close to the hole you couldn't miss.

I scratched the numbers on a sheet, promptly misplaced it, but remembered the basic combinations. If you landed an 8-iron one-third the distance to the hole on a flat green, it would finish near the hole. A pitching wedge that landed half way would result in the same. I figured out the rest by trial and error.

With apologies to Mr. Rogers, my version of the formula follows:

| **The Landing Distance From Ball to Pin** | **Club Selection** |
|---|---|
| Less than 1/4 of the way | 4-5-iron |
| One quarter of the way | 6-iron |
| 1/4-1/3 of the way | 7-iron |
| One third of the way | 8-iron |
| 1/3-1/2 of the way | 9-iron |
| Half-way | Pitching Wedge |
| Three quarters of the way | Sand Wedge |

The procedure:

1. Pick a spot where you would like the ball to land knowing that error is reduced by 'less air-time and more ground-time,' and that bounce is more consistent on a flatter surface. The initial three feet of the green is generally a good place to start. If it is not appropriate - due to slope, firmness or your comfort zone - select another.

2. Move to the side of your line and determine where your spot is in relation to the ball and the hole. Is it half way to the hole? One third of the way? One quarter?

3. Use the formula for the appropriate club selection.

4. Adjust the club and/or landing spot for the speed and slope of the green, the firmness of the turf, the wind (especially on long chips) and shot trajectory.

The same procedure applies to run-up shots where your selected spot might fall short of the putting surface. In these instances, factor in the thickness of the grass and add a club or two for the increased friction the ball encounters. If your execution is clean and the ball lands on or near the spot, it should stop within a few feet of the hole.

The system is so accurate that I can predict the outcome the moment the ball lands. If I miss the spot by an inch, the difference is minimal; by six inches, the result is two feet short or long; and by two feet, the result is 6-8 feet off. The penalty for inaccuracy is magnified at the far end.

Arthur Jones believed that the same magnification process was at work in exercise:

- A slight decrease in the intensity of effort, for example, created a disproportionate decrease in muscle stimulation. If a 70% effort produced no growth stimulation, 80% produced 10 units and 90%, 100 units. The Nautilus® inventor demanded 100%.

- "Increasing the 'intensity of effort' required a disproportionate re-duction in the 'amount' of exercise." Advanced routines demanded less exercise and frequency.
- In certain combinations, it was important to move from one exer-cise to the next in less than three seconds. A five-second rest re-duced stimulation by as much as 50%.

Proper strength training should leave you as "dead" as a good chip.


## SEPTEMBER 26

---

### A Better Tool

I stood at the back of the third green during Monday's practice round of the 2001 Masters tournament in Augusta, Georgia as veteran Darren Clarke approached a ball that had trickled down the slope behind the green. From there, he pitched five balls with a lofted wedge to the top of the slope and watched each race 15-20 feet past the hole. His delicate efforts were no match for the speedy descent to the pin.

But Clarke had a bag full of tools and promptly selected another - a fair-way wood. This time he bumped five balls into the slope and trickled them onto the putting surface where they stopped 3-5 feet from the target. He found the right tool for the job.

Nautilus® inventor Arthur Jones often used a parable to illustrate the same to bodybuilders.

"Imagine you are hiking in the desert and see a figure in the distance - an old, bearded, half-naked man on hands and knees with fingers clawing at the sandy earth."

"As you approach, you ask, 'What are you doing?'"

" 'Digging for gold.'"

" 'How long have you been at it?'"

" 'Weeks - maybe months. It's slow work.'"

"You notice his bloody fingers and raw callused knuckles and suggest, 'Listen! Digging with your bare hands is not a very efficient way to prospect for gold. That hole's only a couple of feet deep. Let me loan you my shovel.'"

"You reach into your backpack, pull out a lightweight, tempered-edge shovel and drive it into the ground. In a few minutes you demonstrate that he can make more progress in moments than he could in months using his bare hands."

"Then an amazing thing happens," said Jones. "The old man's eyes fill with hate and anger. He charges at you, grabs the shovel from your hands and throws it away."

Jones hesitated at the end of the tale and repeated in a hardened tone, "He threw the shovel away."

At that moment, most bodybuilders in the audience shook their heads as if to deny guilt, but they understood the analogy. *They* were 'the old man in the desert' denying a tool that might get them from A to B in a more efficient manner.

From the beginning, Jones described his Nautilus machines as nothing more than a "thinking man's barbell," a logical barbell. Yet, he realized he was up against a strong force - human nature. According to Ellington Darden, Ph.D. who worked with Jones for years, "Old bodybuilders don't change; they just pump away, doing the wrong things over and over. History says that they will never change."

He may be right. I continue to see individuals enter a gym full of great equipment and head straight for the least effective tools (pulleys, barbells, elastic bands and rubber balls). It's not that they don't know how to use the new tools, in spite of the fact that they haven't learned to use their own. It's habit, and habit doesn't budge.

I have used the same putter in golf for more than 40 years. Its crooked wooden shaft and rusted head have survived the test of time, including temptations from the 'latest' technology that I won in tournaments. What did I do with the new? Threw it away.

When asked his age, Jones often replied, "I'm old enough to realize it's impossible to change the thinking of fools. But I'm young and foolish enough to keep on trying."

I appreciate what Arthur endured but will probably go to the grave with that putter.

## SEPTEMBER 27

---

### Hard, Harder and Hardest

From weak to strong, muscles have three levels of strength - lifting or positive strength, holding or static strength, and lowering or negative strength. When muscles can no longer lift a weight due to fatigue, they can always hold it. When muscles can no longer hold a weight motionless, they can always lower it. When muscles can no longer lower a weight in control, the effort triggers the highest stimulus for growth and makes the deepest inroad into the body's reserves.

Lifting a weight to failure is difficult, holding it to failure is harder, and lowering it to failure is the hardest way to train. And the implications are clear - the harder the exercise, the more difficult the recovery.

Mike Mentzer (Mr. Universe, 1978) outlines techniques that utilize this hierarchy in his book, *High-Intensity Training the Mike Mentzer Way* (2003). After a few months of learning proper form, Mentzer urges training to failure - to where "the completion of another full rep is impossible despite your greatest effort." From there, he advocates the use of techniques that take training intensity to higher levels, as follows:

- **Pre-Exhaustion**. Compound exercises that involve several muscle groups suffer from failure at their weakest link. The remedy is to isolate and pre-exhaust the large muscle first, then immediately force it to greater fatigue with the help of a smaller muscle (pull-over, pulldown; fly, chest press; lateral raise, shoulder press; leg extension, leg press). Mentzer suggests six strict repetitions per exercise, not more than two combinations per workout, and only one per week per body part.

- **Peak Contraction**. To activate the greatest number of muscle fibers during an exercise, take a muscle to its full-contracted position and hold it there for a moment (use only on exercises that provide adequate resistance in that position).

- **Forced Repetitions**. At the end of a set, a training partner assists just enough to allow the performance of 4-6 additional repetitions beyond failure.

- **Rest-pause**. Perform one repetition with a maximum weight, rest exactly 10 seconds and repeat for four total repetitions. On the last few attempts, the weight may have to be reduced by approximately 10%.

- **Partial Repetitions**. Lift a heavier-than-normal weight from the mid-range of the movement to the full-contracted position for five repetitions. Menzer recommends the performance of partial repetitions in conjunction with full-range exercise (for the same muscles) to help overcome weak movement angles.

Beyond failure to lift, he also suggests the following: **Static Contractions**. Exercise to static failure in one of two ways: immediately after normal failure or, as a separate entity. In either case, perform one hold for as long as possible, followed by one slow lowering repetition. When executed alone, the weight (20% heavier) should allow a hold of 8-12 seconds (upper body) and 15-30 seconds (lower body). Best results are obtained on single-axis machine exercises that have an adequate resistance in contraction.

- **Negative Repetitions.** The use of negative repetitions results in the deepest level of fatigue and should be limited to advanced trainees. Lower a heavy weight (40% more than normal) until its descent can no longer be controlled. Negative work requires strong assistants and infrequent use - one set per body part per week.

"Growth never comes easy," claims Mentzer, "it must literally be forced."

## SEPTEMBER 28

### Trying to Make a Difference

In the late 1960's, the Soviet national hockey team took to the ice an hour before game time in front of what would be a capacity crowd at Maple Leaf Gardens in Toronto. They skated back and forth in patterns with speed and finesse, with and without the puck, ignoring the hostile environment. There wasn't a weak skater in the bunch. Twenty minutes later, they left as smartly as they had appeared. It was business as usual.

Minutes later, Team Canada took center stage to a standing ovation. They waved, signed autographs and skated around haphazardly in what was *not* Canada's finest hour. The Russians whipped them soundly, which came as no surprise to one man.

Lloyd Percival, a coach and advocate of weight training for all athletes had warned everyone in the 1950's that the Soviets would challenge the best in the NHL within a few years. His 1958 classic, *The Hockey Handbook*, was the guide that Soviet coach Anatoli Tarasov - the Gordie Howe of Russian hockey - used to develop his system of play. To Tarasov, Percival was "the world's greatest hockey theoretician."

To help out, Percival invited Team Canada to train at The Fitness Institute, his state-of-the-art facility in Toronto. The coach rejected the offer, stating, "We are hockey players, not weightlifters." Ever persistent, Percival tested the players individually.

The strongest legs on the team belonged to the stick boy.

Shortly thereafter, Canada withdrew from international competition and refused to play the Russian "professionals" unless they could also use their

437

best, namely NHL pros. The stage was set for the first showdown of hockey's finest.

Canada boasted an easy victory, but Percival saw it differently. In the June, 1972 issue of *Sports and Fitness Instructor* (three months before the event), he wrote, "According to test and evaluation comparisons of NHL and Russian hockey players, they (Russians) are collectively stronger, in better condition, faster, excellent pattern passers and receivers, more agile and mobile at pattern changing - and they are tremendously disciplined."

Winning wasn't the issue with Percival. "We must win big or eat grass," he said, "an event that would cause many of us to choke. A 5-3 edge in the series would be a moral victory for the Russians. We must *dominate* to retain our pride and prestige."

A month before the series, he published a "Sports Power Index" that rated team efficiency in every component of the game: physical condition (cardio-vascular, strength, flexibility, agility), mechanical skills (skating, shooting, passing), psychological and personality factors (adaptability, poise, ability to withstand pressure, discipline) and coaching. Each factor was awarded a numerical score based on how it might 'weigh' in the outcome. Canada had the edge in skills, but was inferior in preparation and condition (618-529). His final tally: Canada, 2,388; Russia, 2,383.

The Index caught the eye of Canadian coach, Harry Sinden, but it was too late. He conducted a three-week crash course that players found boring because it involved few 'playing-into-condition' activities that NHL pros were used to. It almost backfired. When the team arrived for the first game, players were exhausted.

Canada won the series in the final seconds of the last game. A few months before his death in 1974, Percival commented on the state of hockey in Canada. "What did we learn from the Russians?" he asked. "Very little, we are playing the same old game."

You can't reach your potential in a sport without supplemental strength training and without learning from your mistakes. Team Canada did neither.

SEPTEMBER 29

### The Way It Is

The former schoolmarm entered the room with a purpose little known to the majority of the hundreds of adults and children that had gathered. She marched straight to a microphone that served no purpose with her volume, pressed her lips together as if dissatisfied with what she saw, and spoke in a blunt, forceful tone, **"Gentlemen, take off your hats."**

The assembly room of the National Junior AAU Golf Championship at Mission Inn Country Club (Howey-in-the-Hills, Florida, 2001) was a public building, and real men did not wear hats in public buildings. The room fell into silence. The only voice was hers, loud and clear.

She ambled through a litany of problems from past competitions and vowed zero tolerance. The course was too beautiful to spit upon, and the game too noble to allow players and parents to communicate by hand signals.

"If you want to give something to your child during a round," she said, "signal where you will drop it off, and then walk away."

For those who failed to comply, a ride home awaited - and she would drive. On she went, rule after rule.

The kids were antsy - it was practice day - but they were required to sit through another presentation - ours - on 'Conditioning for Golf.' The timing was bad. Not even the names of our distinguished clients, Jack Nicklaus and Jesper Parnevik, could keep tiny buns from wiggling. We felt like P.G. Wodehouse's target in *"The Salvation of George MacKintosh,"* 1924:

"The talking golfer," he said, "is undeniably the most pronounced pest of our complex modern civilization, and the most difficult to deal with. It is a melancholy thought that the noblest of games should have produced such a scourge."

Our efforts were rewarded by a meager interest on the part of the parents. The kids were off and running.

What stuck most about that meeting (in the minds of the majority of the competitors) was the moderator's passion for 'doing things right,' or at least the way she wanted to have it done. Everything had reason - as unreasonable as it appeared - and everything was backed by fact and common sense.

Her performance was reminiscent of the passion that the Nautilus® inventor displayed for what he called "proper strength training" in the 1970's. Arthur Jones first thought things out, performed his own research, backed his ideas with fact and common sense, and delivered his message with the same conviction.

You could ask questions and get answers with Arthur, but you'd better tiptoe around a debate. He could make the best of minds look foolish, if need be; and he embraced conflict. I never once saw him dig a hole, much less one from which he could not escape.

Gary Bannister, B.A., B.P.E., M.Ed.

He often began with shock, then proceeded with fact and opinion. He hit his audience with a brick, and by the time they realized what had occurred, the rules had been both established and modified - and were not to be challenged.

I can only imagine the reaction of bodybuilders to the same in a gym.

**"Gentlemen, take off your hats"** would eliminate the entire male membership, while **"Gentlemen, wear your hats with the brim forward"** would eliminate about 90%.

I liked her style.

## SEPTEMBER 30

---

### All The Moves, Again

He tugged the top of his work boots, sucked in his gut, tightened a wide leather belt and rolled up his sleeves - *my God, a tattoo*. He adjusted his cap to the direction he was headed in life, stroked a hand through his hair - *my God, an earring* - and yanked the base of each glove. He then took a forced breath, merged with the mirror, glanced at the weight a final time and shook his head laterally. This dude was ready.

He jumped and thumped, and barked and arched, and moaned and groaned. It was quite an ordeal. In the end, in plain and public discomfort, he bit and spit, and nearly split - did everything but fail.

And that was only the beginning.

Following the performance, he itched, unhitched, and danced and pranced. He walked and talked with a grin free of sin - right from the text. What next?

Our hero combined every possible bench-press error into one poetic effort. Instead of during, this was a time I might have suggested closing your eyes between exercises. Yet, what would have been a five-minute major in hockey, a two-game suspension in basketball, a fine in baseball, and disqualification in golf was no breach of rules in exercise. The man with all the moves was beyond reproach, if not repair.

The field of exercise rewards such behavior. With it, you suddenly acquire friends. The girl with the plastic boobs takes note. You become a trusted source of information. Teens ask for tips and depart in awe. You have purpose in life. You are *officially* disgusting; and, while only God is the ultimate official, I'm just pointing it out.

I should be hardened to it after four decades, but I'm not - and not alone.

Forty years of correcting seat-heights and body-part positions. Forty years of suggesting that people breathe and relax their head and neck during the lowering phase of exercise. Forty years of watching trainees drop (rather than lower) resistance. Forty years of observing bodybuilders bounce barbells off their chest during bench presses. Forty years of telling people to slow down. Forty years of encouraging them to seek - not fear or avoid - muscle failure. Forty years of waiting for someone to exit an exercise station that provides refuge between sets. Forty years of justifying a pause in a contracted position. Forty years of viewing marathon workouts, one-rep strength competitions and dizzying momentum.

Have I missed anything?

Despite the efforts of those who subscribe to the teachings of Arthur Jones, little has changed. Ignorance, myth, deception and fraud have swallowed the field of exercise - if nothing else, the challenge has kept me off the streets - and there's no end in sight.

"But, not to worry," said Jones, "Joe Weider can provide the solution to all of your problems; or, if not, he will at least tell you some interesting lies."

I wouldn't be surprised if one day I receive a letter similar to that received by a young man in Mobile, Alabama in regard to a debt he had with Charles Atlas. "Mr. Atlas will be in your town within the near future, and he would not like to be forced to come by and personally collect your overdue payments."

A brief time ago, I glanced through the May 2002 issue of *Popular Science*. In the back, I spotted an ad for Charles Atlas.Com:

"No barbells, no..."

*My God*, the nonsense keeps piling up...and up...truly, no end in sight.

# OCTOBER

"When I designed that machine (Nautilus® Lower-Back Machine), I clearly understood that it provided exercise for both the hip and thigh muscles...but I then believed that it also provided meaningful exercise for the lumbar-extensor muscles; an assumption that I now realize was wrong. The machine is misnamed, is in fact a hip and thigh machine, provides meaningful exercise only for the muscles of the buttocks and rear of the thighs.

I founded Nautilus Sports/Medical Industries, Inc., in 1970, and served as chairman until it was sold in June of 1986; selling controlling interest in the company in order to devote my full attention to the continued development of specific testing and exercise equipment for several critical areas of the body, with particular emphasis on the lumbar spine, the cervical spine and the knee.

The project that eventually lead to the development of safe, accurate, specific testing and exercise equipment for those critical areas of the body was started fifteen years ago while I was directing Nautilus; but was not successful until after I sold that company.

This clear statement of fact must not be misunderstood as an indictment of Nautilus or any other product of that company; we all make mistakes, and the misnamed lower-back machine was one of my mistakes, a mistake now being copied by several companies in the field of exercise."

Arthur Jones

# OCTOBER 1

---

## Letting the Air Out

Looks can deceive in exercise. The Neanderthal who disappoints at show time vs. the skinny guy who exceeds expectations is clear proof that output should be taken with a grain of salt - and sometimes two.

A golf-professional named Cindy from Jupiter, Florida recently attended the PGA show in Orlando with her brother. After the show each day, they exercised in a hotel gym on equipment made by a company that had just celebrated 25 years of using air pressure as a source of resistance.

There wasn't much to celebrate.

One afternoon, after their warm-up, a gentleman strutted in with the profile of 'I'm about to set the world on fire.' The gloves, the belt, the shoes and the 'look' matched a series of gyrations performed in front of a mirror - moves that would have embarrassed any mother - all in the name of 'warm-up.'

Cindy shifted to Plan B.

She had worked out several days before and established a resistance on each machine by setting a number on the dial. She was also well aware of how the weight felt at the next notch - and was no slouch when it came to exercise.

She headed for the first machine in the circuit, a leg extension, and kept her brother at bay on the other side of the gym. When she finished her set, she proceeded to the second, a leg curl, and the third, a leg press.

Mr. Set-The-World-On-Fire decided to join in. He swooped in behind Cindy, tugged at his belt and gloves, sucked in his gut and jumped on the first machine, where the aftershock of the mirror gig kicked in. He wiggled up and down, left and right, took two deep breaths, wiggled again and gripped the handles. Ready.

His legs contracted with a mighty effort but the pads barely moved. He braced himself for a more-manly attempt. No dice. The pads wouldn't go. Bewildered, he looked around and gave it one more for the 'Gipper' - nothing. Either this skinny thing ahead of him was stronger than hell, or he was having a bad day.

So it continued, machine after machine - a gallant effort, a lousy result. Cindy and her brother could barely contain themselves as they exchanged glances in the mirror. She had dialed each machine up a few notches before moving on. The victim eventually exhausted his moves, dialed things back, and was still scratching his head when they left.

If there are any advantages to air-pressure exercise, it lies in machine weight, not in results. They are easy to move (but easily move during heavy use) and feature a button that reduces resistance *during* exercise. When properly used, it allows a muscle to lift a reduced load beyond fatigue. Improperly used, it's a panic button.

When you go to a different gym, check your ego at the door and then check the resistance at each station by performing 'trial' repetitions. Machines are different due to friction, manufacturer and age, so go by feel and record what you do, especially if you intend to train there more than once.

Egos thrive on watching heavy weight stacks go up and down, which accounts for few inquiries about 'super-slow' or 'high-intensity' exercise - both of which require an initial reduction in resistance. To date, I've not been asked the location of the nearest gym with air-pressure equipment.

Pumping up is not likely to assume another meaning anytime soon.

## OCTOBER 2

### Ten Steps Ahead

The final slide of my weekly presentation on 'Strength Training Principles' depicted a sleek line of futuristic exercise machines that stimulated interest for the wrong reason. The devices featured something that most overlooked - no weights.

Their creator, Nautilus® inventor Arthur Jones believed, "If you are building strength 'in order to lift weights' then you will have to continue lifting weights to develop the required style if for no other reason. But if you are lifting weights to build strength, then weights are no longer required...better results can be produced without them." *(Strength Training: The Present State of the Art,* 1974).

Jones called the new concept INFItonic - INFImetric exercise, "a form of exercise that requires no resistance source of any kind, yet one that provides all of the requirements for truly full-range exercise...while actually IMPROVING the production of results."

The major difference was in the execution, a change to alternate 'one-limb movement' - lifting one arm or leg while simultaneously lowering the other. The limb that lowered (or performed negative work) provided the resistance for the limb that lifted. Since muscles are 40% stronger lowering than lifting, the source of resistance was unlimited - hence the name.

According to Jones, the advantages over traditional exercise included:

- Improved form. Positive work provided the negative resistance and negative work provided the positive resistance, meaning the weight could no longer be thrown (during lifting) or dropped (during lowering) - a definite plus.
- An unlimited speed of movement, from zero to maximum (then an issue with isokinetics, so-called constant-speed-of-movement exercise).
- The alternate style of performance (limbs moving in opposite directions) ensured good posture, reduced cheating and allowed muscles to move to positions that were normally impossible to reach.
- Easier machine entry (while one movement arm was up, the other was down).

The concept was later hooked to computers. "The machines of the future," said Jones, "won't make you exercise properly, nothing can do that...nobody can do that. All that anybody or anything can do is make it possible for you to exercise properly, and then encourage you to exercise properly, tell you when you are doing something right, and when you are doing something wrong, and the machine can do all of these things, and do them far better than any human supervisor." (*The Future of Exercise: An Opinion*, 1978)

By 1985, Jones had manufactured a complete line of machines with monitors (as seen in my final slide) that told you exactly what to do, how to do it, how hard to push, and how often to perform exercise.

They were slick, but Jones was not satisfied.

The lack of muscle isolation, the inaccuracy of dynamic testing procedures to determine the protocol, and the public's desire to see weights go up and down eventually forced Arthur to adopt the same fate as my slide presentation.

One evening, an elderly couple braved the elements to attend the lecture alone. On the third of 35 slides, I walked to the screen with my laser pointer. When I turned to face them, he was asleep and she wasn't far behind.

The concept was bold - but there was little interest.

## OCTOBER 3

---

### Unholy Wedlock

The ceremony was solemn, the gathering large - athletes, coaches, parents, trainers, owners. The vows were standard, yet stunning in magnitude and message.

"Do you, Miss Danger, *(background music)* take this man, Mr. Nonsense, to be your lawful wedded husband, to have and to hold, until death do you part?" *(cut music)*

"I do."

"Do you, Mr. Nonsense, *(background music)* take this woman, Miss Danger, to be your lawful wedded wife, to have and to hold, until death do you part?" *(cut music)*

"I do."

"I now pronounce you man and wife. *(background music)* Beloved congregation, allow me to introduce our newlyweds, Mr. and Mrs. Plyometrics."

The marriage of Danger and Nonsense represented a new low in the field of exercise. The 'Plyometrics' advocated explosive movements and high impact. Protecting the body from injury through proper strength training gave way to hammering on it. At the same time, sudden movements against resistance exposed the body to high forces (precisely when the weight was jerked) and to little or no resistance the rest of the way. Too much force at one end and too little at the other is what Nautilus® inventor Arthur Jones called, "Danger to no purpose."

Must you practice impact to prepare for it? I think not. The body comes with a limited warranty.

The S.A.I.D. Principle (Specific Adaptation to Imposed Demand) is often used to rationalize the activities in sports performance programs, training the body in a manner that resembles what it encounters in competition. Yet, swinging a 10-pound golf club to increase power in the golf swing, for example, is dumb when you consider that the muscles involved may be capable of lifting 100-200 pounds during isolated exercise. Sharing a 10-pound load with other muscles is like putting a pencil in your hand, curling your arm all day and expecting strong biceps. It won't happen.

But something will. Swinging a heavy club can confuse the nervous system and interfere with skill, especially if its weight is close to that of the club you use. Swinging a heavy club prepares your body to swing a heavy club. Unless you play with that club (or apply the same resistance to your club *as* you swing), avoid weighted movements that mimic sports. As Jones put it: "You can slice it as thin as you can, or pile it as high as you like - but you still end up with cheese; if you started with cheese."

Many of today's trainers are attracted to cheese in a strange way: the lower the order, the greater the attraction. The supposed leg-up provided by Yoga, Tae Bo, Pilates and Tai Chi certifications has all but destroyed the meat and potatoes of fitness, strength training. Exercises in these disciplines feature inferior resistance - rubber bands for leg curls, Swiss balls for abdominal work, bodyweight for grade-school calisthenics - and ignore the very tools that provide full-range exercise. Why pull your car with a team of oxen?

And that's not the worst. Exercises are, in general, poorly performed and monitored - creating a generation of misconception led by one of certified ignorance.

Fifty years from now, when Danger and Nonsense renew their vows, I predict a name change to whatever's "in" and a congregation brimming with therapists, doctors, lawyers, and, until death do 'em part, funeral directors.

What's next - Tai Cheese?

## OCTOBER 4

### A Workout Misconception

A recent article in *Golf Magazine* ("Survival of the Fittest," January, 2001) outlined the training routines of five PGA Tour® players to demonstrate different approaches to fitness. One player was described as the poster boy for plyometrics - "an intense system of jumping exercises designed to develop fast-twitch muscle fibers." His workouts entailed leaping onto benches and over boxes, movements popular in sports requiring strength and speed such as football, wrestling and basketball. Good luck.

As popular as plyometrics may be among athletes, no system of exercise performed in any fashion can *develop* fast-twitch muscle fibers. Either you have them or you don't. Furthermore, it is wrong to assume that muscle fibers can be activated by speed of movement during exercise.

The brain does not preferentially recruit powerful fast-twitch muscle fibers in response to tasks that involve rapid movement against resistance. Nor does it recruit weaker endurance-oriented, slow-twitch muscle fibers in response to slow movements. Muscle recruitment is based solely upon *intensity* of effort, not speed of movement.

During the first repetitions of an exercise when the resistance 'feels' easy, the brain selects the weakest muscle fibers (slow-twitch) for the task. As the exercise progresses, it senses the need for help and engages a stronger order of fibers. For the final repetitions, the brain unleashes the powerful fast-twitch fibers to assist in what is now perceived as an impossible task. When they become involved, all of the fibers are working.

Why are plyometrics so popular? Research shows that they work. Athletes run faster, jump higher and demonstrate more 'power' in their sport after practicing explosive movements. And the reason they work is clear. Trainees become stronger by moving against a resistance that is progressively increased and stronger muscles move body parts more quickly. In the process, however, there are several problems.

To build maximum strength requires the use of *heavy* resistance. To demonstrate maximum speed requires the use of *no* resistance. Placing a pencil in your hand, for example, slows the speed of a biceps contraction. Placing pads on football players disrupts the timing of the offense established during practice without pads - *the heavier the resistance, the slower the speed*. Therefore, any formula that combines the use of resistance for strength and speed (to produce 'power') compromises both.

Unfortunately, doing anything to increase strength in the gym increases speed on the field. Yet, speed of movement during exercise has nothing to do with your ultimate speed of performance - with one exception. Moving quickly against resistance exposes muscle and joint systems to high levels of force that may one day lead to injury and prevent you from moving at all. In the case of plyometrics, the force is magnified by impact.

Jump from your vanity onto a bathroom scale and read your weight upon landing. You'll soon learn that body preparation by exposure to impact makes as much sense as ramming your car into a building to prepare for an accident on the interstate. With explosive training you *will* run faster and jump higher, but you won't do much of either.

As Nautilus® inventor Arthur Jones thought, the only possible result from training performed in such a fashion is injury.

To gain 'power,' reduce your overall body fat and treat the muscles used in your sport to brief, *slow*, high-intensity strength training. An increased muscle-to-body-fat ratio will go a long way in ensuring a safe and effective result.

## OCTOBER 5

---

### History Class

It wasn't "Slammin' Sammy" as I had hoped; it was Mr. Sneed. And he ran his 10th grade class with an iron fist. History used to be a piece of cake.

One peep, one chew of gum, one wavering eye - and we were out in the hall. The rest of the time (and there wasn't much of it), we analyzed the rise and fall of the Roman Empire and were expected to know how it formed, worked and unraveled.

There's a lesson in everything but we rarely learn from the past, unless it leads to ruin, at which point it's too late. And even then, few are willing to admit they made a mistake.

Beginning in the early 1970's and every few years thereafter, Nautilus® inventor Arthur Jones published his 'State-of-the-Union' address on exercise. In 1983, he wrote a three-part version called "Exercise, 1983...The Possible and The Impossible" in which he reviewed his mistakes along the way and lessons learned. The purpose: to "start a few people in the direction of a logical approach to exercise" - a start he never had.

*The following is a list of mistakes he included:*
- "Believing that somebody knew something of value on the subject of exercise."
- "Believing that most people were capable of producing any possible degree of results" and then "trying to produce results that were impossible, while ignoring possible results of great value."
- Failing to "understand the cause and effect relationships involved in exercise."
- "Looking for a simple, step-by-step guide to success."

*And a list of what he learned:*
- "You cannot learn much of value on the subject of exercise by reading."
- "Question the motives of people, particularly when seeking their advice; and, even when their motives appear to be aboveboard, never forget that advice is really only somebody's opinion."
- "Most of us fall into the much larger group of people who find it fairly easy to build some body parts, but very difficult to build others."

451

- "The fact that somebody else can produce a certain degree of results does not mean that you can do the same...and it does not mean that the method used to produce those results was the best method, or even a good method."
- "The results of exercise are not produced in proportion to the amount of time devoted to exercise."
- "Very little in the way of exercise is required to stimulate a rapid rate of growth."
- "More (exercise) is not necessarily better, and is usually worse."
- "Your body only needs a certain amount of food, that anything extra in the way of calories will simply be wasted if you are lucky, or converted to fat if you are not."
- "You cannot judge your progress on the basis of changes in your bodyweight; since it is easily possible to gain weight while losing muscular mass, or lose weight while gaining muscular mass."
- "Do not compare your progress, or your results, to the progress or results produced by somebody else; instead, compare yourself now to yourself at a later point in time."

Somebody once said, "The only thing we learn from history is that we don't learn from history." Maybe I didn't miss a thing in the hallway.

## OCTOBER 6

---

### Presbyterian Pass

As a teen, I gave no thought to the fact that my first set of golf clubs consisted of wooden-shafted hand-me-downs, my brother's paper-route Christmas bonus from a prominent Judge in town. Despite the hockey-tape that held them together, one club, a putter made in the mid-1920's performed nobly enough to keep. To this day, it retains its stature in an upgraded set, ignoring sneers of "old-fashioned" from its victims.

At the same time, I gave little thought to the proposed modification of the golf course we played. The Board of Directors claimed a few holes were unfair - the greens were not receptive to good shots and often rewarded bad ones. They were right to some extent, but dead wrong in the case of the eighth.

It wasn't length or degree of difficulty that made the eighth a world-class hole. At 150 yards from the lower tee and 185 from the tip of the upper, it could play anywhere from a feathered nine-iron to a screaming driver, depending on the wind. It was "character."

The Lookout Point Golf Club in Fonthill, Ontario was built in 1922 on the edge of the Niagara Escarpment, a rock formation that left dramatic rifts in elevation throughout the area. The clubhouse sat atop "the highest point on the Peninsula" and overlooked the spray from Niagara Falls in one direction, the Toronto skyline in the other and seven holes below. Only two challenged the escarpment. The par-four eighteenth abandoned its attempt half way up, from where a much needed cable-car ride intervened. The par-three eighth, aptly named *Presbyterian Pass*, provided no such ease.

The narrow path that climbed to the eighth began at the base of a dense-wooded hill. At the tee, the bush succumbed to an array of grassy sumac-strewn hills that intertwined as fingers in a clasp of hands. The tee itself cut into the left side of the first hill that ushered in a series of progressively ascending slopes cascading from left, then right, then left - neither side friendly to an errant shot. At their feet, a swath of fairway wound its way to an elevated green nestled between two final mounds whose grassy tops hovered 30 feet above the putting surface. The green was flanked by a shallow bunker etched into the face of each hill, a craggy sumac protruding above the one on the right.

The climb was steep, the shot dangerous. Anything short rolled back 20-30 yards. Long flirted with a deep but elevated grass bunker from which there was no reasonable escape. In the summer months, when the grass was dry, a wayward shot bounded from the hillsides toward the green. It was the only way to get close.

In the end, they leveled the hill left of the green, enlarged the putting surface to uncharacteristic proportions, gently sloped its entrance and filled in the grass bunker.

*Presbyterian Pass*, once in a class with the *Postage Stamp* at Royal Troon, the 9th at Jupiter Hills and the *Alps* at Prestwick, was built by U.S. and British Amateur champion, Walter Travis, author of his own (Schenectady) putter controversy in 1904. Remodel it? As Bernard Darwin wrote in *The Golf Courses of the British Isles*, 1910, about proposed changes to Royal St. George's Golf Club (England), "Why do they want to alter this adorable place? I know they are perfectly right, and I have even agreed with them that this is a blind shot and that an indefensibly bad hole, but what does it all matter? This is perfect bliss."

To walk its path in the fall, to set spikes on its tee in a breeze, to behold its rugged beauty and challenge its rigors was indeed "perfect bliss." One day, someone will see fit to restore the eighth to its original state and I'll be first to donate a shovel.

## OCTOBER 7

---

### On Second Thought

If given a second chance, I wouldn't change much, but it would be a battle.

In the early 1970's, the introduction of Nautilus® machines sparked a boom in the field of exercise. Gyms became fitness centers overnight, many using the name 'Nautilus' to attract clients. For the first time in the history of exercise, a brand name represented more than a product. It was not just something new to sit on, or someone new to instruct you - it was a system that explained 'why.'

Many centers adopted the philosophy in its entirety, either trusting the source or believing it wise commercially. Others were less receptive, providing separate rooms or circuits as options. Some ran new clients through the system the first few months and let them loose from there. Regardless of how it was done, a gym without 'Nautilus' was doomed...and so were its workouts.

While trucks delivered equipment, the system delivered law and order to an unruly field. It focused on form, intensity and progression - concepts long gone from the gym scene. It drew supervision to the forefront, trainers to the 'what' and 'why' - and it kicked butt. Properly performed, no one viewed the workout as inferior, except bodybuilders, who generally moaned that it was "too brief" as they basked in a pool of homemade fluid following only minutes of training. The hype attracted people and, for the most part, they got their money's worth.

Times changed.

Nowadays, a typical facility adopts *no* philosophy for fear of treading upon the right to choose. Thus, most trainees are left in the dark about the potential benefits of circuit training, if they know it exists. And young trainees have never heard of Nautilus, let alone that it once stood for something. The handful of centers that feature a designated set of machines for circuit training allow clients to wander around unsupervised, doing things that in no way relate to the production of best results. What remains of the oversized NUMBERS on such machines says nothing more than 'BIG DEAL.'

Yet, the rest of the clients are no better off. They are forced to tolerate questionable orientations, forge results from intensity levels they are unwilling (or unable) to produce, and join the list the trainer eventually calls to 'renew.'

The Nautilus inventor was once asked what part of his life he would change if given a second chance. "Damned near all of it," he said. "But in order to do that, I would have required the knowledge that I now have at the start of my life; which, of course, was impossible...if we could look accurately into the future, I doubt that we would have done most of the things that we actually did."

Arthur Jones was not easily satisfied; rarely did things turn out the way he thought. But gyms are satisfied, to the point that they have fallen into complacency and reduced their efforts. I don't think they care.

I once owned a Nautilus gym in Caracas, Venezuela that followed the philosophy of Jones to the letter for 10 years. It was a successful and satisfying struggle.

If I could do it all again, I'd take the same stand, and revive something that was in the best interest of the client - everyone fully attended, every time, staff on the same page, a philosophy, an education. I don't pretend to have all the answers (then or now), but if I couldn't do it my way (really Jones' way), I wouldn't try.

And if I couldn't make it work, I would at least have no regrets.


## OCTOBER 8

---

### Arthur and The Scientists – Part 1

Throughout the 1970's and 1980's, Arthur Jones wrote a series of articles titled *"Strength Training...The Present State of the Art"* in which he expressed little faith in the exercise and testing tools of the day. In the 1986 version, he added, *"...Now a Science"* to the title after developing equipment that could accurately measure parameters that were supposedly being measured.

One of his creations, a low-back machine he called "the closest thing to a miracle I have ever seen," was nominated for a Nobel Prize in medicine, an honor at which he scoffed. It wasn't the first time he refused association with the scientific community.

"And why do I hate scientists?" he said. "I don't, but I clearly recognize them for just what they are: idiots. Arrogant idiots. Exceptions? A few, damned few, but even these few have learned nothing from their own efforts and generally refuse to look at the results of other people. If you mention something of value that is 'new' to one of these people...their usual response is something along the lines of ... 'Oh, where did you read that? Which long-haired, dope-smoking, scrawny, jogging, Ph.D. published that in which eminent, peer-reviewed, scientific journal?' My usual response to this being to tighten their necktie by several inches, grab them by the crotch and the throat and offer to drag them out into the alley and 'explain things' to them; that is kick their ass."

According to Jones, few scientists were involved in the field of exercise 30 years ago. When financial reward and academic gain were introduced, however, science suddenly abandoned its 'search for the truth' and became "an almost desperate attempt to get 'credit', to become a 'recognized expert' in a particular field."

He regarded the scientific process as nothing more than a review of literature in which "some idiot reads the publications of earlier idiots and then tries to combine a lot of little lies into a big lie," and remained convinced that "almost all of the truly valuable ideas and inventions have come from people who were totally outside the scientific community, people like Edison, Tesla, the Wright Brothers and a long list of others."

Jones' discoveries, nonetheless, thrust him into the spotlight.

"During the last 25 years, I have been approached by several thousand scientists; all of them trying to get me to give them money for research, and they generally made it very clear that their 'results' will 'prove' my current opinions, regardless of what they are."

Arthur refused to associate with anything he did not consider honest or truthful and soon found himself the victim of published attacks. Yet, instead of submitting or publishing articles in scientific journals, he invested his money, time and energy in medical research that led to the development of his own tools.

In 1997, Jones replied to an effort to nominate him for a post on the Sports Science Committee as only he could. "Since I am not a 'member of the club,' that is do not wear a white coat and call myself 'doctor,' such people (scientists) almost invariably reject anything that I have to say...because I do not 'follow the rules,' do not find it necessary to at least mention every single one of the seemingly endless list of stupid theories that somebody else has published."

He then concluded, "Having already published everything that needs to be said, or that can truthfully be said on this subject (exercise), I am no longer willing to even attempt to meaningfully communicate with fools, liars and other such people. As Rhett Butler said 'Frankly, my dear, I don't give a damn.'"

## OCTOBER 9

---

### Arthur and The Scientists – Part 2

Arthur Jones tiptoed onto the exercise scene in 1970 with his book, *Nautilus Training Principles: Bulletin No. 1* - "a serious attempt to apply the basic laws of physics to the field of exercise." It was also an attempt to attract scientists to a field that, until then, offered little financial reward. Jones used his most effective weapon, although sparingly at first, to pull it off.

"Quite frankly - and this is perhaps an admission that I would be well advised to keep to myself - I have purposely been critical of some scientists; in an effort to attract their attention to a field of study which I consider important - and if this can only be done by arousing their indignation, sobeit. As the kindness-expert said after he hit the mule across the head with a club, 'first you must get their attention.'"

That he did.

Jones had money, and scientists showed up at his door to offer their services in exchange. But he had something else - integrity. While the majority of scientists were willing to perform the needed research, they were just as eager to conclude exactly what Jones had in mind. The Nautilus® inventor would have none of it.

He decided to perform his own research and "let the chips fall where they may."

If 20 sets of curls were required to build an arm, then sobeit. His brutal system of exercise and harsh treatment of people were offset by his honesty - a first in the field.

Jones refused to publish his research through traditional channels - he self-published. His curiosity led him to test the accuracy and reliability of tools in current use by a strict control of variables. When he found them inadequate, he built something superior, creating enemies and troops along the way. Some devices took weeks and months to build, others decades. Most were scrapped. When the final tally was in, he would proclaim his discovery to the world.

His first 'breakthrough' in the medical field came when he announced that isokinetic exercise and dynamic testing (in common use) were useless and dangerous. The medical and scientific communities didn't take the kindness-expert's comments kindly.

"Remember," said Jones, "these are the same people who are still trying to test strength with isokinetic devices, years after it should have been obvious to a goat that isokinetic tests are worthless for any purpose. But, then, I have met very few scientists who were as smart as an average goat, so I guess I should not be surprised."

He could expose the faults of dynamic testing in minutes, yet was repeatedly ignored - which only added fuel to a raging cauldron.

"They (scientists) cannot bring themselves to admit their own ignorance," he barked, "which provides clear proof of their stupidity, or even insanity. For my part, I may be insane (after all, just how can we meaningfully judge our own stupidity?), but I am not utterly stupid; ignorant of many things, yes, but stupid, no. I am at least aware of simple physical laws that many others continue to overlook, or even attempt to deny."

Jones eventually put an official stamp on his work by establishing the Center for Exercise Science at the University of Florida - with his equipment and strict guidelines. Yet, despite (or because of) the fact that the 'official' research only confirmed what Jones had already discovered, it failed to satisfy the skeptics.

Today, most orthopedic and physiological evaluations are performed with tools that remain useless for their intended purpose. And it's still just as obvious to a goat.

## OCTOBER 10

### Fluff

For years I entertained the thought of professional golf and did everything possible to improve performance, including physical preparation beyond the call of duty. In the end, I was ready to play any sport, but didn't have the talent to pull it off.

In golf, talent is more important than condition, despite the recent surge in fitness that has left the average tour player in better shape than his counterpart 30 years ago. For each player that has taken the plunge, however, there are many others that don't get the idea, are too lazy to start, or have tiptoed in. And they may be better off - the field of exercise has become a vessel for nonsense, a target of commercial interest.

I will state it clear, *golfers do not need a special conditioning program -* they have only been led to think so, and the field of exercise has accommodated that desire.

I was once caught up in the curiosity of learning from other trainers, watching how they worked certain muscles. And while it increased my repertoire of choices and helped fill the hour, I was generally left with the thought, "Why am I doing this dumb thing when I have a 'Cadillac®' in the room?"

The majority of 'dumb things' were copies of basic exercises, limited in range-of-motion, performed with a source of resistance inferior to what was available, and had little or nothing to do with the sport - some detrimental to skill.

Nonetheless, clients were happy and trainers were covered. The inferior gains in strength were enough to produce a slight increase in performance, and where they did not, the program was justified by consolation: "Give it time, things will improve."

Most athletes have entrusted their physical progress to 'experts' who have become as good at following trends as their clients - doing something because somebody said so, and doing it because everyone else is. Forget the basics.

What ever happened to strengthening major muscles, prime movers? What happened to the notion that proper strength training was the window of access to things that serve only to support movement once it has been initiated by the strength of muscular contraction? Functional, core, cardiovascular and flexibility training have overshadowed the only productive factor in physical preparation - muscle strength.

My beefs are these:

- Hours of stretching with results that can be accomplished in minutes.
- Sport-specific training that has nothing in common with proper Preparation, other than an ointment I've used.
- Lengthy core training that can be more effectively achieved in minutes.

I hear the slings and arrows of outraged fortune. Small muscles need strength. The abdomen may be too weak to connect torso and lower body, to twist the trunk and to protect the lower back; it's the muscle most likely to fail. A set of chin-ups fatigues a stomach more than a round of golf. A strong back - not a strong stomach - protects a weak back, and what trainers perceive as low-back exercise is a waste of time. What's left for golfers? To strengthen muscles that rotate the spine in a slow, careful manner.

Old school? Unattractive to athletes convinced they need something 'special?' Behind the times? Hauntingly familiar from sport to sport? Try it: identify the muscles used in your sport, strengthen them with proper full-range exercise, perform 20 minutes of cardiovascular exercise, stretch a few minutes, and leave. Twice a week.

Then spend more time at your profession, instead of wading through hogwash.

## OCTOBER 11

### Does Anybody Really Care?

It's not easy to help someone in a gym nowadays. Men pretend to know everything, women are immune to hard work, and youth have been misled by magazines, coaches and peers. Getting the message across is further complicated by having to disarm the 'perpetrators of bad form' of their cell-phones and CD players.

The gym business is a service business and information that improves the production of results and safety should form part of that service. The battle against 'bad form' during exercise is what clients pay for. Yet, the reaction to 'help' is often alarming.

Some trainees take it as an affront; others as an attempt to shove a philosophy down their throat (which is what they get when they opt for personal training). Some are threatened by what they perceive as verbal abuse, sexual harassment or an intrusion upon their leisure time. Many listen out of respect; but few truly hear.

It's time to set the record straight.

In 1980, I operated a gym in Caracas, Venezuela with an exercise philosophy born of Nautilus® inventor, Arthur Jones - a philosophy I believe to this day. Back then, clients did things my way or not at all, a stance that made an impact on those who stayed - and there were many - but took a heavy personal toll. My intent was to give them the best of exercise, and nothing less.

Ten years later, I returned to the United States and modified my stance. Rather than dictate what people did in regard to quantity, I focused on the quality of performance - from *what* to do, to *how* to do it. I didn't care if they came everyday and did 10 sets of exercise; I cared only about how they performed each repetition, the heart of the workout. The new approach reduced the personal toll, though I spoke my mind when asked. There was no asking in Caracas.

My current approach is even more relaxed.

I now plant seeds of change in regard to philosophy and execution, and let them grow. I sight current research, quote those who adhere to the ideals of high-intensity training, and inject stories from past athletes who produced their best results from hard, infrequent exercise.

The aging process has worked both for and against. To many, my information is reliable, experienced; to others, it's ancient. What does exercise in the 1970's have to do with exercise today? Plenty. Step off a building today and 30 years from now - and note the direction of your fall. The Nautilus philosophy is based on logic, sound physiology and the laws of physics. Gravity hasn't changed.

But I have.

In Caracas, I spent hours attempting to educate clients about the 'why.' When they didn't listen, I'd review things another time. If they still didn't get it, I approached them with a checkbook in hand.

"How much did you pay me?" I'd cut a check and tell them to train elsewhere.

When today's trainees show no interest, I greet them at the door, that's it. I won't bang my head on a wall with anything less than the shock absorption system of a woodpecker.

Those who construe (or construed) my efforts to assist as anything less than the best of intentions can heed the advice John Kerry's wife spewed to a group of reporters in the recent presidential election. Any donkey can hand out a towel.

...with apologies to those who listened, learned and appreciated.

## OCTOBER 12

### Hasta La Vista, Baby

An ad from *The Daily Journal*, an English-speaking newspaper in Caracas, was clear.

*Six years ago, I established Venezuela's first Nautilus® gym, and apparently its last. Since then, an avalanche of 'Grand Openings' has occurred, each claiming to be cast from the same mold. Yet, all have proven nothing more than rooms of equipment in which you supply the philosophy. The well-documented Nautilus system has been ignored, lost or mutilated in a cloud of ignorance, commercial interest and outright fraud, resulting in a decline in the average production of results from improper use of equipment.*

*And don't hold your breath for things to improve.*

*Our dedication to the Nautilus philosophy has never waned, and never will. An advanced degree in exercise physiology, complete library of Nautilus*

*literature, frequent visits to the home base and sincere desire to apply it all to*
*your program have kept us where we are - #1 in Nautilus training.*
  *Gimnasio Multicentro - no one's got it right since.*
  *Gary Bannister: B.A., B.P.E., MEd.*          *TLF. 32-53-42.*


Despite the chest pounding, Nautilus never really caught on. After its initial thrust, no one was willing to stand up and dictate philosophy, just as no one
tells you what to eat in a restaurant. It was viewed as commercial suicide.

There are many ways to get the job done, but probably one 'best' way. I
believed then, as now, that high-intensity strength training was that way. To get
the message across, exercise had to be controlled - just as it should be now.

Recently, a Venezuelan business-associate invited me to participate in a
project he has cultivated for five years. It involves establishing exercise/reha-
bilitation centers in Spain and other European countries, and then hitting the
US market. All of his centers are equipped with MedX® medical machines -
Lumbar Extension, Cervical Extension and Knee - and MedX commercial
exercise equipment, versions of which he's upgraded with computers. The
facilities also feature tools that measure bone density, a problem among women,
the elderly and heart-transplant patients.

The value of strength training as a primary exercise choice, the value of
high-intensity within that realm, and the presence of an instructor who creates
progress have long been ignored. From the timing of each repetition to the
accurate measurement of results, each person is controlled, measured and prodded to produce best results (in strength, flexibility and cardiovascular health)
every time in.

Why MedX? When your facility is truly service-oriented, you buy the best
for your clients and don't just pamper them, you push them - a serious approach, not a social visit. Twice a week, maybe three - in and out.

The cost? A fee far less than the cost of personal training with a clown who
talks about the weather.

My contribution? To train a staff and certify MedX technicians by means
of a rigorous educational process - an international school.

The effort is likely to make no more than a small ripple in a large pond. It
will, however, assure the exposure of some people to safe, productive exercise
and, at the same time, provide the punch line to a joke often told by MedX
inventor, Arthur Jones:

"What do you have when you find 1,000 lawyers lying on the bottom of
the sea?"

"A good start."

# OCTOBER 13

## Learning and Unlearning

I'm not sold on swing mechanics in golf. During a one-time, rooftop lesson in downtown Caracas, the professional had me in a knot in five minutes. The change he proposed felt drastic; my body wasn't willing to give it a go.

The same occurred when I attempted a swing change in mid-season. Tired of hitting balls that finished short and right, I decided that a club-path modification would curve the ball the opposite way and create more distance. The arduous task was pressed into action all too soon by a club championship where, under pressure, I couldn't pull it off. The 'new' swing shot 86, while the 'old' fashioned 73 the next day. It was too late.

Most tour pros who attempt swing changes are plagued by the same, a process Robert Singer aptly described in *Coaching, Athletics, and Psychology* (1972): "When a new response is to be made to a familiar stimulus, negative transfer (interference) will probably occur" and "The most prominent cause of interference in transfer is competition between responses."

When the 'old' competes with the 'new,' the nervous system struggles to decide which muscles it will use and when - and seldom gets it right.

This explains why professionals whose swings *appear* to need a major overhaul - Jackie Cupit, Miller Barber, Moe Norman, Mason Rudolph and Jim Furyk - don't mess with them. And explains why others (some hailed as the next Jack Nicklaus) take the advice of peers, attempt long-term change, disappear for years and return - having scrapped the 'new' for what worked in the first place.

Nautilus® inventor, Arthur Jones ran into the same in the field of exercise. Trainees were reluctant to change, especially if they were doing well with the 'old.'

Ellington Darden, a case in point, experienced success on the national bodybuilding scene in the early 1970's and felt he was on the right track. Then he met Jones.

"After talking with me about strength training for 10 minutes," said Darden, "Jones confronted me with the following: 'You think you're pretty smart, don't you?' Jones asked as I nodded my head. 'If you can unlearn everything you've learned about exercise - and if you can do this unlearning before you reach age 40 (Darden was 28) - you'll be headed in the right direction. At age 40, at the zero level of learning - then, maybe you can learn something of value. If so, you'll indeed be smart.'"

The words, meaningless at the time, proved prophetic. Jones challenged bodybuilders to adopt a more logical and physiological approach to strength training. In the process, he got them to think and change more than their training practices.

"I always admired Jones for his brutally realistic and honest approach to bodybuilding...and to life," said Darden. "It helped me unlearn and relearn more efficiently."

One way to relay a message in the field of exercise is to clear heads of existing nonsense - you can only cram so much into a full head. A better way is to start with a clean slate and then teach the next generation open-mindedness and logic. Otherwise, you deal with negative transfer.

Most trainees are beyond hope - their heads stuffed with sources of inferior resistance, speed and core training, plyometrics and the commercial bias that smothers the field. And those in positions of influence - coaches, trainers, therapists and doctors - are no better off. Victims of the same, many sadly believe in what they do.

Nowadays, when the 'old' competes with the 'new,' the 'new' seldom gets it right.

## OCTOBER 14

### Harry Krishna

There's only one thing worse than spotting a guy with a shaved head, ponytail and robe in your parking lot after a six-hour drive - and that's seeing a half dozen of them. The trip from Hilton Head Island, South Carolina to Greensboro, North Carolina was tedious, especially after walking a golf course all day in the heat and sleeping in the car the night before. My college roommate and I were beat.

"Watch this," I said as I opened the car door.

"Hari Krishna," hollered an approaching skinhead.

"Hi, Harry," I replied, extending a hand. "Nice to meet you - Gary Bannister."

"Oh, no. Hari Krishna is a greeting. It means..."

I didn't care, or recall how I made it upstairs without being 'saved.' And if Harry was at all aware of the 'animals' in that dorm, he would never have shown in that outfit.

Everyone has an agenda, and the field of exercise is no exception.

For the most part, agendas are driven by money - as Nautilus® inventor Arthur Jones discovered when he entered the field - and many are steeped in ignorance. 'New' trainers are bombarded by chaotic theory based on so-called research performed in this country over the past 30 years or on the mystical practices of some Eastern-block county. Add to that the interpretation of veterans and characters in this field (those who were once introduced to a smaller but equally confused pile), and it's tough to distinguish fact from fiction. The latter has devoured the former and the public gets the tail end.

What used to be a sane and logical approach to exercise - proper strength training as defined by Jones - now sports a ponytail, shaves its head and wears a robe. It has become the minority, old school.

The field of exercise has always been blessed with a handful of people of good intent, but burdened with truckloads of bad. When the bad outweighs the good, we find ourselves immersed in a pile of nonsense, with physiology and common sense at the bottom, and the term "strength training" fast becoming nothing more than a greeting.

Jones' retirement was timely. Sixty years of wading through heavy manure was enough. Each year, despite his efforts, the pile grew thicker and deeper as he unveiled one outrage after another, issues he chose to confront, head on, with perseverance, truth and honesty. It eventually wore him out.

I recently spoke with Dr. Michael Fulton, an orthopedic surgeon who worked with Jones for 30 years. Our conversation wandered to the latest crazes in the field of exercise. He referenced an article on his desk that hailed the virtues of a new product called "Water Wings." Somewhere between the laughter and the roar, all you had to do was strap a set of wings to your arms and head for the beach where the wind (or water) provided the necessary resistance for "exercise." To add credibility, the article was accompanied by a photo of a gathering of winged idiots, in full gear, on some beach like an outdoor aerobics class. It redefined the term 'safety in numbers' and reiterated the fact that lunacy came in a multitude of colors.

Good luck.

If I were to advise Arthur Jones, a man who does not lightly take advice, I'd say, "Stay retired." The pile that so raised his ire has deepened, and the wind is blowing harder than ever - this time, in color.

How about neon pink for Harry?

## OCTOBER 15

---

### Letters

While leafing through early 1970's *Ironman* articles, I came across several letters to the editor that shed light on Nautilus® inventor, Arthur Jones.

"Mr. Jones' personal devotion to work and his careful attention to detail is almost legendary. He seldom if ever works less than eighteen hours a day, seven days a week. His investment in both time and money in the development of the new machines is simply enormous, yet he is never satisfied with halfway measures. One of his machines has now gone through more than twenty models, and the final result of so much work is almost literally a masterpiece."
- Coach Bill Bradford, Deland Public High School

"...Totally apart from his activities in the field of physical training, Mr. Jones has made a number of very significant contributions to the field of motion picture production. Among other things, he invented and developed a motion picture camera mount which totally removes the vibration from films made with such equipment; this camera mount makes it possible to film from moving platforms (helicopters, landrovers, boats, trucks - any vehicle) with no slightest trace of vibration. A truly revolutionary development.

He has also made significant developments in the field of optics for motion picture work, especially in the field of anamorphic lens systems.

His film credits include 'Wild Cargo,' 'Capture,' 'Call of the Wild,' "Professional Hunter'...as well as a number of special films for television, the most recent being the top-rated 'Free to Live: Operation Elephant.' ... This film detailed the progress of a major conservation program planned financed and carried out by Mr. Jones; the capture and relocation of entire herds of elephants, a type of undertaking that was considered impossible before he did it. While the present widespread interest in conservation is a fairly recent development, Mr. Jones has been quietly working in this field in a very practical manner for more than twenty years - and so far, utterly refuses to publicize the results of his work. Even giving credit in his films, in many cases, to individuals who contributed nothing apart from unnecessary problems.

I'm not an expert in the field of physical training, but I do know Mr. Jones very well - and if he says that his new machines work, then they work better than he says."

- Robert Glenn, Manager, General Music Corporation, Hollywood (Post Production Supervisor for 'Daktari,' 'Gentle Ben,' etc.)

"I have personally known Mr. Arthur Jones for a period of twenty years; during that time I have had the opportunity to closely observe his activities in a number of varied fields, international airline operation, motion picture production, the importation of tropical fish and wild animals on a large scale, and a number of projects in the field of conservation. His credentials are in order, his status beyond doubt. While I sometimes failed to agree with his ideas at first - in the end I always did. Visionary, he certainly is - but careful almost to a fault, and always practical. In short, his ideas work."

- R.C. Demers

Most bodybuilders, scientists and medical doctors failed to get the message.

OCTOBER 16

------------------

### One for the Ages

Arthur Jones and his wife showed up for what he called his "Flirty Thirties Reunion." The comments were many, and expected.

"Oh, I see you brought your granddaughter."

"It's not my granddaughter," replied Arthur. "It's my wife, Terri."

They looked at the gorgeous teen, glanced at their wives and mumbled under their breath, way under.

For a man who looked like a dried toad on the edge of a highway, he sure attracted a slew of stunning women. He married five of them (when they were young) and divorced most not long after. It kept him in touch with youth.

Jones had three stock responses to inquiries about his age: "Twenty-nine and many months;" "Only the Devil knows for sure and, as my competitors would have you think, I just might be the Devil;" and "I'm old enough to realize it's impossible to change the thinking of fools, but young and foolish enough to keep on trying."

And try he did.

He began by engineering better tools for resistance exercise, Nautilus® machines. Yet, the majority of bodybuilders and athletes he trained were too stubborn or stupid to believe that best results could be produced by brief exercise. They were addicted to long, frequent workouts, and couldn't comprehend the meaning of "time off" or "get a job."

The problem was magnified by the leaders in the field, who were interested only in their bottom line and warned Jones early, "Don't mess up a good thing."

But Jones sided with the victims, believing that his discoveries would one day alter physical training. By 1986, he developed tools that could isolate and accurately measure physiological parameters, and delivered his message in typical fashion.

"In very plain English," he said, "it is my firm opinion that these facts constitute the most important discoveries in the history of exercise, by far. To those of my readers who disagree, I can only say...laugh now, and cry later."

With this, Jones entered the medical field and encountered a wall known as isokinetic technology - the established, reliable source of information on muscle strength.

His solution was unique. He built an airport at his home in Ocala, Florida and flew doctors in for education. Seven days a week for 10-12 hours a day, he showed them what worked, what didn't and why. In the end, the medical community refused to abandon its tools and the tradition of insurance companies paying their bills.

Finally, with nothing more to say, Jones threw in the towel:

"During the last thirty years, most of the worthwhile characteristics of civilization, no small part of the Earth itself, and practically all of the benefits of progressive exercise have been so perverted that almost nothing of value remains; the problems are known, but ignored - the answers are available, but denied - primarily, it seems, because far too many people are interested only in avoiding controversy or are unwilling to face up to difficult solutions."

His solution was difficult, yet simple - seek the truth.

Jones once paused in the middle of a long article to speak his mind: "...and while you may or may not appreciate or agree with my opinions," he said, "you will be forced to live with the facts I present."

Only the Devil knew for sure.

OCTOBER 17

---

## High Tech for Low Backs

It's remarkable what 90 seconds of low-back exercise once a month will do I thought as I muscled the golf bag to my shoulder. I had carried it 18 holes for the first time in 20 years. My back was back.

According to medical estimates, 80% of people suffer low-back pain at some time in their lives and 80% of back problems are muscular in nature. I was a statistic at 30 - two operations from years of running, weight training and sports.

To complicate matters, both attempts at recovery drew me near additional surgery. During the final crisis, a myelogram revealed excess scar tissue and a 90-degree bend in the needle used for the photo, an error that could have led to paralysis. I picked up my back support and limped to the exit. The search for an alternative was on.

As a physical educator and fitness enthusiast, I understood the value of exercise and recognized the limited effectiveness of what was being medically prescribed. On the recommendation of an orthopedic friend, I quit running and began using the Nautilus® Low Back and Abdomen machines. Four years later, I visited the Nautilus inventor to thank him for his contribution to my health.

I had read of Arthur Jones' efforts to isolate muscle function in the lumbar spine but was not prepared for his announcement. "My low-back machine doesn't work (fails to access the appropriate muscles) and the abdomen has *nothing* to do with low-back pain." The more he talked about the device that would ultimately save the day, the MedX® Lumbar Extension machine, the more he made sense. I returned to Venezuela where I was living at the time and put his theory to the test by removing both Nautilus machines from my work-out. It was no loss.

I devoured every article I could find about the MedX device. Its premise was clear - to meaningfully access the muscles of the lumbar spine, the pelvis must not be allowed to rotate during torso extension (traditional exercises - calisthenics, swimming, commercial back machines - were ineffective for that very reason). Initial studies at the University of Florida (Gainesville) produced excellent results with an infrequent exercise protocol. Regardless of diagnosis, 80% of patients responded with a reduction in pain perception. Thirty-three percent became pain-free in 12 weeks.

When my MedX machine finally arrived in Caracas, I performed two minutes of exercise once a week for 20 weeks and increased my strength and mobility dramatically. Ninety seconds of exercise once a month has kept me pain-free for 17 years.

Not everyone is as fortunate. Despite a large statistical base, the medical community cannot predict a patient's outcome - which does little to dampen their confidence. Dr. Vert Mooney, professor in the Department of Orthopedics at the University of California in San Diego states, "The MedX strength program is a must before making further decisions about back surgery."

Despite its success, MedX has spread slowly since its introduction in 1986. At that time, the medical community was inundated with isokinetic technology and reluctant to invest in a costly alternative. Today, many physicians remain unaware of, or continue to ignore the need for pelvic stabilization in back strengthening.

Many clinics in the country have the MedX machine. Find one. It's as close to a non-invasive cure for chronic low-back pain as there is. And who knows, it may improve your golf.

## OCTOBER 18

### Proper Evaluation of the Lumbar Spine

You wouldn't embark on a weight-loss program without first measuring your weight. Nor would you rehabilitate the muscles of the spine without first evaluating their status. All of which implies having the proper tool - a bathroom scale in the first case, a MedX® Lumbar Extension machine in the second.

Figure 1 features three curves that represent a complete evaluation of the isolated muscles that extend the low back. The numbers on the left are measures of force in foot-pounds of torque; along the bottom, of position in degrees. The top curves are static strength tests: #1, conducted *before* exercise; #2, immediately *after*. Curve #3 represents a dynamic exercise (work-capacity test) conducted between the static tests.

The information provided by the testing sequence (#1, #3 and #2) is significant. Curve #1 quantifies the level of fresh strength as high, low or normal. Its shape indicates the position and extent of an existing abnormality; its slope, the subject's response to exercise - specific or general.

A comparison of the shapes of Curves #1 and #2 reveals the subject's cooperation. If they differ radically, one (if not both) is invalid. A comparison of their strength levels is a measure of the effect, the momentary loss in strength, produced by the exercise. The magnitude of the effect indicates the subject's muscle fiber-type or fatigue rate, crucial to the determination of an appropriate exercise protocol.

According to MedX inventor Arthur Jones, the information gleaned from a static test of muscle strength is not only more accurate and meaningful than that from other test protocols, it is safer. By slowly pushing into a fixed pad during a static test, the subject can gradually increase the intensity of the effort and "back off" if discomfort is felt before maximum force is attained. As can be seen from the chart, forces are higher during a test of fresh strength than a test of exhausted strength. In both cases, they are much lower than that encountered during tests on isokinetic machines.

But," says Jones, "as important as the information provided by these strength tests is, and as safe as these (static) test procedures are... the work-capacity test (exercise) is even more important, and much safer."

During a work-capacity test (#3) on a MedX machine, the subject leans slowly into a pad positioned at the mid-back. A sensor records the force applied and traces the effort via computer (the line ascending from the bottom of the chart at 72°). The line climbs and moves a bit to the left (due to unavoidable slack in the system) until the effort reaches a level slightly higher than the resistance (in this case, 75 foot-pounds, half the force produced during Test #1). The gradual increase in force to a lower maximum triggers the exercise and ensures a safer scenario than that of *either* static test.

"But that," you say, "is an exercise - a test of endurance, not strength."

Wrong. The relationship between muscle strength and anaerobic endurance (how long a muscle lasts during exercise) is constant in any one individual. Once known, you can determine strength by measuring endurance - and endurance by measuring strength.

A strength test (Curves #1 and #2) means exposure to high force; an exercise (Curve #3) does not. A comparison of any two exercises over time provides all the information needed to identify progress. If performance is up 20%, strength has increased 20%. The actual strength level may remain unknown, but the degree of progress will not.

When in doubt, take the safe route for testing strength - perform an exercise.

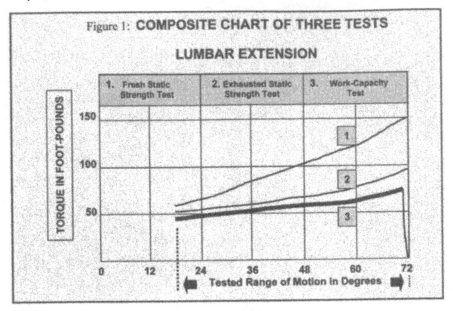

Figure 1: COMPOSITE CHART OF THREE TESTS
LUMBAR EXTENSION

OCTOBER 19

## Low-Back Strength Is Not What It Appears

In the early 1980's, a man from Seattle named Stan Bigos tested the low-back strength of thousands of Boeing Corporation employees and charted their health for several years to establish a relationship, if any, between back strength and spinal problems. The conclusion was unexpected - stronger subjects were *more* likely to suffer back problems - but also correct...

...for the wrong reasons.

First off, there was no tool capable of measuring low-back strength at the time - Bigos might as well have used a kettle. Second, a factor far more important than strength, the rate of muscle fatigue, was ignored.

It seems only logical that a corporation would hire the *strongest* candidate for a job involving extensive use of the low back. Yet, if other factors are equal, judging work capacity from an accurate test of strength is misleading - at least, used to be.

Isolated muscle testing with the accurate MedX® Lumbar Extension machine recently established a relationship between low-back strength and pain perception, and between muscle fiber-type and the risk of having back problems.

The tests revealed that stronger individuals possessed an abundance of fast-twitch (fast-fatigue) muscle fibers that tire rapidly when faced with repetitive tasks. On the other hand, weaker individuals possessed an abundance of slow-twitch (slow-fatigue) muscle fibers, a built-in advantage during prolonged work.

If a fast-fatigue and slow-fatigue worker were placed on an assembly line, the stronger one would fatigue more rapidly, change his posture within minutes and be on Worker's Compensation in weeks. The weaker one could perform difficult tasks (relative to his strength) all day long with little or no fatigue.

On October 8, 1987, MedX inventor Arthur Jones introduced the potential benefits of pre-employment screening for low-back problems in the *Washington Post*. He claimed that a brief MedX fiber-type test and subsequent rehabilitation could save "at least 50 to 80 percent" of the then $40 billion cost of low-back problems in the United States.

He was ignored...and not for the first time.

Years before, Nautilus Sports/Medical Industries® (founded by Jones) sent orthopedic representative, Dr. Michael Fulton to Washington to participate in a Senate hearing on the rising cost of low-back care. Fulton had just completed six years of research on the effect of low-back strength on pain perception with thousands of chronic patients. Among the 'experts' on the panel was actress Linda Evans, who had recently completed a book on exercise. To make a long story short, the press and the Senate committee doted on her every word while Fulton was ignored.

Pre-employment screening for the fatigue characteristics of low-back muscles has enormous potential for industry, government and insurance. It could assist with job placement, identify false claims, re-build millions of ailing backs and save a lot of money in the process - if there was interest. Yet, current discrimination laws prohibit the hiring or firing of individuals based on race, religion, creed, gender and now, muscle fiber-type. How refreshing it would be to rid of politics long enough to make a significant change in the physical and financial health of the nation.

Stan Bigos was recently appointed to head a committee of 'experts' to evaluate everything associated with the treatment of spinal pathology. Save your kettles.

## OCTOBER 20

---

### Isolation and Stabilization

When the idea finally popped into his head, it was so obvious that he never bothered getting out of bed to write it down. Years of effort were resolved in seconds. Jam the thighbone into the pelvis to prevent pelvic rotation. It worked.

For a man who often appeared "in a ratty, tan sports jacket," Arthur Jones didn't mess around when it came to physiological measurement. He refused to talk about a muscle unless it was all of that muscle, and only that muscle. Isolation was the goal...but his mentors would have nothing to do with 'ratty' suits.

"During prohibition in Chicago," he said, "some of the guys had a rather quaint habit that prevented movement of any kind, to the point that it was even impossible for you to wiggle your toes; not difficult, impossible.

If they failed to approve of your movements, or your actions, they would take you down to the dock at night, seat you in a chair and stick your feet in a large bucket of fresh concrete. Then, after the concrete set, they would give you a halfway trip across Lake Michigan. Believe me, you literally couldn't move your toes.

But since we had no interest in preventing you from moving your toes, and since that method offered certain disadvantages for practical applications in the field of exercise physiology, we had to devise a faster, a better and a far safer procedure...although it had to provide an equal degree of restraint. And it does.

I promise you, you will be able to move with almost no restriction in the desired direction, and to the desired degree; with absolutely no restraint except the very small amount of unavoidable friction involved in any sort of machine...

And, I promise you, you will not be able to move in so far as your position is concerned; so you will have the best of both, with the problems of neither...much more freedom of movement where it is required, and no movement where it is not desired."

The result was a contraption *Business Week* (December, 1987) called, "a La-Z-Boy recliner designed by the Marquis de Sade." To Jones, it was much more.

"This is the first machine that truly isolates the muscles of the lower back. My competitors who say otherwise are liars or fools - or both. Let them sue me. I can't wait."

He was so confident that his creation blocked unwanted pelvic movement that he installed a free-moving circular pad firmly against the pelvis during testing and exercise. If the pelvis moved one millimeter, the pad moved two. If it moved at all, it was tightened. The MedX® Lumbar Extension machine was as foolproof as concrete.

When clinical trials began at the Center for Exercise Science (University of Florida), its director, Michael Pollock, Ph.D. said, "What we're finding is so astounding, we're having trouble believing it ourselves. Our test subjects are showing 300-400% increases in back strength." The norm in strength research was 30-60%.

Not everyone was a believer. Bob Bowen, the director of sales for Cybex® (which manufactured three back machines at the time) said, "The research shows that our machines work. I don't believe his (Jones') can give an accurate measure of back strength." He then pointed to the common use of Cybex tools in clinics and testing centers for professional athletes across the country - proof to Jones that ignorance and stupidity were indeed widespread.

Joseph Densen, CEO of Ward International®, summed up the belief of those who had crossed Arthur's path, "If he says something works, you'd better listen."

## OCTOBER 21

---

### The Lumbar Spine and Uncommon Sense

"In order to solve any problem," said MedX® inventor Arthur Jones, "you must first understand the problem." It wasn't easy in the case of the lumbar spine.

Testing lumbar function requires an understanding of lumbar function. The small and relatively weak muscles located alongside the rear of the lower spine move the lumbar vertebra in the direction of extension and in relation to the pelvis, which is connected to the lowest vertebra. Because of that connection, any movement of the pelvis produces some movement of the vertebra.

The pelvis also moves in relation to the legs when the larger, stronger muscles of the hips and rear thigh (buttocks and hamstring) contract. If the pelvis is free to move during tests of lumbar extension strength, the contraction of hip and leg muscles pulls it forward and upward with a force that is easily confused with that of the lumbar muscles. For that reason, the pelvis had to be anchored during testing and exercise - a process that proved a challenge.

Jones first applied force to the front of the pelvis through various means, but the legs were in the way. His first success involved suspending a subject in the air and forcing the thighs into a position where they could not move to the rear in relation to the pelvis. "When the thighs are locked in that position," he said, "then any additional movement of the femurs is impossible, and thus any involvement of either the muscles of the buttock or the thigh-biceps is also impossible...and that position will certainly anchor the pelvis to the required degree." But it was not a practical solution. Few people returned.

One night the light came on:

"You cannot provide a stabilizing force against the front of the pelvis to prevent the unwanted pelvic movement...but you do have access to the femurs, and the femurs are joined to the pelvis... Thus the key to anchoring the pelvis in a practical manner proved to be anchoring the femurs."

Jones applied an upward force through the feet at an angle of 30° in relation to the midline of the femurs by means of a foot board (A in Figure 1). At the same time, he blocked the upward movement of the femurs by using a thigh-restraint belt (B) that acted as a fulcrum, rotating the hip-end of the femur downward. The combination (foot board and belt) prevented the pelvis from moving up and forward.

It still wasn't enough.

"Believing that the pelvis is not moving during testing or exercise is not good enough," he claimed, "you must know that the pelvis is not moving."

That certainty was provided by a round, free-rotating pad (C) installed at the rear of the pelvis. The pad restrained the pelvis from the rear without restricting lumbar function and acted as a watchdog for good form and muscle isolation.

"Under proper compression," said Jones, "the radius of the pad is only about half the radius of a normal-sized pelvis in an average adult...which means that a one degree rotation of the pelvis will produce a two-degree rotation of the pad." A rotating pad, in plain view, instantly revealed the existence and degree of undesired movement.

Meaningful test results in regard to muscle function were impossible without total isolation. For Jones, that meant all of a muscle and only that muscle - something previous tests had ignored.

First things first.

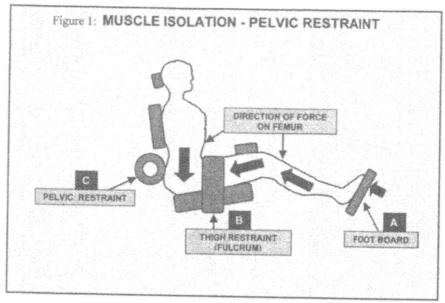

Figure 1: **MUSCLE ISOLATION - PELVIC RESTRAINT**

DIRECTION OF FORCE ON FEMUR

C PELVIC RESTRAINT

B THIGH RESTRAINT (FULCRUM)

A FOOT BOARD

## OCTOBER 22

------

### Front vs. Back

Many people who suffer low-back pain have returned from the doctor's office with a sheet of exercises designed to eliminate the symptoms. The pre-scribed 'home' remedy generally reflected one of two approaches. The first targeted abdominal muscles by means of trunk-flexion movements called William's exercises. The second focused on the muscles that extend the spine, movements called McKenzie's exercises.

While the medical community understood the cause-and-effect relation-ship involved in flexion, few, if any, understood the mechanics behind exten-sion, including Dr. McKenzie. Extension exercise represented a direct avenue to the problem of low-back weakness and produced the same positive result, but no one understood 'how' or 'why' - until Arthur Jones came along.

The MedX® inventor was a grade-school dropout with a passion for prob-lem solving. He began his quest by examining the basic positions of the lum-bar spine in dynamic X-rays: flexion (bent forward), lordosis (standing up-right) and extension (bent back). He concluded with an article - "Lumbar Func-tion" (*Risks and Benefits Management*, October, 1987) - in which he described the mechanical workings of the lumbar vertebra as they moved from flexion to extension.

When you stand in a normal upright position (lordosis), there is a slight curvature in the lumbar spine toward extension. In this posture, the disc spaces are reduced in the rear (of the vertebra) and increased in front because the axis of rotation is located somewhere between the vertebra's front and rear faces, where it acts like a teeter-totter.

When you bend forward to flexion, the axis of rotation remains between vertebral faces and disc spaces become more even, front and back (Figure 1). There, the vertebrae are stacked in a straight line and any compression force on the rear of the discs present during lordosis is reduced. This common knowledge provided physicians a sense of security in using flexion exercises for the treatment of back pain.

It also laid the groundwork for a great misunderstanding.

Because of the reduction in disc space at the rear of the vertebra when the spine moves from flexion to lordosis, it was generally assumed that further movement toward extension increased the compression forces on the rear of the discs.

"Quite the opposite is true," according to Jones. "Rather than compressing the discs in the rear, hyper-extension actually increases the disc space along the rear face of the lumbar vertebra...instead of increasing the forces on the discs, hyper-extension reduces the force on the discs."

This occurs because the axis points of rotation of the lumbar vertebrae change during extension. They move far behind the rear wall of the vertebrae, into the facets. This opens the disc spaces in both front and back (Figure 1), hence the success of extension exercises for back pain - with one exception. Extension movements can aggravate conditions of local bone loss or facet weakness.

"Doctors have been looking at X-rays for 50 years," said Jones, "and never noticed (disc-space changes during extension)." He didn't stop there.

Jones developed a way to measure the changes and shared, by phone, his information on spinal mechanics, on isolating back-extensor muscles and on a practical method of quantifying the degree of movement from X-rays. After 90 minutes, Dr. McKenzie finally understood the cause-and-effect relationship behind the success of his approach.

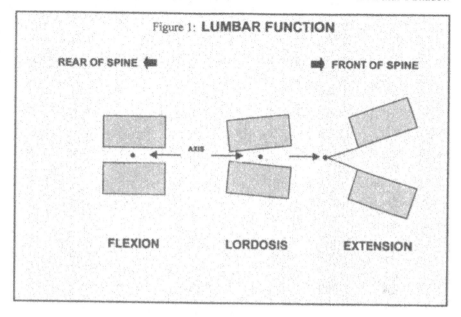

Figure 1: **LUMBAR FUNCTION**

REAR OF SPINE ⬅    ➡ FRONT OF SPINE

AXIS

**FLEXION**         **LORDOSIS**         **EXTENSION**

## OCTOBER 23

### Determining Lumbar Function From X-Rays

The 'Grand Opening' of South America's first MedX® low-back rehabilitation center in Caracas, Venezuela was a two-evening event that featured MedX orthopedic surgeon, Dr. Michael Fulton. It attracted a number of local physicians including the neurosurgeon who had twice operated on my back, Dr. Rafeal Lara Garcia.

As Dr. Garcia toured the facility, he stopped by a poster depicting the mechanics of the lumbar spine and asked if I had more information. I had plenty.

MedX inventor Arthur Jones had not only unraveled the dynamics of the lumbar spine, but had created an accurate method of determining the degree of movement from one vertebra to another from a simple X-ray. It was not the first attempt, but was by far, the first meaningful and accurate one.

According to Jones, "The primary problem with attempts to measure vertebral movement results from the lack of a fixed reference point." The exact position of the top and bottom of a vertebra was confused because X-rays provided a picture of both near and far sides. The corners of the vertebra were

479

too irregular in shape for accurate comparison, the rear face was confused by the facets and the front face was concave in the center. This made it difficult to measure motion by comparing front faces in different positions. To complicate matters, the perspective changed as the vertebra moved.

Jones noticed that the only part of a vertebra that maintained the same perspective in all positions was the front face. It was also the clearest part of the X-ray.

He began by scribing a thin straight line that barely touched the two most forward bumps on the front face of each of the vertebra (Figure 1). Together, the five lines (on the X-ray) provided an almost perfect method for measuring the movement of each vertebra, though they revealed nothing about changes in the disc spaces between. In the same manner, he scribed a straight line along two of the bumps that appeared on the front face of the sacrum to measure angular changes between the sacrum and L5.

Jones next selected a point along the line on the front face of each vertebra - a point below the top and above the bottom of the vertebra - and scribed a line at right angles to the first. The new line was approximately one inch long (25 millimeters) and did not extend as far as the rear face of the vertebra. Its exact length didn't matter as long as it was consistent (he added a short line to indicate its end); its exact position didn't matter as long as it was between the top and bottom of each vertebra.

The system made it possible to measure changes in disc space, not the precise degree of change, but the direction of change one way or the other (Figure 2). It also revealed that such change affected the length of the spine. "The overall length of the spine changes during extension, changes in both directions," he claimed, "first becomes shorter than the length in the straight starting position (flexion), then becomes longer. The greatest overall length of the lumbar spine occurs in a position of maximum extension." (Figure 3)

The problem of measuring changes in disc space and locating axis points of rotation still existed. When the vertical distance between the two lines increased in both front and back (during extension), the precise location of the axis of rotation and the relationship between the disc spaces could be determined by mathematical calculations and geometric relationships. But all of that, according to Jones, was unnecessary.

"The more I study the lumbar, the more impressed I become by its design."

The more I study Jones, the more impressed I become by his insight.

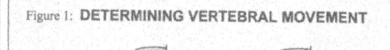

Figure 1: **DETERMINING VERTEBRAL MOVEMENT**

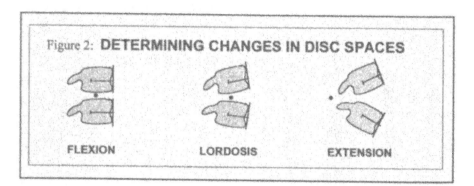

Figure 2: **DETERMINING CHANGES IN DISC SPACES**

FLEXION          LORDOSIS          EXTENSION

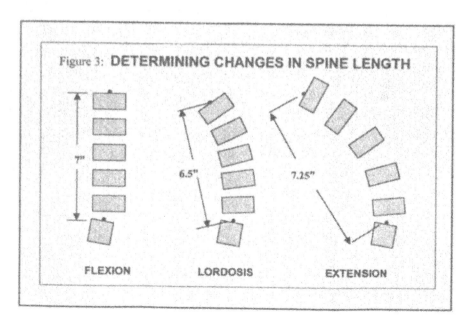

Figure 3: **DETERMINING CHANGES IN SPINE LENGTH**

7"          6.5"          7.25"

FLEXION          LORDOSIS          EXTENSION

## OCTOBER 24

---

### MedX, Golf and Chronic Back Pain

Ignorance, reluctance to change and old-fashioned politics are denying professional golfers sidelined by low-back pain access to a machine that can solve their problems.

Ironically, the solution originated on the doorstep of PGA Tour® headquarters in the neighboring town of Ocala in 1986. Yet, despite its success, the MedX® Lumbar Extension machine remains unknown among touring pros, and worse, the PGA Tour appears to have little concern.

Golf is tough on backs. According to orthopedic surgeon Dr. Michael Fulton, "Spinal discs do not tolerate the forces of rotation well." He sees (in his practice) greater degeneration among golfers than non-golfers, a direct relationship between frequency of play and injury risk, and a high incidence of weak musculature. Throw in torso extension, impact and the demands of competition and it's no wonder that, of the golf-related injuries studied by Centinela Hospital in the PGA Tour fitness van (1990-95), low backs led the way with 24%.

"The profile of injury is simple," says Fulton. "If the force imposed on a muscle or joint system exceeds the breaking strength of that system, injury occurs."

Which leaves golfers two choices: decrease the force the system is exposed to, or strengthen the system. Many address the first by modifying their swing, but few address the second in a meaningful way. As Fulton suggests, "The focus is still on flexibility and cardiovascular improvement, not on the critical issue of strength."

Some pros, like Fred Couples, are afraid to lift weights. "I'm a bit leery of doing anything as far as lifting weights that might hurt my back, so I take it easy and stick to the stretching exercises." Others, like Davis Love, suggest "a lot of sit-ups" to those in need. But MedX inventor Arthur Jones, who understands the cause-and-effect relationship of lumbar pain as well as anyone, disagrees. "The stomach has nothing to do with low-back pain. The problem is weakness in the muscles that extend the spine."

Those who elect to 'do something' may be no further ahead. Traditional low-back exercises (including health-club machines) fail to target the involved muscles because they allow the pelvis to rotate during back extension of the torso.

Only the MedX machine provides the degree of pelvic stabilization needed to access these important muscles. Related research shows dramatic strength gains with a protocol of infrequent exercise - gains that correlate well with a reduction in pain perception.

In 1986, Dr. Fulton successfully introduced MedX to a PGA tour pro disabled with back pain, but that's as far as he got. Tour directors were too caught up in the exploits of Jack Nicklaus who, at the time, was not on the same page.

The introduction of 'fitness vans' to the three pro tours appears to bring a glimmer of hope. According to Barry Sommerville, the HealthSouth® representative who operates the program, "Each van is equipped with an exercise tool for strengthening the spine." Not quite. The Cybex® machine in current use confirmed its inability to strengthen low-back muscles in research at the University of Florida 15 years ago, which renders the vans nothing more than first-aid facilities for acute, not chronic, back pain.

The solution is clear: (1) Pray that "HealthSouth remains open to the latest technological advancements," as Sommerville suggests; (2) install a MedX machine in each van and have players use it once per event; and (3) don't hold your breath about (1).

HealthSouth has an equipment affair with Cybex that won't soon help anyone.


## OCTOBER 25

---

### Oh Canada!

The Canadian health-care system looks great on paper, but has its problems. Years ago, I sought an appointment with world-renowned back specialist, Dr. Ian McNab in Toronto, only to find a nine-month waiting list. Now, an attempt to locate less-renowned physicians may prove as difficult, as a recent case in Welland, Ontario demonstrated.

A popular pediatrician in the town where I was born was overloaded with patients due to a shortage of doctors. Every day was a struggle, yet everyone appreciated his efforts - everyone but the government.

According to them, the doctor spent too much time with patients and made more than the cap allowed. He was fined $135,000. There was nowhere to go. His nature refused to turn patients away (there was no one to take the overflow) and his pride rejected inquiry into his integrity. The doctor drove to Lake Erie one morning and kept walking.

Gary Bannister, B.A., B.P.E., M.Ed.

A recent trip to Canada revealed that the fields of exercise and rehabilitation are not far from the same fate. MedX® machines were as scarce as MRI centers; good form as scarce as in the US. The only coed gym in the local phone book had a charm that dated back to the Dark Ages, and a visit to the alma mater was much the same.

I hadn't seen the grounds of McMaster University in Hamilton, Ontario - perched on the western tip of Lake Ontario midway between Niagara Falls and Toronto - in 15 years, and only twice since graduation in 1971. Things had changed.

There were new additions to old structures, an indoor eatery that rivaled ritzy shopping centers, a maze of streets that defied entrance, yet shorter distances between buildings than I recall. The PE edifice appeared worn despite a new wing of rooms and labs for graduate students, sports psychology, kinesiology, physiology, rehabilitation, evaluation and sports medicine.

The original gym (probably now a broom closet) and its successor (what I saw 15 years ago) had been replaced - along with a centerpiece Nautilus® Pullover machine - by a larger facility shared by the student body and athletic teams. The new wing housed another extensive room dedicated to the rehabilitation of spinal cord injuries.

Several graduate students toured us through the physiology lab where my favorite professor, Dr. Digby Sale, was still active. I missed him by a few days. The lab housed a Biodex® machine (an isokinetic device) and other familiar tools. The gyms were stocked with Magnum® equipment; the rehab center with everything but MedX.

The students spoke of biopsy research to determine muscle fiber type, which reminded me of a letter from a research scientist (in the Department of Rehabilitation Medicine at another Canadian university) to MedX chairman, Arthur Jones in the late 1980's.

"I very much enjoyed my stay with you and found it most stimulating, exciting, but also - to a certain degree - disturbing... My electromyographic work on the identification of muscle fiber types in lumbar muscles, although it appears to generate valid findings, would have to be verified with physiological parameters. Sampling muscle biopsies would be one way to confirm the findings; however, a functional and therefore better way would be an assessment similar to the one developed by you. I only wonder, how much the electromyographic work will contribute to our understanding of the lumbar muscles or if this work becomes increasingly academic and removed from applied clinical research?"

Jones had discovered a better way. It just never found its way across the border.

## OCTOBER 26

---

### Guarantees

After lecturing all day to a group of medical doctors, Arthur Jones escorted me across the runway of "the world's largest private jetport" to a prefabricated building that housed his manufacturing facility (in Ocala, Florida).

It was quite an honor. The MedX® inventor trusted only a small core of people and had more enemies in the field than friends. His incessant 'potshots' at the establishment left more people waiting for his demise than for the next idea to copy.

Once inside the building, we stopped by the soon-to-be-painted frame of a MedX Lumbar Extension machine, the third off the assembly line - one at the University of Florida for research, the other in the conference center from where we came. The structure was a maze of cross-supports held together by thick bolts.

"We were tightening the seatbelt one day," he said, "and noticed the frame bend. We doubled it up so it wouldn't." What started out as a basic Nautilus® machine (built like a battleship) turned into something hardier by necessity.

The only thing stronger was its warranty.

At a time when the 'standard' for commercial exercise machines was one year, Jones offered a 10-year written guarantee adding, "under heavy gymnasium use, you won't touch it once for 50 (years)." When asked about the warranty on his medical device - the frame of which stood before us - he replied, "This machine should last out the century - not this one, the next."

They were built to last - which is more than can be said of his competitors' tools.

In 1994, I trained on 12 brand-new BodyMaster® machines. Besides a few lousy cams (the device that changes the resistance), parts began to fall off the equipment within a month. In another gym, I watched clients abandon 11 LifeFitness® pin-selector machines within weeks of delivery. They didn't like their 'feel,' which frustrated both the sales rep and the owner.

Unfortunately, 'guarantees' with exercise fall in the same category - unpredictable - and the reasons why are clear. Exercise only *stimulates* change; your body makes the change. If your body is genetically superior, the change is fast and dramatic. If it is average, some change occurs. If it is a dud, little happens, regardless of input.

But there's 'good' news. Everyone can increase muscle strength significantly with regular, progressive training. And 'bad' news: the corresponding increase in muscle size produced by strength gains varies enormously. Most trainees don't have the potential to look like anyone in the magazines.

In the same way, proper rehabilitative exercise - perhaps the closest thing to a cure-all there is - only *stimulates* change. The body has the final say.

When Jones sold Nautilus in 1986, he sent a core of workers to Dallas, Texas to ensure a smooth transition for the new owners. After a year, some returned (by agreement) to Jones' next venture, MedX. One employee, Scott Koch (sent to install my MedX equipment in Venezuela, 1988) revealed that the new Nautilus owners requested at least three estimates for any expenditure - large or small. When he returned from Dallas, Koch approached Jones about a minor purchase.

"Scott," said Arthur, "go out there and buy the best damn bolt you can and put it on the machine." His prime concern was quality.

If people would only exercise with the same conviction...

## OCTOBER 27

### The Genetic Crap Shoot

I was formally introduced to golf high atop the Niagara escarpment on a Monday, the single day Lookout Point Golf Club (Fonthill, Ontario) allowed caddies to play 18 holes. Yet, what was always a glorious day for those who carried was a tough one for head professional, Gord McGinnis, Sr. Famous for his work with Marlene Stewart-Streit, the best female amateur in the world, 'Senior' was torn between finding a successor and visions of "Caddie Shack®." No wonder he suffered migraines.

Approximately 80% of our ability to excel in sports is genetically determined. The rest is sound coaching, good practice habits and, among other things, a positive psychological environment. Everyone has the potential to reach his or her summit, but most don't have what it takes to get to the top of their sport. And as often as superior athletes boast of the sacrifices made to get where they are, the fact remains - they were lucky, and some of that luck can be measured.

In the mid-1980's, Nautilus® inventor Arthur Jones tested the front-thigh strength and fatigue characteristics (muscle fiber-type) of a world-class tri-athlete from Canada. He then had her perform leg extensions at set intervals using different percentages of her peak strength. The endurance of her quadriceps was outstanding. Months later, he tested her nearest rival, an identical-twin sister, in the same manner and got exactly the same result - great genes in the right place.

On another occasion, he measured the front-thigh strength of the current world-record holder in 'squats' and found it "pitiful" compared to subjects that had gone before. Jones then tested his muscle fiber-type and discovered an abundance of endurance fibers. Embarrassed, the champion refused to acknowledge the results and allowed no further testing. "Given slow-twitch (endurance) fibers in all of his muscles," commented Jones, "he would not be setting records in the squat."

In 1989, I tested the back strength of two world-champion water-skiers on a MedX® Lumbar Extension machine. Anna Maria Carrasco (current champion) was 'average' in strength and 54% stronger than her retired sister, Esperanza. Both were then exercised to fatigue using 50% of their respective peak strengths. Anna performed 13 repetitions (122 seconds) and fatigued at a normal rate, while Esperanza completed 10 repetitions (105 seconds) and displayed no fatigue in a post-exercise test. *Following* exercise, Anna was only 19% stronger than her sister. If either had possessed an abundance of fast-fatigue muscle fibers in the low back, she would not have been a champion in that sport.

But not all luck is good luck - or necessarily passed on.

In the early 1990's, Jones tested a former Chicago Bears' linebacker and his eldest son, a college football player. The father's front thigh, left in a state of atrophy, pain and restricted mobility by a career-ending knee injury, was *much* stronger than the healthy leg of his son - due to muscle fiber-type. The father had power; the son, endurance.

You never know with genes, and you're stuck with what you get. The best you can do is test the fatigue characteristics of a muscle and use an appropriate repetition scheme to strengthen it.

'Senior' spent a lot of time searching for a successor, which was smart. A female could more easily climb golf's ladder and, more discerning, you can't train a donkey for the Kentucky Derby®. One Monday, a fellow caddy and I played 63 holes before we got the boot - more, I hope, for the divots we dug than the potential we had.

## OCTOBER 28

---

### The Greatest Show on Earth

A group of orthopedic surgeons strutted into the Medical Research Center of MedX® Corporation in Ocala, Florida. Following greetings and coffee, they were seated in a semi-circle. Without fanfare, a short, be-speckled and balding ringmaster (who resembled a janitor imitating Napoleon) strolled methodically toward them. Nine AM, June 11, 1987 was an appropriate hour for a roast.

"Gentlemen, today we're going to take grade-one math and grade-two physics. I hope you can stay with me."

There was no middle ground with MedX chairman, Arthur Jones. You either liked him or you didn't, and it never took long to decide. Arthur exploded from the blocks and really didn't care where you stood. He was there to educate and market his equipment.

The education was superb; the marketing, questionable.

My visit was born of curiosity. I had read many of Jones' articles, purchased his equipment and followed his exercise system in my business and personal life for years. But I had yet to follow up on one suggestion: "If you think his writing is good, you've got to hear him speak. He's 10 times better."

His writing was brilliant. His presentation, well...I arrived for one and stayed for seven. It was the greatest show on earth.

Every day was unique. Arthur kept his guests on the edge of their seats; some through intrigue and reverence; some because they *were* on edge; and some because they may have wanted to leave. No one dared. When Jones moved left, *every* eye moved left. When his voice jumped, the room jumped. When he whispered, you could hear the "whisp." One minute close; the next, distant. One phrase soft; the next, intense. Fact, opinion, conjecture - Jones had them all. It was education with passion.

By the end of the week, Arthur had covered a gamut of topics, slain every rehab dragon out there and provided a lifetime of entertainment.

One day, he tested the strength of a therapist on the Rotary Torso machine. When he saw that the young man was extraordinary in flexion and pitiful in extension, he soared into delirium. The potential for improvement was astronomical and Jones loved numbers - big numbers when it came to strength gains.

"I want you to come work for me," he blurted.

"I don't know that I can," fumbled the youth. "I've got a job I'm content with..."

"Then I'll fly you here every Friday and pay you double what you lose in wages."

One weekly exercise on the rotary device would produce an increase in strength in the thousands of percent - and great ammunition for lectures.

The following day, it was my turn. I tested on the Lumbar Extension machine during a break and took the results directly to Jones, hoping that I, too, was a genetic freak. I'd have worked for him in a heartbeat.

Glancing at 14 three-digit numbers, Jones replied. "Well, you're down (in strength) 18% here, 27% at 36', about 14% in extension..." I was disgustingly average.

Years later, I returned only to be forewarned as I mounted the bus in Orlando, bound for Ocala, "Focus on the message, not the messenger." It was a daunting task.

No greatest show on earth was complete without elephants. Arthur harbored more than 100 (salvaged from slaughter in Africa) behind the research complex.

Like his guests, they would not soon forget the ringmaster.

## OCTOBER 29

### Muscle Testing

There are two ways to test muscle strength: dynamically, as a muscle moves; and statically, without movement. Only one is accurate. Only one is safe.

Muscle testing began in the late 1960's with the advent of isokinetic (motorized) machines that allowed a muscle to contract at a constant, pre-selected speed. Resistance was provided by mechanical or liquid friction.

In 1980, Nautilus® inventor Arthur Jones built an isokinetic leg-extension device to compare the accuracy and safety of the two test methods. His protocol was threefold: (1) a dynamic test of lifting strength (a maximum effort against a mechanical arm that moved upward); (2) a dynamic test of lowering strength (a maximum effort against the same arm as it lowered); and (3) a static test of strength (maximum isometric efforts against a fixed arm set in various positions throughout the range of motion).

He performed this protocol on thousands of subjects - before, during and immediately after exercise - and identified several trends. ONE, before exercise, a fresh muscle was 40% stronger lowering than lifting. TWO, during sub-maximal exercise (e.g. the first five of 10 repetitions), both lifting and lowering strength declined gradually. THREE, as intensity increased, lifting strength dropped rapidly while lowering strength increased. When lifting strength declined by 100%, lowering strength had declined by only 14%. FOUR, static strength *always* fell midway between lifting and lowering values.

With three apparent levels of measurable strength (lifting, lowering and static), the first problem of dynamic test accuracy was identified. The difference between lifting and lowering output was the result of internal muscle friction. A dynamic test of lifting strength always produced a value lower than it should have because friction decreased lifting output. A dynamic test of lowering strength was too high because friction helped lowering. 'How much' too high or low could never be determined (friction increased with fatigue and speed of movement), nor accurately added to, or subtracted from, the result.

A second problem emerged when force values were too low in the first third of a dynamic test due to the muscle's inability to recruit fibers instantly or too low in the last third due to fatigue. Stronger subjects (with predominantly fast-twitch fibers) recruited quickly but fatigued toward the end of each test. Weaker subjects (with an abundance of slow-twitch fibers) recruited slowly but displayed little fatigue. Most subjects (and their test results) suffered from one or the other, but not both.

Jones identified a third variable that challenged the safety of dynamic testing. To move from zero to any selected speed, the machine had to accelerate and then "brake" to maintain that speed. The moment it braked, subjects were exposed to an impact force against the movement arm, and many reduced their effort when they saw the spike in force. When they resumed their effort, they produced another spike (again, the result of impact) that increased the risk of injury.

None of these problems existed with static testing. "Fifty years from now, when all the research is in," said Jones, "every company in the field of muscle testing will test the way we do (statically), because *there is no other way*."

Sadly, the field of rehabilitation was saturated with isokinetic tools when he revealed his findings. Most doctors were unaware of, or worse, ignored the facts.

To determine the strength of a muscle, isolate it and test it without movement. After all, muscles have only one *true* level of strength - static.

OCTOBER 30

---

## When Peers are Dumb, Too

You can't believe everything you read or hear, even if the source is 'reliable.' The other day, an astute physical-therapy assistant with a 'certified training' text in hand was confused by a statement (about resistance and speed of movement during exercise) that appeared to deny the laws of physics. She was right. The statement was dead wrong, the opposite of what it should have been.

There are degrees of reliability in journalism. While most magazines have their own agenda and publish only what their readers want to hear, an article in *Time* or *The Wall Street Journal* is considered more credible than one in *The National Enquirer*. And research articles published in medical journals that are written, edited and reviewed by peers are generally regarded as even higher on the scale. But don't be fooled.

For the past 30 years, the output of muscle function has been measured primarily by isokinetic machines (motorized tools that claim to establish and maintain a constant speed of motion). They test strength in a dynamic fashion, as a muscle moves. When first introduced, the methodology complemented the bias of the day - that a test of dynamic strength was somehow more 'functional' than a test of static strength. Medical facilities were quick to jump on board - it was the only thing out there.

Soon, thousands of tests and hundreds of research projects flooded the journals. No one questioned the validity of the tools; no one questioned the results - until Arthur Jones came along. "We settled on static testing for the good and simple reason that no other method works," concluded the MedX® inventor who spent 14 years and $88 million in the process. "Static testing is far more than the best method of testing strength, it is quite literally the only meaningful method of testing strength."

In the November issue of *Risk and Benefits Management*, 1987, Jones exposed some of the fallacies of isokinetic research as reported in medical journals. One issue of *Spine* magazine, for example, reported higher levels of strength during dynamic lifting tests than static holding tests, a result Jones called "utterly ridiculous, simply impossible." The relationship between the three levels of strength - lifting, holding and lowering - had been clearly established. Under fresh conditions, muscles are 20% stronger holding than lifting, and another 20% stronger lowering. With fatigue, the relationship amplifies (holding and lowering percentages increase). Lifting strength is *always* the weakest of the three.

He also pointed out that most isokinetic studies report higher levels of force at faster movement speeds, a lie that has lured coaches and athletes to 'explosive' training.

Perform a bench press as quickly as you can with 50 pounds. Film and time the movement by counting the number of frames it takes to get the bar from your chest to extension. Repeat the same with 100 pounds, then 150 pounds, and so on. The speed of movement declines as the resistance increases. Nothing else is possible.

The higher force levels at greater speeds recorded during isokinetic tests are measures of impact force added to muscle output. "All of which," claims Jones, "should be obvious to anybody, but certainly is not obvious to some people; the problem being that a lot of other people are encouraged to perform meaningless tests in a dangerous fashion by reading published statements that are simply ridiculous." And peer reviewed.

Muscle function is still primarily measured using isokinetic tools; and many athletes are encouraged to train in a senseless and dangerous fashion.

## OCTOBER 31

### The Retention Factor

Some muscles retain strength longer than others for the following reasons:
- *Frequency of use.* A muscle can maintain its strength (and size) if exposed to an adequate resistance on a regular basis; if not, it declines in as little as a week and can eventually reach a state of atrophy. Judging from soreness produced during initial workouts (and upon return from lack of use), chest, calf and inner-thigh muscles are not stimulated in a meaningful way nor moved through a complete range of motion by normal daily activities. They lose strength rapidly. For the same reasons, rear-thigh muscles lose strength faster than front-thigh muscles, but their return from decline does not produce the discomfort encountered with the chest and calf. They appear active enough to keep out of trouble.
- *Length of time taken to produce the result.* A muscle that trains for one month and then stops loses strength quickly. A muscle that trains for 10 years and stops loses only a small percentage of its strength (the body adjusts to a higher set point). When exercise resumes, the muscle remembers where it once was and, depending

on the amount of time it has trained, facilitates the return to its former level - another reason to make exercise a long-term commitment.

Nautilus® inventor, Arthur Jones used an analogy of twins as proof of the latter. If identical twins doubled their strength in 12 months by progressive-resistance exercise and then quit, their retention would differ if:

- Twin A reached the goal (double strength) within the first three months and maintained it for nine.
- Twin B gradually reached the same goal just in time for the re-test.

Which twin would retain more strength if tested months later?

Unlike the hare and tortoise, Twin A. His system had nine months to adapt to its new level of strength and establish a higher *normal* point for a longer time. On the other hand, Twin B's system had only a few days to adjust to its newly acquired strength and would lose its final gains rapidly. If training were resumed, Twin A's muscles would display better memory (in relation to prior strength levels) because they were in an elevated state for more time.

Unlike twins, however, muscles differ.

In the mid-1980's, Jones measured the strength of the isolated muscles that extend the lumbar spine in approximately 10,000 subjects and found the majority (90%) in a state of atrophy. He declared that daily activities and participation in sports and traditional low-back exercise failed to stimulate these muscles in a meaningful way. Only the use of a MedX® Lumbar Extension machine produced a dramatic increase in strength.

Then came the real surprise.

A cessation of low-back exercise should have placed the 'unused' back muscles in the same category as the chest and calf. Yet, research at the University of Florida's Center for Exercise Science indicated that the strength loss following a 12-week protocol of specific (MedX) exercise was minimal. There was no loss after four weeks of disuse and only a 10% loss after 12 weeks. Furthermore, the same muscles required only one brief exercise (60-90 seconds) per month to *maintain* strength.

If the rest of the body were that efficient, we'd be swamped with infomercials.

# NOVEMBER

"When your back is out, you won't care how big your arms are."

Arthur Jones

## Presto! Your Back is Better

The TV room on the second floor of the dorm buzzed with astonishment and laughter as 6'4", 230-pound defensive-end Greg White sat with a puzzled smile in a chair that, moments earlier, he was unable to lift. The chair weighed two pounds. Greg looked like he could hoist the room.

On command, a friend sat in front of him and started a conversation while another lit a match directly beneath his forearm perched on the arm of the chair. Greg was not the kind of guy to mess with, let alone torch. He didn't budge. Another match, no reaction - no scar, no burn - just a friendly conversation about football.

It was all part of an incredible evening. Greg had been hypnotized.

I went to school with one of the greatest magicians of his time, if not of all time, Doug Henning. Doug roomed a few doors down the hall in one of the men's dormitories at McMaster University in Hamilton, Ontario in the late 1960's. From time to time, he'd execute a 'trick' that would leave a small gathering bewildered in spite of (perhaps because of) the fact that we were at times only inches from the performance.

When asked the secret to his illusions and feats of escape, Henning would invariably reply, "It's all in the equipment."

Things are not much different with low-back care in this country. Despite the fact that the cure is right under their collective noses, the major players (insurance companies, doctors, therapy and exercise technicians, patients, equipment manufacturers, coaches and athletes) continue to ignore the facts. The only device capable of strengthening the muscles that extend the lumbar spine is the MedX® Lumbar Extension machine.

Commercial low-back machines in health clubs, isokinetic tools in rehab clinics and traditional exercises *do not, cannot* and *will not* strengthen back muscles. Because they allow pelvic rotation, they strengthen muscles of the rear hip and thigh (buttocks and hamstrings). Only the MedX device offers the degree of pelvic stabilization necessary to access the important muscles of the low back, a fact clearly established by research at the University of Florida in 1986.

When Nautilus® inventor Arthur Jones first introduced the MedX machine that year, he made the following bold claims:

- Fifty to eighty percent of the $40 billion cost of low-back pain in government, insurance and industry could be eliminated by a simple, specific test.
- The MedX device was a lie detector - could confirm or refute the existence of a claimed injury with a high degree of probability.
- Prior studies that pointed to a negative correlation between low-back strength and injury probability measured the wrong muscles (hip and leg muscles impose high forces on the weaker lumbar area) and the wrong factor (they should have measured *rate* of muscle fatigue, not strength).

Jones' exercise protocol was equally unique. "Use it (MedX) once a week. If you don't get a good result, try it once every two weeks."

Following two low-back surgeries, I have used the brief, infrequent, research-based protocol for 17 years, and the feeling I get after each session is no illusion. It's all in the equipment.

Find a MedX Lumbar Extension machine for your back...and leave the matches at home. The machine comes with its own kind of burn.


## NOVEMBER 2

---

### Low-Back Muscle Challenge

MedX® inventor Arthur Jones was eccentric, but brutally honest. When he discovered that infrequent stimulation of the low-back muscles was required for best results from exercise, many thought it was a continuation of his Nautilus® philosophy. Not so. The muscles that extended the spine were as eccentric as he.

Jones believed that most back problems were caused by the inability of traditional exercise to stimulate the appropriate muscles. The only way to meaningfully access the muscles that extend the lumbar spine was to prevent pelvic rotation during torso extension.

He was so confident in his findings that he challenged non-believers with the following: "Measure your isolated low-back strength on a MedX machine. Then, strengthen your back however you choose and return when you're ready. If you re-test one ounce stronger, I'll give you five-hundred bucks."

It was Arthur's way of making a point.

One day, a young therapist who believed in traditional exercise (and an isokinetic back device he used with his patients) called Arthur's bluff. He tested on the MedX machine and promised to return.

When he showed up for the easy money, his re-test revealed a 20% loss in strength. He stormed away and returned months later, only to test the same as he had during the initial effort.

His loss of time, however significant, proved less than that of a man I tested in Coral Springs, Florida. Steve Z, at 43, looked the role of reigning world-champion weightlifter. The back of his thighs and butt were thick with muscle, yet a test of his isolated low-back strength on the MedX machine revealed a level only 10% above average for males his age, weight and size. It also showed that he couldn't stand much exercise (by birth). A lifetime of competitive lifting had done nothing for the strength or endurance of his low-back muscles.

Because of his quick rate of fatigue (predominance of fast-twitch muscle fibers), Steve required infrequent exercise (approximately one minute every two weeks or *less*) to improve his strength. The news did not sit well with "the strongest man in the world." We settled on a protocol of once a week. When his re-test revealed a strength loss of 20% at four weeks, I insisted on once every two weeks. Within months, he regained the strength he had lost and added another 18%.

Years before, I tested a Venezuelan athlete with similar genes. Martin Materano (ranked 10th in the world in karate) claimed that the fatigue he felt during an all-day tournament was limited to his low back. A MedX test revealed a rate of fatigue twice that of the norm - a rate that required (as above) brief, infrequent exercise. Because of a busy schedule, Martin performed only eight exercises in five months (once every three weeks) yet increased his back strength by more than 100% at several angles. Four months later, at one session per month, his strength increased another 15%.

His symptoms disappeared.

I have used the MedX Lumbar Extension machine once a month for what seems forever and my back is no longer an issue.

Trainers and therapists must recognize the unique nature of the muscles that extend the spine, measure the risk factors involved and prescribe appropriate solutions. Until then, a great deal of unnecessary effort and suffering will likely continue.

# NOVEMBER 3

---

## Requirements for Testing Specific Muscle Function – Part 1

According to Arthur Jones, much of the confusion on the subject of measuring work-capacity revolved around the attempt to compare mechanical and muscular work.

"No such relationship exists," he claimed. "Mechanical work is one thing, and muscular work is an entirely different matter...mechanical work requires movement, muscular work does not. Muscles produce force...nothing more and nothing less."

The problem was further magnified by decades of muscle testing with tools that could not accurately measure force or even identify its source. As Jones put it, "It is possible to measure the level of force produced in a leg press movement; but it is not possible to determine just which muscles produced that force." Compound movements were valuable for exercise, but "utterly worthless" for testing.

Meaningful testing first required total isolation of the muscle in question. "In careful tests of the strength of the muscles involved in torso-rotation," said Jones, "we have found that an error in position of as little as one degree may produce an error in strength of as much as 11 percent. And if the pelvis is free to rotate even slightly during such tests, then errors in position of as much as 20 degrees are almost unavoidable, with a resulting error in the strength test in excess of 200 percent." (*The Lumbar Spine*, 1988).

Total isolation meant more than good form, posture and position. It meant the creation of equipment that eliminated the contribution of other muscles to the output of force. To add to the challenge, Jones chose the lumbar spine.

"During tests of lumbar strength in the direction of extension," he said, "the pelvis has a natural tendency to tilt forward; that is, the bottom of the pelvis moves forward. Is pulled forward by the buttocks and (rear) thigh muscles."

The pelvis had to be anchored from the front to eliminate input from the muscles of the hip, but the legs were in the way. He eventually used them to solve his problem and anchored the pelvis by means of four restraint systems (see Figure 1):

- A force imposed on the bottom of the feet (A) was conveyed to the pelvis by the legs.
- Large pads located above the knees (B) limited their ultimate height and set the knee-end of the femur slightly higher than the hip-end.

- A wide belt (C) prevented upward movement of the thighs and pelvis, and acted as a fulcrum, rotating the hip-end of the femur down (as the knee-end was forced up).
- A round pad at the rear of the pelvis (D) indicated pelvic rotation and prevented pelvic movement toward extension. The radius of the pad was half that of an adult-sized pelvis; if the pelvis moved one millimeter, the pad moved two.

Besides the built-in audits *during* exercise and testing, Jones had a practical way of reviewing the degree of isolation *before* exercise. He'd suggest that the subject was out of position and ask him to move. If he could, all restraint systems were further secured.

Ultimate muscle strength and meaningful testing require single-axis movements (combined with compound movements in the case of exercise only) and total muscle isolation - something that not everyone 'gets.'

"The owner of one company intends to introduce a line of strength-building exercise machines," Jones wrote in *Ironman* (April, 1994). "But having been hoodwinked by two idiots that are associated with him into believing that single-axis exercises are dangerous, he intends to market only compound exercise machines."

Good luck.

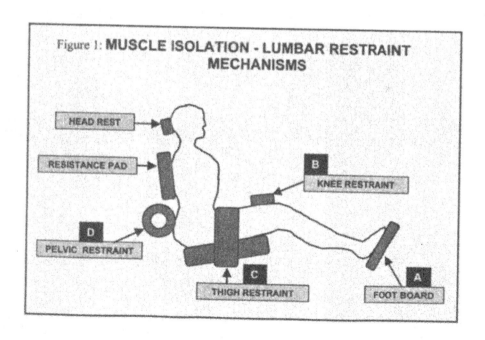

Figure 1: **MUSCLE ISOLATION - LUMBAR RESTRAINT MECHANISMS**

# NOVEMBER 4

---

## Requirements for Testing Specific Muscle Function – Part 2

Golf is a high-skill sport requiring a complex series of movements around an axis of rotation; movements muddled by high-speeds at impact, action/reaction and an urge to view the results. The axis can only remain fixed in a relative way.

But not so with muscle testing. The axis must be *determined* and *fixed* (as in concrete) to produce accurate and meaningful results - a fact that left Arthur Jones scratching his head when he first looked at the five vertebrae of the lumbar spine.

As the vertebrae moved back into extension, their axis points moved in different directions in relation to each other. And the overall length of the lumbar spine changed - first shortened, then increased as much as an inch beyond its normal length at standing.

Jones was determined to build a machine to isolate the muscles that extend the spine, a process, "So simple that it only took us about fifteen years to figure out how to do it."

In the end, compensation for the changing axis points of rotation and the changing length of the spine were built into the resistance pad. The computer was always aware of the exact length of the moment arm of force produced by the subject, in every position regardless of individual differences in lumbar function. The margin of error was less than 1%, "an error so small," said Jones, "that it is almost impossible to measure."

He counterbalanced the machine's moving parts, as he had done with Nautilus® machines, so that the force output was not biased. He next counterbalanced the subject's torso mass (head, torso and arms) as it moved through its range of motion by first determining its centerline (a factor that varied as much as 18° among individuals, see Figure 1). If the centerline of mass was out of line with the torso-mass counterweight on the machine, the resulting measurement of force could vary by as much as 100 percent.

He then weighed the torso mass - a variable of 30-150 pounds - and counterweighted its effect throughout the range.

Figure 2 shows the effect of the torso mass on the measured output of force for a six-foot tall, 200-pound man. In an upright position (B), there is no effect. In a position of flexion, 72°, (A) on the right side of the chart, the subject has to lift a torso weight of 111.47 foot-pounds against gravity. That amount must be added to the subject's output to not understate his tested effort. In full extension on the left side of the chart (C), gravity helps the subject by providing 61.01 foot-pounds of downward push. That amount must be subtracted from the subject's output to not overstate his tested effort.

To verify the accuracy of his counter-weighting mechanism, Jones built a lumbar extension machine (for research only) that tested from a lateral position where gravity was not a factor. Volunteers were secured in an upright, seated position and then rotated sideways like a barbecue. He realized that perfect counter-weighting was impossible (the machine had one axis; the spine, five) but pointed out, "the unavoidable difference in torso mass and counter-weight torque has no effect on the accuracy of test results; because it is subtracted from the tested level of torque along with the torque from stored energy."

He went on. "Regardless of your purpose, you must have a tool that is capable of providing you with the ability to do what you are trying to do... Don't try to drive nails with a saw, or cut wood with a hammer."

Arthur Jones left nothing to chance and, in that regard, was much like golf legend Walter Hagan, who often approached the first tee with the comment, "Well, boys, who's going to be second?"

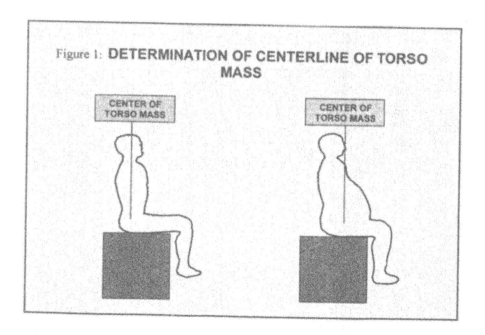

Figure 1: DETERMINATION OF CENTERLINE OF TORSO MASS

CENTER OF TORSO MASS

CENTER OF TORSO MASS

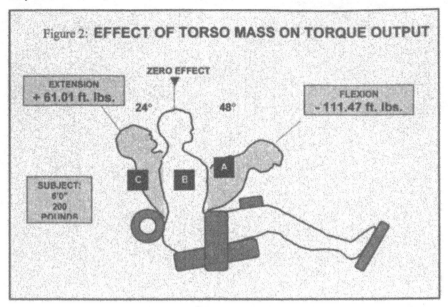

Figure 2: EFFECT OF TORSO MASS ON TORQUE OUTPUT

NOVEMBER 5

---

## The Requirements for Testing Specific Muscle Function – Part 3

The laws of physics are undeniable: Movement creates friction; and conversely, no movement means no friction. Yet, the existence of friction as it relates to dynamic muscle testing has long been ignored (and even denied) in the field of exercise and rehabilitation. "The result," according to Arthur Jones, "is that test results are biased to such an extent that they are worthless for any purpose."

Friction during exercise appears in two forms: friction within the tool itself, and internal muscle friction produced *within* the muscle by soft tissue movement.

Both reduce the ability to lift (concentric output of force) and increase the ability to lower a weight (eccentric output of force). Compare a normal arm curl with a barbell to the same in a neck-deep swimming pool and you'll find that you can't lift as much in the pool due to increased friction created by the thicker medium. But you can lower more in water because the additional friction acts as a braking mechanism.

Muscle friction can be measured, but the process is confounded by two factors: speed of movement and fatigue. As they increase, internal muscle friction increases, and both can influence the results of a muscle test by several hundred percent.

In one study by Jones, the ratio of lifting to lowering strength changed from 1:1.4 (in a fresh state) to 1:54 (in an exhausted state). In other words, the muscle was 40% stronger lowering when fresh; and 5,300% stronger lowering when exhausted.

Despite its influence in dynamic strength tests, friction has been totally ignored by the scientific community and by most 'experts' for decades.

Why? "Because most of these people were not experts," says Jones. "Having been taught by an earlier generation of people who in fact knew little or nothing about exercise, they simply accepted what they were taught without question... Remember, fewer than 100 years ago the scientific community believed that heavier-than-air flight was impossible. Which raises a question: Were these people unaware of thing like birds? Or did they believe that birds were inflated with helium?"

Jones solved the problems associated with internal muscle friction by eliminating movement during tests. In the end, he was convinced that the only way to produce accurate and meaningful results was to test in a 'static' manner. Jones locked subjects into positions that isolated movements and had them gradually apply maximum efforts against a pad that did not move. Static testing allowed more accurate testing positions, eliminated the bias of friction, and allowed subjects more control of their immediate environment. That is, they had more time to generate a full effort and more time to back off if there was pain - safer and more accurate.

Only the problem of friction within the machine - a non-factor with static testing, but a factor with exercise - remained. Jones reduced it to a minimum by the use of ratios on his cams and leverage systems. A movement of 72° of the isolated lumbar spine, for example, moved the weight stack only six inches, which helped eliminate kinetic energy. Friction was reduced to such a negligible level that, if the machine was supposed to provide a resistance of 50 pounds at angle X, it was within 2.7% of that weight at worst. The average variation in any one position "was something less than one percent above or one percent below the desired level of force."

By comparison, a car is 30% efficient, and one of the most efficient things known to man, an airplane propeller, approximately 70%.

## NOVEMBER 6

---

### The Requirements for Testing Specific Muscle Function – Part 4

A test of functional strength (the output of torque during a maximum effort) can be misleading because there is no relationship between functional strength and true muscular strength. Functional strength is influenced by muscle friction, joint-system leverage, stored energy and the torque produced by the mass of the involved body parts, all of which serve to understate or overstate true muscular input.

According to Arthur Jones, "For meaningful test results, true muscular strength must be measured: the torque actually produced by the forces of muscular contraction, Net Muscular Torque, NMT. In order to determine NMT, all nonmuscular-torque factors must be measured and considered in relation to the levels of tested torque."

The first time I performed a strength test on a MedX® Lumbar Extension machine, one of the neglected variables stared me right in the face - stored energy. Once I was secured in the device, the technician slowly moved my torso from a seated upright position to a fully flexed one (chest to knees) and asked me to relax. A column indicating torque appeared on the right side of the screen *before* I was instructed to push (Figure 1). This 'non-muscular torque' (from a combination of body-mass, counterweight torque, gravity and stored energy) was registered for future reference.

I then exerted a maximum effort against the resistance pad located about mid-back. The column rose (Figure 2), a measure of functional strength - the one unrelated to true muscular strength. What, then, was the input from the muscle alone at that angle? Easy. Subtract the non-muscular torque (Figure 1) from the peak functional torque (Figure 2) to determine the true level of muscular strength.

The same two-step procedure was performed at other angles throughout the range of motion - first, a relaxed measure of non-muscular torque followed by an all-out test of functional strength. The results were summarized by the computer (Figure 3). Curve #1 is a compilation of seven measurements of gross torque or functional strength. Curve #2 represents true muscular strength, NMT, while the area between the curves designates non-muscular torque that was subtracted from the gross values.

Stored energy (part of non-muscular torque) produces changes in functional output due to variations in body-part position and the influence of antagonistic muscles. When lowered to a flexed position, chest to knees, low-back muscles are stretched beyond their norm and, like a rubber band, rebound in protest. At the other end, the abdomen is compressed into the thighs and rebels in the same way, creating an upward force against the resistance pad, a force called stored energy. It can have an unbelievable effect on the measurement of true strength.

In one study conducted by Jones, three errors were introduced by stored energy: the first, 13%; the second, 30,000%; and the third, more than 240,000%. Errors of this magnitude are common in muscle testing yet remain ignored by the scientific community and by health insurance companies. They pay by code, not accuracy.

Jones once commented on the magnitude of ignorance surrounding the omission of stored energy in testing. "If the fresh corpse of a large, dead man was restrained in this machine in the lateral position (via a MedX Lateral Lumbar Extension machine in which test results are biased only by stored-energy), with the body pulled into a position of full flexion of the lumbar spine, then the output of torque might exceed 300 foot-pounds; torque that obviously would not be a result of muscular contraction."

I'm not dead yet, but you might have thought so from that first test.

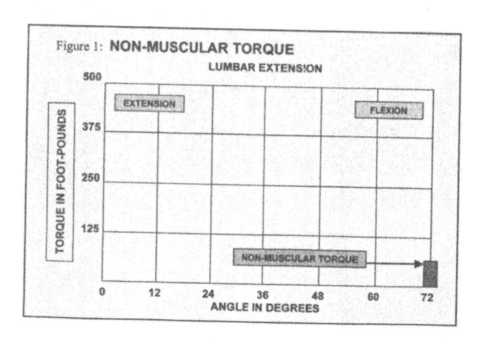

Figure 1: NON-MUSCULAR TORQUE

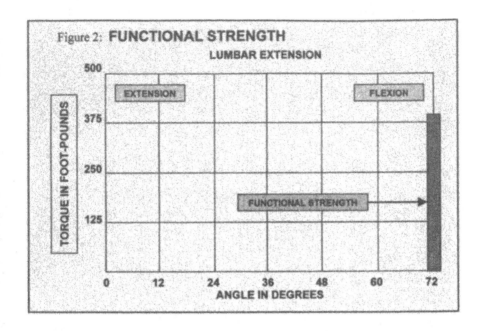

Figure 2: **FUNCTIONAL STRENGTH**

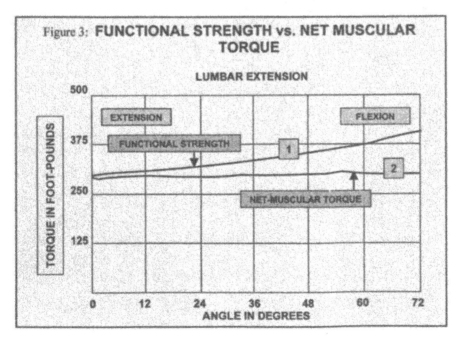

Figure 3: **FUNCTIONAL STRENGTH vs. NET MUSCULAR TORQUE**

NOVEMBER 7

---

## The Requirements for Testing Specific Muscle Function – Part 5

If there was one thing I learned from the MedX® certification course at the University of Florida, it was the Commandment hammered home by professor, David Carpenter, "Thou Shalt Standardize."

The idea behind standardization was obvious - to eliminate as many variables as possible in order to produce an accurate, meaningful and consistent result - but it never struck home until I witnessed it first hand on the gym floor.

Standardization errors in an exercise setting fall into two broad categories: lack of familiarity with equipment, and refusal to use a workout chart. I don't know how many times I've heard trainees exit a leg press with the good news, "Today, it wasn't all that bad," only to find that their seat position was incorrect. A slight error in position can have an enormous effect on how the resistance 'feels' during exercise and a greater effect on the results of a strength test.

One afternoon in Ocala (Florida), I witnessed a therapist from Philadelphia test the strength of the muscles that rotated his torso. When MedX inventor Arthur Jones examined the results, his heart rate shot skyward. There was such a vast discrepancy between the subject's strength in flexion and extension that Jones strongly urged him to go through a 12-week exercise protocol. His potential for gain in extension was infinite.

To that point, tests of torso rotation had revealed large differences from one end of the range of movement to the other, but nothing of this magnitude. From a position 60° rotated to the left of neutral to one of 60° to the right, his strength varied as much as 2,424:1 - an average change of more than 200% per degree of movement. Furthermore, the test was conducted in a static manner on a horizontal plane, meaning that the results were not biased by muscular friction or body-mass torque (gravity).

Jones' elevated heart rate was short-lived. He was unaware, at the time, of 'stored energy' (described in Part 4). When the subject's functional strength values were adjusted for stored energy, the results changed to a ratio of 7:1. His true strength values (net muscular torque, NMT) varied by 5% per degree of movement.

Precise positioning presented Jones with the greatest challenge in the development of accurate tools. "An error in position of five degrees (on the rotary torso machine) would make it appear that strength had changed by 25%, when no change had occurred. Some machines now in use consistently produce errors in position exceeding 30 degrees" ...and that "errors in excess of 60 degrees are not rare." The machines mentioned are currently used to evaluate the results of rehabilitation - another reason not to break a leg.

When positions are standardized and the requirements for specific testing are in place, how reliable are tests with MedX machines? According to Jones, "When two such tests (of static strength) show a difference in excess of two percent of the area under the curve, then the subject was not cooperating in one or both of the tests." Subjects unable to produce results within that range were not selected for research.

Despite the superiority of MedX medical tools for testing and rehabilitative exercise, they have been largely ignored. As Max Planck, the inventor of the quantum theory in physics (1900) put it, "A new scientific discovery does not prevail by convincing its opponents and leading them to see the light, but only because its opponents will eventually die and then a new generation will grow up who are aware of the truth."

Jones will have to wait it out.

## NOVEMBER 8

### The Requirements for Testing Specific Muscle Function - Summary

Some of the greatest inventions in the history of mankind have come from people outside of the scientific community and foreign to the field. The Wright Brothers, two bicycle mechanics from Ohio, sat on their front porch with a pocketknife whittling what would eventually become a propeller for a contraption they flew six years before scientists would accept that heavier-than-air flight was possible.

Years later, a man with no brother in sight kicked down the door of the 1970 Mr. America Contest in California with a contraption and barrage of theory that no one had heard before. In 1986, in the same brash manner, he kicked down the door of the medical field by introducing a rehabilitation device for low backs built around ignored concepts. Was the boisterous, bold intruder a scientist, visionary or a mere blowhard? Who was this Arthur Jones?

Those who sat on the thrones of either field (exercise or medicine) soon wished he'd disappear as quickly as he appeared. It's tough for a doctor to listen to someone who, by choice, didn't make it to high school.

Like the Wright Brothers before, however, Jones had done his homework - more than fifty years of whittling in Africa, South America and on porches he created along the way, the last at his home in Florida.

His first discovery in the field of medicine rubbed the establishment the wrong way. Jones claimed that the technology then used for the functional testing of joint and muscle structures made, "just as much sense as trying to weigh yourself by jumping up and down on a scale; while in the air you will weigh nothing, but when you come back down the scale may record a force of over a thousand pounds; so which is your weight, zero or 1,000 pounds?"

By 1970, Jones had identified 10 ingredients for a perfect form of exercise; and by 1986, five ingredients required for accurate muscle testing.

"Meaningful testing of strength requires total isolation of the joint being tested, requires careful counter-weighting in order to remove the effects of gravity, requires a static (isometric) testing procedure to remove the effects of friction, requires the measurement of torque produced by stored energy so that it can be factored into the test results, and requires an accurate measurement of the relative positions involved in the test, such positional requirements being required because changes in position produce changes in strength; until all of these requirements are provided, any attempt to measure strength is an exercise in futility at best.

With very few exceptions all of these critical factors have been ignored in the thousands of supposedly scientific studies that have been performed during the past 50 years; so all of that research was worthless, and any theories based upon that research are misleading at best."

Then he added, "Now all we have to do is shove it down the throats of the scientific community, and this will eventually be done. The truth cannot be ignored forever."

Arthur held the bicycle mechanics from Ohio in high esteem. The propeller they carved on the porch that day was so close to perfect in shape and function that modern technology has improved it by less than two percent.

Pocketknife anyone?

## NOVEMBER 9

---

### Net Muscular Torque – Your Real Strength

Short of inserting a strain gauge into a muscle, strength cannot be measured directly. Muscle strength must be determined in an indirect fashion, by measuring the output of force - which is where the problem begins.

Muscular strength is a result of only one factor, the force of muscular contraction. But tested torque (strength output) is a result of four: muscular

Gary Bannister, B.A., B.P.E., M.Ed.

force, the effect of gravity on the mass of the involved moving parts, stored energy and muscular friction (if the testing procedure is dynamic). A brief look at each will help clarify the issue.

If you sit on a bench in an upright position, gravity has no effect on the mass of your torso other than to keep you on the planet. If you lean forward so that your chest is near your thighs, the force of gravity pushing down hampers your ability to return to a seated position. If your torso, head and arms weigh 75 pounds, your low-back muscles must generate 75 pounds of force plus that exerted by gravity to return to upright. A 75-pound torso bent 42° forward, for example, produces 100 foot-pounds of torque.

If you lean backwards, however, gravity has the opposite effect - it helps you extend. The same 75-pound torso leaned back 30° produces a torque of 75 foot-pounds.

Any device purporting to measure true muscle output must counterweight the mass of the involved body part(s) throughout the range of motion to compensate for the changing effect of gravity in different positions. To assure an accurate result (above), you would have to add 100 foot-pounds of torque to the output at 42° of flexion, and subtract 75 foot-pounds from the output at 30° of extension.

Besides the influence of gravity on the measurement of torque, there are other non-contractile forces at play. The move to a bent-forward position (above) compresses tissue in the front and stretches tissue in the back of the torso. Like a springboard, this creates 'stored energy' (a combination of the compression of soft tissue surrounding the spine and muscle elasticity) that produces a force in the direction of extension.

MedX® inventor Arthur Jones was the first to determine its magnitude and effect. A large person with a protruding abdomen is difficult to pull to a position of flexion and invariably produces a large amount of stored energy in the process, even in a machine that counterbalances the weight of his torso. To complicate matters, stored energy changes as the body moves to a new position and must be added to, or subtracted from, any measure of muscle output to secure a true strength reading at that position.

Another source of error is produced by muscular friction, but only during dynamic tests. Muscle fibers slide over each other and create friction that hinders lifting, but helps lowering. In a dynamic test of strength, where the machine registers torque as the muscle moves, the output of lifting strength, decreased by friction, is always *understated*. The output of lowering strength, increased by friction, is always *overstated*. Both must be adjusted, up or down, to ensure accurate test results - not an easy task. Muscular friction constantly

512

changes with speed of movement and fatigue. The greater the speed and fatigue, the greater the friction.

Fortunately, the friction issue and the accurate determination of non-muscular torque can be resolved by performing 'static' strength tests. With static testing (where involved body parts are counterweighted), true and accurate muscle output can be reduced to a simple formula: Net Muscular Torque = Total Torque - Stored Energy.

Net muscular torque is your *real* strength.

## NOVEMBER 10

### If Bones Could Fly

If bones could fly, they would. They'd 'ping' off windows, bounce off carpets, whiz by peers and generally increase the range of motion of those dumb enough to continue. Torso rotation, one of the most dangerous exercises in gyms, is also the one most poorly performed. Yet, the fact that so few injuries result from improper use of rotary machines remained a mystery until Arthur Jones came along.

According to Jones, the ability to rotate the spine occurs from just above the lumbar area (vertebra T10 and upward). "The lowest seven vertebra and the sacrum are locked together by the facets (lateral protrusions of bone) in such a manner that rotation is nearly impossible without damage to the bones."

With that in mind, he designed a torso-rotation machine for rehabilitation (MedX®) that matched (or limited) the range of motion to that of its user, to avoid the danger of moving too far. Nonetheless, he found that most people increased their range of motion by using the machine and concluded that bones were not the limiting factor.

"When you twist your torso," he said, "you are compressing the soft tissue on one side of your body while stretching the soft tissue on the other, which compression and stretching produces stored energy that will then produce torque that will try to twist your body back toward the neutral, relaxed, straight-ahead position. And the further you twist your body, the greater the resulting level of stored energy."

Logically, when the level of stored energy increases to that of the torque produced by the contracting muscle, movement becomes impossible. And equally so, when the torque of the muscle increases through proper strength training, it's ability to increase its range of motion improves - more strength paves the highway to greater flexibility.

Yet, as much as the cushion of soft tissue protects you from injury during normal, controlled movement, the picture is different in gyms. There is no gravity working against moving body parts during the lifting phase of a rotary torso exercise, which makes it possible to generate more speed than with other movements. In doing so, trainees often exceed their existing, or safe, range of motion.

So, why are there not more injuries?

The saving grace lies in a factor few suspect - bad equipment. Commercial exercise tools fail to properly isolate the movement, thereby making it safer.

Sit upright in a chair and check the position of your knees in relation to each other. Now, slowly twist your torso to the left and watch your knees. Your right knee moves forward. The reason? Your hips rotate to 'soften' the *amount* of spinal rotation.

The same occurs in a gym. Your pelvis rotates in the direction of movement to ease the blow to the spine from an overzealous effort. Most gym machines (at least those with a tight chain) feature a range of motion of 90° to the left and right of neutral. The MedX Rotary Torso machine, which does not allow pelvic movement, depicts a more accurate portrayal of range of motion - 60°, both left and right.

With either device, don't rely on structural mechanisms or equipment to protect you from injury. Count on good form. Use slow movements that don't bang against the end of the machine, and pause in a full-contracted position.

"The vertebra and their related facets," concluded Jones, "are simply a masterpiece of structural engineering."

Don't transform them into an archeological puzzle.

# NOVEMBER 11

## Dead or Alive

"I'd like you to meet your host. Excuse his limp handshake and pasty smile - Bernie died a few days ago. Despite that, his low back is still stronger than yours."

The introduction was less than flattering, but true. The last 30 years of research related to low-back strength shows that you might be better off dead.

The movie, *Weekend at Bernie's*®, depicted a party sponsored by a corpse who was propped up (to avoid suspicion) by two students who rented the place for the weekend and found him in that state. The result was as laughable as the research.

In 1986, Arthur Jones revealed the ideal strength curve of the isolated muscles that extend the lumbar spine from a position of full flexion to that of full extension, a range of motion of 72°. At the same time, he revealed normative values for healthy men and women of different age groups, based on approximately 10,000 tests.

The ideal curve - straight and descending from flexion to extension - demonstrated a flexion/extension strength ratio of 1.4 to 1. That is, the muscles of the spine were 40% stronger in flexion (bent over pushing backwards) than in extension (bent back and pushing back). Females were closer to the 'ideal' than males, who were generally stronger in flexion and weaker in extension than they should have been.

The average level of torque measured by a static test *in flexion* for men (18-35 years old) was 337 foot-pounds; for women (same ages), 180 foot-pounds. The average torque measured *in extension* for men was 171 foot-pounds; for women, 97 foot-pounds. With the exception of a few professional water-skiers, peak torque values (denoting peak strength) occurred in the position of maximum flexion.

In the early 1990's, a large man visited the MedX® complex in Ocala (Florida) and performed the same low-back test as that above (a static test at seven different angles through a complete range of motion). He registered a torque of 352 foot-pounds in flexion, a value slightly above average, but expected considering his size. The real surprise came when the technician realized that the subject hadn't begun to exert force in that position.

In the words of Arthur Jones: "A much larger man that we later tested produced 352 foot-pounds of torque from stored energy alone, and would have produced the same result if he had been dead; and since 352 foot-pounds of torque is higher than the level of total torque produced by an average untrained man (see above), it would have appeared that he was stronger than average even after he was dead."

Jones described 'stored energy' and its effect as follows:

"Moving forward into the fully flexed position of the spine compresses soft tissue in front of the spine while stretching soft tissue behind the spine, and this compression and stretching of soft tissue stores energy which will then produce torque that tends to return the spine to a neutral position. Thus a test that ignores stored energy torque tends to overstate the strength levels that are measured." (*Ironman*, December, 1995)

In the past 30 years, other than that of Jones, not one test conducted by the scientific or medical communities considered the existence of stored energy, let alone its effect on test results. Now that they are aware of it, they continue to ignore its existence.

Next time you go to a funeral, rest assured that if the corpse weighs more than you, he or she is probably stronger than you in flexion on a lumbar test conducted by one of today's scientists. Just another reason to respect the dead more than the living.

## NOVEMBER 12

### What Is and What Should Be

The definition of a 'perfect' back or knee may depend upon whom you ask. From "breaking a world record" to "getting out of a chair" to "something that doesn't ache," the answers have a common thread. The muscles that surround the joint system(s) must be proportionately strong throughout their range of motion.

Yet, specific muscle tests using machines developed by MedX® (Ocala, Florida) indicate that only a small percentage of untrained subjects have a 'perfect' functional relationship. Most have strength deficiencies in flexion and/or extension.

In some cases, the weakness can be directly attributed to lack of proper exercise. Gym equipment that features resistance changes (by cam or leverage) out of sync with 'ideal' changes in strength potential can result in disproportionate gains, as can poor use of equipment (partial-range or fast-speed movements).

In others, deficiencies mirror the movement patterns common to the joint. Elite water skiers, for example, have strong lower backs in extension but not in flexion - a function of their activity. In contrast, daily activities, sports and so-called 'low-back' exercises fail to meaningfully stimulate the muscles that extend the spine.

In all cases, and to no one's surprise, disproportionate strength relates to genetics.

Figure 1 demonstrates three strength curves of the isolated muscles that extend the spine. The top curve shows the 'ideal' relationship between functional strength in flexion (bent forward, right side of chart) and extension (bent back, left side of chart), a numerical ratio of 1.4:1. That is, low-back muscles should be 40% stronger in flexion than extension, regardless of strength level. They rarely are.

Eighty percent of healthy, untrained subjects produce the bottom curve (Type S) when first tested. "Type S" refers to a muscle response limited only to the range of motion in which it works - a genetic factor, not subject to change. As such, typical "Type S" subjects demonstrate less than 40% of their 'ideal' strength in full extension - if they can get there - and a strength ratio greater than 2.5:1.

In contrast, "Type G" subjects (20% of those tested) respond throughout the range of motion regardless of where work is performed. As such, they demonstrate less deficiency in extension (middle curve) and produce a strength ratio closer to 2:1.

The curves in Figure 2 reflect the functional strength of isolated quadriceps (front thigh) muscles. The 'ideal' curve (top) reveals a flexion/peak torque/extension strength-ratio of 1.3:2:1. As before, "Type S" subjects (72% of those tested) are weaker in flexion and extension than "Type G" subjects who demonstrate a more proportionate distribution of strength throughout the range.

"Specific" or "General" response to exercise can be determined by testing. Regardless of which you are and unless you are restricted to limited-range exercise, both "Type S" and "Type G" subjects respond to full-range exercise in the *same* way. Proper exercise improves *both* curves in the direction of 'ideal.' How? A 'cam' in the machine provides an exact and appropriate resistance throughout the range of motion, forcing the muscle to work hardest where its needs are greatest - in essence, the ideal curve. All you have to do is show up, plug in the effort and your strength becomes proportionate in approximately 12 weeks (according to studies using MedX equipment).

Muscle response to exercise cannot change, but strength curves can. When resistance is properly applied, and strength proportionate, things will *feel* close to 'perfect.'

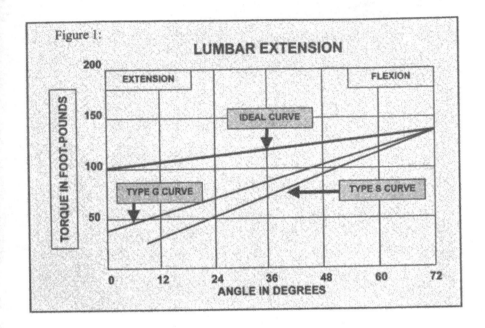

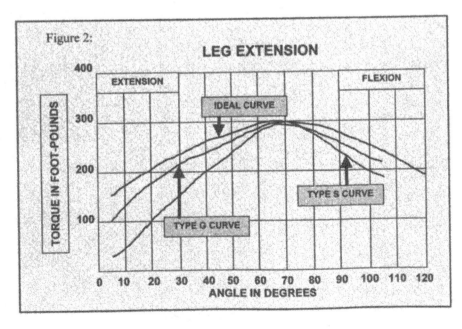

NOVEMBER 13

---

## Arthur and the Magnificent Five

There was no gunslinger in town, no town to save and no point to make. But there was a "bad guy," and he made his point anyway.

When Arthur Jones introduced his latest creation in 1986, he did so amid controversy. The medical profession thought he was in too deep - the muscles that extend the low back were impossible to isolate because of their close functional association with rear-hip and thigh muscles. Little did they know that Jones was driven by the word "impossible." He persisted in spite of the skepticism around him, eventually succeeded and tested the new device - the MedX® Lumbar Extension machine - on five subjects selected from his research staff "to learn what to expect from later and much-larger-scale research."

The results of the initial testing were as follows:

- **Subject One** increased the strength of his lumbar extension muscles in a position of full extension by 180% as a result of 10 exercises performed over a period of 10 weeks (one brief exercise per week).
- **Subject Two** increased his strength 450% as a result of one brief exercise every two weeks for a period of five months.
- **Subject Three** performed one exercise approximately every 14 days for a period of 27 weeks and increased his strength by 877%.
- **Subject Four** increased his strength 1,460% by performing one exercise every 14 days for 11 weeks.
- **Subject Five** performed one exercise every 14 days for five months and increased his strength in extension by 7,300%.

The gains were astounding. Untrained subjects using progressive resistance exercise in previous research increased strength by 30-60% in 6-12 months. High increases (such as those above) clearly indicated the existence of muscle atrophy. If you break your arm and put it in a cast for months, you can increase its strength dramatically because its starting level is abnormally low. All five subjects apparently *began* the study in a pitiful state despite the fact that four had performed regular exercise on a Nautilus® Low Back machine for 2-6 years prior to the study.

I once owned the Nautilus Low Back machine in a gym. No one used the entire 250-pound weight stack in seven years. Subject Four (6'4", 250 pounds) regularly exercised on a custom-built version of the same with two adults standing on top of a 450-pound weight stack. When he first tested on the MedX machine, everyone assumed his strength curve was good. An increase of 1,460%, however, indicated otherwise - his muscles were atrophied from lack of use. Something was strong in lifting 850 pounds, but not the muscles that extended his spine.

Subject Five, an orthopedic surgeon, performed heavy, high-intensity training for years. When he first tested the strength of his back on the MedX tool, he produced a force of only four foot-pounds of torque, 6° shy of full extension. Five months later, he produced 296 foot-pounds of torque at the same angle (6°), an increase of 7,300%.

When the smoke cleared, several points were apparent:
- Traditional low-back exercise proved useless for its intended purpose because it allowed pelvic rotation, leaving its users in a state of atrophy.
- Isolated, lumbar muscles were unique in their response to exercise.

Even at that, Arthur and the Magnificent Five had to shoot their way out of town.

## NOVEMBER 14

### The Big Search

It could have been the butcher, the baker and the candlestick maker - or Curly, Larry and Moe. By the time the three professors arrived at the gates of the Grandfather Golf Club in North Carolina, it didn't matter. The trip from Averett College in Danville, Virginia was far behind; the thrill of a one-time shot at a 'gem' was on.

The trio played a lesser course the day before, an event best put into perspective by Bernard Darwin's description of the final train exchange preceding his arrival at a famous links in Britain (*James Braid*, 1952). "For a change just before the last lap, by delaying our arrival and lengthening our rapture of expectation, does add something, and it so happens that some of the best and most famous of links possess just such an exciting halt, on the very verge of paradise."

Paradise it was. Every turn in the fairway was a feast of sparkling streams, rolling hills and rugged boulders set in a backdrop of mountains that made it hard to keep your head down - and private.

First up, the tall, distinguished history teacher, to whom golf was a science, smacked a ball down the middle. As he did, the short, distinguished art teacher, who fancied golf an art, accidentally dropped his ball down *into* his bag.

His first reach came up short, so he began removing clubs one by one. I took to the tee to pacify a stream of carts forming behind and hit a ball up the middle. By then, he had removed his bag from the cart, turned it upside-down and shook it over the cart path. The first thing that popped out was a crushed Coca-Cola® can; the last, a ball. Between, about every confection wrapper you could name, half a newspaper, a bruised hat, tees, a second ball and some dirt.

As we steered the mess to a nearby receptacle, I yearned for two things - an eclipse of the sun and no eye contact. Finally, the last of the Triumvirate smacked it *not quite* down the middle. It mattered little by then.

First-tee jitters are as common as the search for relief from chronic back pain.

In October of 1987, Arthur Jones introduced his solution through an ad in *The Washington Post* - pre-employment or job-placement screening.

"Within five years," he said, "screening for lumbar problems will be one of the most frequently performed testing procedures in the field of medicine...may soon be an insurance requirement for many occupations...a requirement for employment by nearly every large corporation in the country...and a routine but very important part of the physical examination for every branch of the military service."

Despite his optimism, six years later he wrote, "Total costs of health care in this country are now estimated to be in excess of $830,000,000,000, and about 12 percent of that cost (around $100 billion a year) is a result of chronic lower-back pain; and here we sit with both the equipment and knowledge that are required to reduce those costs by about 80 percent...and in general the so-called 'experts' in this field are not even aware of what we have done, refuse to even look at the facts." *(Ironman*, Oct. 1993)

His solution was further stagnated by cries of 'discrimination,' which led him to add, "When talking to lawyers, politicians, or 'experts' it is a damned good idea to keep one hand on your wallet and the other hand on your gun. Better yet, avoid them entirely."

I say turn them upside down and shake them over a cart path.

# NOVEMBER 15

---

## Legitimizing Exercise

Arthur Jones was in a good mood and why not? It was lunchtime on Friday and his bi-monthly medical lecture at the University of Florida was far behind.

He sat down at an oversized, round table - his 'new' forum - and wasted no time. He spewed numbers, names and statistics as he had all morning - relentless, but never dull. In a rare moment of silence, a military dentist from Caracas spoke up.

"Mr. Jones," asked Bernie Maurovich, "have you ever flown to Venezuela?"

I was curious. In the mid-1980's, a client (who was a pilot) told me that Jones had landed in the city's jetport - a tale I could not confirm.

"Nope," barked the Nautilus® inventor with disdain. "And I never will. Back when I was flying animals to and from of Brazil, I was tempted. But rumor had it that when you landed, you were always one document short of what they required. And while you were in the city sorting things out, they'd steal your damn airplane."

He was probably right in not chancing it, but he was dead right about something else. The medical community was the best venue through which to send his message. "The real importance of exercise" he said, "will be recognized when, and only when, a high percentage of medical doctors become truly knowledgeable in this field...then they can, and I believe they will, help to educate the public."

Despite his optimism, Jones was not impressed by what he had seen. In the early days, he encountered only one physician out of 100 - a specialist in reconstructive surgery - who knew the primary function of the biceps. He was equally lukewarm to those involved in exercise. "Many weight trainees are medical doctors or members of other professional groups who should have the educational background to at least understand basic physiology - but who, in practice, still seem to unhesitatingly accept the outright stupidities recommended by muscle-heads who aren't even literate."

In the summer of 1983, he announced plans to connect with the medical school of a major university to educate doctors on not only the importance of exercise, but on the 'how to' - a brief but comprehensive course in exercise physiology. "Every week, fifty-two times a year," he said, "a Nautilus Jumbo

Jet will depart from Atlanta for a round trip to the location of our upcoming research project, with a passenger load of 100 doctors."

Jones looked at Latin American countries - Brazil and Puerto Rico among others - and settled on Mexico for three reasons: distance, availability of subjects, and cost. Why not the United States? Standard of living. "Believe me," he said, "people living under such conditions (of poverty) can be motivated, and they are available in large numbers."

The plan was as grandiose as its importance.

"Additional research may or may not be the answer," he continued, "but if the existing literature resulting from previous research in the field offers any reasonable criteria for judgement, then I think we can look forward to at least another century of confusion, missed opportunities, and largely wasted effort. Or worse; the present confusion could easily lead the medical profession, as a whole, into an almost outright rejection of exercise. And if so...many centuries could pass before exercise will even be afforded the courtesy of another look. In which case, the loss to everyone would be enormous."

The project never came to fruition in Mexico. Jones hooked up with the University of Florida in Gainesville and flew doctors to his 'home school' in nearby Ocala.

The venue had changed but the mission remained the same.

## NOVEMBER 16

-----

### Risk Factors for Spinal Injury

According to medical estimates, 80% of low-back problems are muscular in nature. Yet, until recently, little was known about the muscles of the low back. In 1972, Nautilus® inventor Arthur Jones set out to investigate the situation and, by 1986, developed a tool to isolate, test and strengthen the muscles that extend the spine.

Jones first tested 10,000 people before donating his MedX® Lumbar Extension machine to the University of Florida for 'official' research. By 1993, 45 studies involving 3,339 subjects, 18,540 functional tests and more than 100,000 exercise procedures identified three muscular factors related to the risk of developing low-back problems: chronic disuse atrophy, specific response to exercise, and muscle fiber-type.

The first was expected, but not to the degree to which it was found. Research reaffirmed what Jones had discovered, that "99% of people on the planet are walking around in a state of chronic disuse atrophy." The muscles that extend the spine were inaccessible when the pelvis was allowed to rotate, as with traditional exercise.

The case of Jim Flanagan was proof.

After years of heavy exercise on a Nautilus Low Back machine, Jim (at 6'4", 250 pounds) tested his back strength on a MedX machine. He then trained (on MedX) once every two weeks for 11 weeks and re-tested. His strength increased 1,460% at its weakest point, demonstrating an initial state of atrophy from lack of use. There was some solace: Jim was among the majority.

The second factor was unexpected, specific muscular response to exercise. Eighty percent of subjects produced limited-range fatigue and limited-range results from limited-range exercise. That is, they fatigued or increased in strength *only* where they 'worked' and showed no change where they did not - a specific *(Type* S) response to exercise. Since most exercise provides little or no work for the spinal muscles in full extension, the majority of subjects demonstrated a disproportionate low level of strength in that position - a condition that increases the risk of back problems.

In contrast, 20% fatigued and gained strength equally throughout the range of motion, regardless of the range in which they 'worked.' A general *(Type* G) response to limited-range exercise put them at less risk.

The third factor, muscle fiber-type, surprised many with the magnitude of its variance. Sixty percent of subjects displayed an average mix of fast-fatigue (fast-twitch) and slow-fatigue (slow-twitch) fibers that resulted in a strength loss of approximately 2% per repetition. Muscles of predominantly one fiber-type were unique.

To demonstrate the variance, Jones measured the strength of two subjects on a MedX machine at "The Challenge of the Lumbar Spine" (New York City, 1987). One subject was twice as strong as the other, yet both were exercised with the same weight for six repetitions and tested immediately after. The stronger subject lost 54% of his strength; the weaker gained 11%. In subsequent tests, the fast-fatigue subject always lost his shirt while the slow-fatigue subject always gained. Approximately 30% of low-back muscles fatigue quickly (a high-risk situation); 10% fatigue slowly, if at all.

Taken together (Figure 1), the muscle-related risk factors for spinal injury go a long way to explain why injury is so common in the lumbar spine. All three can be identified by MedX testing and two can be improved by specific exercise. While muscle fiber-type cannot change, functional and structural strength can increase regardless of fiber-type...and doing so will greatly reduce the risk of injury.

Figure 1: RISK FACTORS FOR SPINAL INJURY

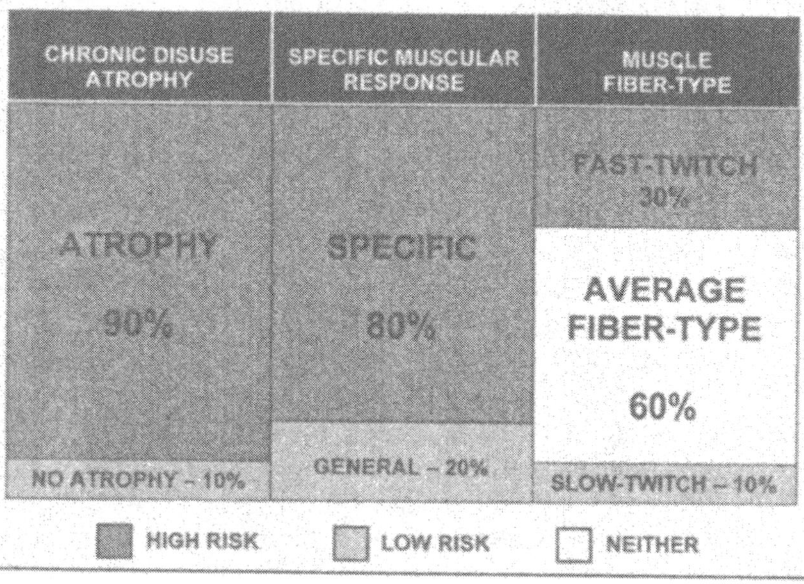

| CHRONIC DISUSE ATROPHY | SPECIFIC MUSCULAR RESPONSE | MUSCLE FIBER-TYPE |
|---|---|---|
| | | FAST-TWITCH 30% |
| ATROPHY 90% | SPECIFIC 80% | AVERAGE FIBER-TYPE 60% |
| NO ATROPHY – 10% | GENERAL – 20% | SLOW-TWITCH – 10% |

HIGH RISK    LOW RISK    NEITHER

## NOVEMBER 17

### Major and Miner Problems

The PGA Tour® should consider Colstrip, Montana. While the barren remains of a pit-mine appear unsuitable for competitive golf, it provides an ideal setting for a lesson in longevity. To prolong their careers, a handful of workers at the Rosebud Coal Mine dug a little deeper than golf's touring elite in their search for a long-term solution to chronic low-back pain.

Strip mining is tough on backs. In the early 1990's, the incidence of torso injury on a national level was about 63% (most classified as "lumbar strains"), while low-back injury comprised approximately 25% of *all* injuries to miners. Golf statistics weren't far behind. In a Centinela Hospital study conducted in the PGA Tour fitness van from 1990-1995, the incidence of torso injury was 47%, with low backs in the overall lead at 24%.

The situation at the Rosebud mine, however, was far more critical than that of the PGA Tour. From 1991-1993, the U.S. Department Interior Bureau of Mines reported 1.09 back injuries per 200,000 employee hours worked in strip mines. The nine-year average at Rosebud was 2.94. During that time, management was approached three times by the government to implement accident-reduction programs. Four hired consultants arrived at the same conclusion - "poor performance and a deep-seeded resistance to change."

One State Worker's Compensation specialist was blunt. "If we were a private insurer, we would give notice of cancellation. However, since we are the insurer of last resort, we can only continue to raise your premiums in relation to your loss ratio. In time, you will become non-competitive and fail as a business."

In July of 1992, the Western Energy Company, which operates the Rosebud mine, hired Pat Rummerfield as safety coordinator. He quickly recognized the need for back-injury prevention and suggested a revolutionary approach in the form of an exercise device called the MedX® Lumbar Extension machine.

The program officially began on August 2, 1993 with 30 volunteer employees. By year's end, with nothing in the way of promotion other than word of mouth, 180 workers (approximately 45% of all employees) were involved.

The results of the once-a-week, two-minute exercise program were outstanding. Low-back strength increased 54-104% during the 20-week protocol. In a pre-program survey, 90% of the participants reported mild to severe levels of low-back discomfort. After 20 weeks, 80% reported a reduction in pain perception; 40% were "pain-free." The average monthly worker's compensation liability for the 40 months prior to initiating the program was $14,430.00. The monthly *total* for the first nine months of the program was $389.

From August 2, 1993 through March 31, 1994, the incidence of injury in the exercising group was .52 per 200,000 employee hours worked (with one back injury report). Among non-exercising workers, it was 2.55 (with four injury reports). Last, but not least, only two workers dropped out of the program. According to Rummerfield, "The Lumbar extension machine had a greater positive impact upon 'how employees perceived their employer' than any other programmatic activity preceding it."

PGA Tour directors would do well to exchange their golf caps for miners' helmets to shed some light on their own plight. Their workers can't be happy. The so-called "low back machine" in the fitness van is, as the MedX inventor often described, "worse than worthless" for its intended purpose. Worse, because it is dangerous with heavy weights.

The PGA Tour needs to dig a little deeper.

NOVEMBER 18

---

## The Need For Surgery

The first time I crawled into a neurosurgeon's office, he combined flexibility, strength and neurological-response testing with a myelogram and promptly added my name to a list of 'immediate' low-back surgeries. I was dumb enough to agree.

The second time I crawled in, he ordered bed rest for a month and again put me on the list. I was still dumb enough to agree.

The third and fourth times, he elected therapy. Two operations were enough. I agreed.

In a 1992 book, *Breakthrough for Back Pain*, William Zucker, Ph.D. and Brian Nelson, M.D., outlined five rules related to the decision to opt for low-back surgery based on "information gathered from authoritative orthopedic surgeons:"

- Don't have surgery until you're sure it's required. "Frequency of lumbar surgery in the USA is 2-10 times higher than in other countries whose positive health-care statistics and lumbar health are about equal to or better than ours."

- Don't elect surgery until you have participated in an active exercise program, and received professional, multidisciplinary help (therapists, psychologists, social workers, etc.). "In short, do not let surgeons play God with your back pain."

- Allow sufficient time to heal (three months to a year). In general, after a year, a delay in surgery may jeopardize the potential outcome. When in doubt about performing surgery, Dr. Alf Nachemson, M.D., Ph.D. says, "If the patient can sleep through the night, I lean heavily towards not doing anything. If the patient wakes-up because of the pain, then I begin discussing surgery with him."

- Never elect surgery primarily on the results of MRI or CAT scans. Significant spinal abnormalities (that may have nothing to do with the symptoms) appear in 30-50% of MRI images (in 90%, over age 60). Before what the authors called "an expensive disservice to the public," physicians generally used a 12-week guide (by 12 weeks the repair process was likely to set in and diminish the symptoms).

- Get 2-3 independent opinions regarding the need for 'immediate' surgery.

My initial problem was "three herniated discs," the most common reason for surgery. Discs have poor blood supply, few cells per unit area and don't recover well. Yet, doctors routinely tell disc-surgery patients that the chance of at least some pain relief is about 80-90%. They don't relay the high price of a weaker spine, an increased load on surrounding vertebra (if the disc is removed) and, often, additional surgery.

According to Vert Mooney, M.D., "One percent of back injuries are protruded disc herniations that lead to unremitting sciatica." In such cases, surgery may be indicated and is generally performed within 6-12 weeks of the onset, so as not to diminish the rate of post-surgical recovery. Yet, even in stubborn cases, say the authors, "they (disc herniations) may be static for a while, or improve very slowly, but they rarely get worse." Statistically, in the 12-week *pre-operative* recovery stage, approximately 60% of patients improve within the first 4-6 weeks, while another 30% improve before 12 weeks.

The authors concluded, "You almost never cure a back through surgery," and recommended the closest thing to a cure, the MedX® Lumbar Extension machine. Strengthening the muscles that support the spine takes a load off the discs, which is why the MedX tool has enjoyed widespread success in the relief of chronic back pain.

There are too many needless surgeries performed in this country, or as someone put it, "If you're a hammer, everything looks like a nail."

## NOVEMBER 19

---

### Peak Torque

"Worse than worthless" is what MedX® inventor Arthur Jones called the use of peak torque as the accepted measure of strength; and the reason was clear. Peak force - the highest tested force on a strength curve - when measured accurately does not provide the total picture; and worse, can mislead.

The first accurate strength test for the isolated muscles of the low back was performed by a man expected to do well. He had performed heavy exercise for more than 20 years, including seven on a Nautilus® Low Back machine and, in prior quadriceps testing, peaked at more than 400 foot-pounds of torque, well above average. He didn't disappoint. On the back test, he produced a peak torque of 340 foot-pounds in flexion.

Jones was not surprised but thought the reading was high considering the size of the spinal muscles relative to the quadriceps. He rechecked the strain gauge by exposing it to a known torque and concluded, "The error was less than one tenth of one percent." The result must have been due to the subject's long history of exercise.

It wasn't.

After five months of training, the subject's strength increased to such an extent that his starting level was no longer considered high. When norms were later established, his initial strength was *well below average for a man his age and size* - with one exception, it was slightly above average in flexion. In full extension (seated, bent back and pushing back against a pad), he was 60% *below* average.

Strength must be measured, and ultimately developed, through a complete range of motion. Good strength in one position doesn't mean the same in others.

Figure 1 shows the strength curves of three subjects who produced a similar output in flexion (right side of chart), 340-360 foot-pounds of torque. In extension, however, Subject C produced 343 ft-lb.; Subject B, 125; and Subject A, only 26. Following the initial test, each subject was exercised with an 'appropriate' weight - approximately 50% of the peak torque - one that would allow the performance of 8-10 repetitions.

Subject C performed 15 repetitions with 175 foot-pounds. The weight (175 in flexion) was only 125 in extension because of the effect of the cam, while the subject possessed 343 foot-pounds of strength in that position. The selected weight was too low.

Subject B performed nine repetitions with 200 foot-pounds (200 in flexion = 143 in extension, similar to the subject's strength in that position). The weight was proper.

Subject A completed less than half of a repetition with 150 foot-pounds. His strength was so low beyond mid-range that he was unable to continue. When the weight was reduced to 100, he could barely reach extension. One hundred foot-pounds in flexion equals 71 in extension...and 26 units of strength cannot lift 71 units of weight.

Subjects B and C were exercised for 10 weeks. B increased his peak torque (in flexion) by 68%; by 180% in extension; and by 100% throughout the range. C increased his strength by 22% at his angle of peak-torque (18°); by 33% in extension; and by 60% in flexion. In both cases, the change in peak torque did not tell the whole story.

Jones believed that Subject A, not available for exercise, had the potential to increase his strength 60% in flexion and 1,000% in extension (because of his low initial level).

The muscles that extend the lumbar spine are unique in their response to exercise. The changes brought about by specific exercise are dramatic and quick, but are not properly quantified by the measurement of peak torque alone.

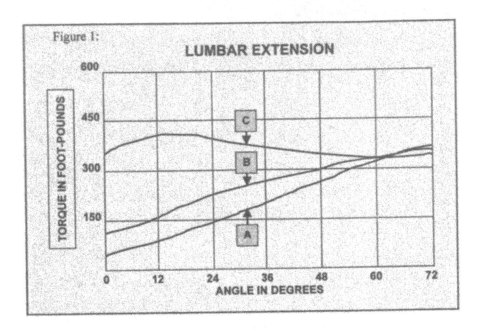

Figure 1:

NOVEMBER 20

---

### Genetics 101

Andres and I never did see eye-to-eye. As a 10-year gym member, he took an approach to exercise that opposed my Spartan philosophy. When he showed up, he rode a bike a few minutes, did a handful of machines and took a L-O-N-G sauna. My idea of a workout was to eliminate the bikes, exercise to fatigue and blow up the sauna.

So, expectation that he would cooperate during a test of low-back strength on a MedX® Lumbar Extension machine was lower than his output - the lowest I had ever measured. In flexion (bent forward, pushing back), he produced 150 foot-pounds of torque, pathetic for a man his size (6'3", 190 pounds). In full extension (extended back, pushing back), he mustered 13 foot-pounds, the equivalent of a mosquito landing on the pad he theoretically pushed.

Immediately after the test, I exercised Andres with a resistance that, under normal conditions, would lead to fatigue at about two minutes (10-12 repetitions), though I was certain he'd abandon ship before then. With only 13 foot-pounds of strength in extension, he faced the problem of reaching the back of the machine (a position of full extension) where the resistance would be approximately 50 foot-pounds. Thirteen pounds of strength can't lift 50 pounds of weight.

But Andres was unique. He touched the back of the machine on his first, second and third repetitions. It was obvious that he had not put forth his best effort during the test, which rendered the weight inadequate for the exercise, so I thought.

A second surprise came when I instructed him to move slowly, and he did. His 35-second-per-repetition speed made the exercise 'brutal' - and Andres was into anything but brutal. I said nothing as he plodded on.

At six minutes, I asked if he felt fatigue in the muscles of his back. None.

At thirteen and a half minutes (the previous record was three), Andres raised his head and asked, "How long do I have to do this? My wife's waiting downstairs." Tired of watching him go back and forth, I stopped the exercise and immediately tested his remaining strength. In flexion, he recorded 168 foot-pounds of torque (an increase of 12%); in extension, 33 foot-pounds (an increase of 150%).

Prior to his performance, I had only read of subjects who, instead of reaching fatigue slowly, gained strength during exercise. Andres' pre- and post-exercise strength curves were similar in shape, indicating that the test was valid. He had cooperated.

"Did you feel fatigue in your low back during or after the ordeal?" I asked.
"None."

"Did you have difficulty touching the back of the machine?"

"Only at the beginning. It got easier as I went along."

Andres was born with a predominance of slow-twitch (slow-fatigue) fibers in the muscles that extend his lumbar spine. As such, he will never demonstrate great strength, only great endurance. According to MedX creator Arthur Jones, approximately 10% of people possess a similar genetic tendency and, as strange as it seems, are less likely to suffer back problems than stronger candidates who fatigue more quickly.

Andres had never had a back problem in his life.

While he basked in the revelation that his uniqueness had been confirmed by cold, hard fact, I took a few days to put the puzzle together. When all was said and done, his lack of strength was something to celebrate.

## NOVEMBER 21

---

### Low-Back Exercise

There's only one way to strengthen the low back - and it's being ignored. Traditional medical recommendations such as Williams' flexion exercises (for abdominal muscles) and McKenzie's extension exercises (for low-back muscles) are limited by the weight of the body segments involved and do not provide resistance through a complete range of motion. They also fail to access the muscles of the low back due to lack of isolation.

Other solutions, such as torso hyperextensions and low-back machines in gyms, are equally ineffective regardless of how they feel.

Research at the University of Florida's Center for Exercise Science clearly shows:

- If the pelvis rotates during backward movement of the torso, the muscles of the hip and rear-thigh receive the benefit, not those that extend the spine.
- Only the MedX® Lumbar Extension machine provides the degree of pelvic stabilization necessary to meaningfully access the muscles of the lumbar spine.

A few case studies lend support:

A. After seven years of heavy training on a Nautilus® low-back machine (that allows pelvic rotation), Jim F. tested the isolated strength of his back muscles on a MedX machine (that prevents pelvic rotation). He then exercised once every two weeks for 11 weeks (with MedX) and increased his strength in full extension by 1,460%. Such a dramatic increase is possible only if the muscle has atrophied through lack of use.

B. After 20 years of bodybuilding, an orthopedic 'back specialist' tested the strength of his isolated low-back muscles on a MedX machine. His effort, judging from the color he turned, was maximum; his strength, 5.6% greater than that of my secretary who did nothing but smoke cigarettes. His exercise regimen, generally performed without specialized equipment, had little or no effect on the strength of his back.

C.  Scott L. performed a series of muscle fiber-type tests on a MedX machine using a three-step procedure: a 'fresh' strength test, an exercise to fatigue, and a re-test in an 'exhausted' state. He consistently demonstrated a strength loss of 18-20%. Scott then performed the same three-step procedure substituting a Nautilus Low Back machine for the exercise phase. His pre- and post-exercise tests showed no loss in strength from the eff<sub></sub> In Arthur's Shadow at the low-back muscles were not involved.

D.  The low-back strength of 12 sets of identical twins was tested on a MedX machine. One twin exercised on a Nautilus machine for six weeks, the other on MedX. They then re-tested and switched equipment for six more weeks. Final testing revealed a significant increase in strength among those who exercised in the Nautilus-to-MedX sequence, and a loss among those who exercised in reverse.

E.  Researchers at Syracuse University measured the low-back strength of 18 elite male rowers on a MedX machine. At 6'3" and 195 pounds, their average strength was the same as an 'untrained' male. Years of rowing had no effect on low-back strength.

The MedX Lumbar Extension machine continues to prove itself superior to anything out there. If you try it, don't be surprised by the results. Low-back response to valid exercise is often dramatic...and now, reliably measurable.

## NOVEMBER 22

---

### Art of the State

I was late the day state-of-the-art Tomfoolery became Art-of-the-state fooltomery.

By the time I entered the conference room ("Exercise Rehabilitation of the Spine: Update '93", Orlando, Florida), someone was in the middle of a slide presentation. I shuffled along the back wall in the dim light and stood beside a man who had worked with MedX® inventor Arthur Jones for 20 years, Dr. Michael Fulton.

As I fumbled through my conference packet to identify the speaker, my attention was drawn to a man pacing back and forth immediately in front. He was deep in thought, intent on the words of the speaker. Back and forth, back and forth, like an elephant swaying at the zoo, he paced and paced then paced again, until it was time to strike.

Like a hawk, the blow was swift and final.

He slipped to the microphone in the center of the room, politely interrupted the speaker and prefaced his comments with insight and insult.

It was clear. Arthur Jones was in the building.

With the same silent efficiency, he slithered back and waited for the next opportunity. With a new speaker every 30 minutes, it didn't take long.

Later that morning, a member of the seminar staff spotted a guest with no ID badge and an 'active' camera. The young man (I'll call him Tom for the sake of semantics) worked for *David*, an exercise equipment company, and was 'gathering' information. Arthur got word and, despite a crew of available bouncers, stormed out of the conference hall on the longstanding belief that "a committee never solved a damn thing."

"Where the hell is he?"

Well, Tom was about as close to Hell as you could get - tightly secured in a MedX Lumbar Extension machine in the middle of a test. The device that provided a first haven for low-back muscles during exercise was the last place from where you'd want to defend yourself. Arthur went for the jugular and by the time they peeled him off, two firsts had been established. The MedX machine had saved more than a back and, much to Arthur's dismay, a committee had indeed resolved something. Tom and his bent suit were removed from the building.

Arthur did not protect his Nautilus® patents with any ease or proficiency but he intended to with MedX - even if it involved a scuffle or two.

"Violence is not something to joke about," he said. "Toughness is fake. The real tough people in this world don't go around bragging about it. If you've been there, telling you about it is unnecessary, because you know. And if you haven't been there, you're not capable of understanding."

Jones' penchant for 'adventure' put things into perspective.

"In the Forties, I was doing something that had never been done, something that no one believed was even possible at the time: capturing adult crocodiles. I made a trip to Africa and captured 189 of them in excess of 11 feet and thousands smaller, and I brought them back to this country. I made a film of that for my own amusement and later sold it to ABC. It was used and rerun and became something of a classic."

I once saw a video of Jones talking to and poking a 17½-foot Australian crocodile at his home in Ocala, Florida with a stick the length of a golf club - just reminding it to be judicious in distinguishing 'fake' from 'real' toughness.

The scenario matched one of his favorite phrases, "If you think I'm joking, try me."

## NOVEMBER 23

### "To Cut or Not to Cut, That is the Question"

"Let's do four months of exercise," said Dr. Fulton to one of his patients with chronic low-back pain, "and then we'll decide." The MedX® orthopedic representative hadn't operated on anybody for a decade.

An aggressive exercise program can prevent spine surgery, but you'd never know it by the number of surgeries performed each year. How do physicians define adequate conservative care? Are patients informed of *all* viable alternatives?

Only a small percentage of patients account for a high percentage of the cost in most health-care systems - mainly because they've had some form of surgery (with low-backs currently ranked third). Yet, despite poor long-term outcomes and a minimum failure rate of 15%, the number of surgeries is on the rise.

In 1994, the average cost of an industrial back injury was $24,000 and a worker's compensation lumbar fusion, $168,000 (in some cases, more than $500,000). The amount is absurd in light of the cost incurred in a recent study (conducted by Dr. Brian Nelson, orthopedic surgeon) that recommended aggressive and specific exercise as a solution for chronic spine pain. Research shows that multi-disciplinary approaches have enjoyed success when they include aggressive exercise, and that non-invasive treatment strategies that include intense exercise are more successful than those with low-intensity exercise or passive modalities. It also shows that exercise must effectively target the muscles that extend the lumbar (or cervical) spine.

Dr. Nelson's study was unique. No one had documented the effects of aggressive strengthening on patients recommended for spinal surgery. From May 1993 to December 1995, Dr. Nelson tracked 651 cervical or lumbar patients referred to his clinic for 'rehabilitation' by physicians familiar with his program, by patients treated at the clinic and by insurance companies. Ironically, there were no referrals from surgeons.

Sixty-two patients (of 651) were told (by one or more physicians) that they were 'candidates for surgery' (581 were not and two decided not to participate). Forty-six of the 60 that started the program completed it under the following diagnostic categories: degenerative disc disease (lumbar, 17; cervical, 4); disc syndrome (lumbar, 15; cervical, 9); and Spondylolisthesis (lumbar, 1).

The 10-week program (one hour, 2x/wk.) included use of a MedX Lumbar or Cervical Extension machine, a series of Nautilus® machines for major muscle groups, and aerobic exercise. Patients were encouraged to push beyond their initial pain to achieve symptomatic relief and were discharged when they reached 'normal' functional levels (or approached 'pain-free'). Upon discharge, they were encouraged to perform an aggressive home maintenance program with recommended devices.

Approximately 16 weeks after their last visit to the clinic, the patients were contacted and asked, "Since you completed the program have you had surgery for your spine?" If yes, "What kind of surgery did you have?" Only three of the 38 located for follow-up required surgery (2 lumbar laminectomies and one fusion; no cervical). The average cost of the program was $1,950 - 86 times less than the cost of an average WC lumbar fusion.

Dr. Nelson's study brought out the good ("Even patients recommended for spinal surgery can tolerate intensive, specific exercise") and the bad ("Adequate conservative care is defined however a physician wishes it to be defined") of the health-care system.

It doesn't take a rocket scientist to fill in the blanks.


## NOVEMBER 24

---

### *What if...*

I never climbed a mountain, but ran one when I got the urge. I once took a car to its top, put it in neutral and watched the speedometer race to 60 miles per hour at the bottom - something I refused to try on a bike. The long, steep hill that led to Effingham, Ontario was a challenge. Going down was scary; going up, downright brutal.

The route I ran to its base wandered, without notice, downhill, past gently rolling hills, a golf course, orchards, vineyards, open fields and an old cemetery. All the time, I conserved for what lay ahead. It was never pretty or quick, but when I reached the summit there was instant joy, despite the time it took to return to normal.

No doubt, it takes a long time to climb a mountain - hours, days, weeks, months. Yet, once there, glory is brief. Following his party's conquest of the Matterhorn in 1865, Edward Whymper described it as "one crowded hour of glorious life."

*What if* you could climb a mountain in hours and enjoy the peak for weeks or months? *What if* I could have conquered that hill in minutes and enjoyed it for hours?

*What if* a car lasted a lifetime? *What if* brief exercise produced a quick and permanent result?

It takes a long time to get somewhere in exercise. An untrained subject generally feels better in a month and sees results in three or four; but the loss is quicker. "Seven days (or less) without exercise makes one weak." One exercise begs to differ.

Figure 1 demonstrates the results produced by the first group of subjects to use a MedX® Lumbar Extension machine for exercise. The gray columns (left at each angle) represent the average static strength of the isolated back muscles measured *before* an exercise protocol that lasted from 10 to 27 weeks. The black columns represent strength levels attained *after* the protocol. Eighty percent of the subjects had a two-to-six-year history on the Nautilus® Low Back machine.

The average increase in the level of peak torque (right side of chart) was 87%, while the average increase in extension (left side of chart) was 686%. The average overall increase throughout the range was 142%. The MedX machine was used infrequently: at most, once a week; the least, once every two weeks. The subject who exercised for 27 weeks performed only 13 exercises and produced an increase in extension of 877%. The time per exercise was brief, less than two minutes. "To say that we were surprised by the results," said one of the subjects, "is to put it mildly indeed, we were stunned."

Figure 2 demonstrates staying power. The black columns represent the average strength level of a larger group of normal subjects following a 12-week program of specific exercise. The gray columns represent strength levels following an additional 12 weeks using a frequency of only one exercise every four weeks.

There was no change in the first half of the range (right side of chart), a 1% increase at mid-range, and a 7% decrease in extension (left side of chart). The conclusion: "Having increased the strength of the spinal muscles with specific exercise, very little in the way of additional exercise is required to maintain the peak level of strength." Amen.

Brief, infrequent exercise can produce quick, long-term results in the muscles that extend the lumbar spine, and the implications for industry, government and insurance companies are huge. The MedX protocol is time-efficient, and could save billions of dollars and prevent a mountain of unnecessary suffering, if it were not for one thing. The political rhetoric in its path is longer and steeper than any Matterhorn.

*What if ...*

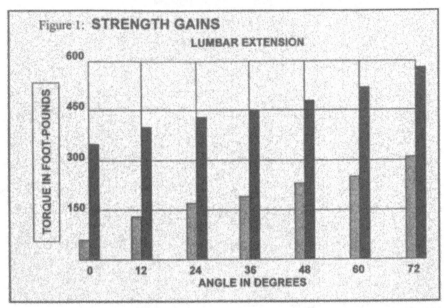

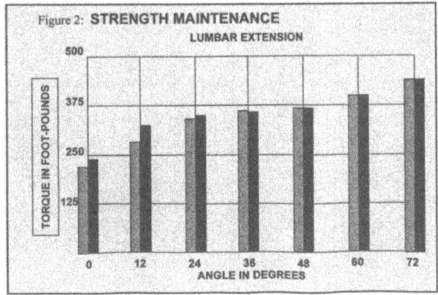

NOVEMBER 25

---

## Eureka

Dr. Fulton received a telephone call late that night.

"Where are you, Mike?"

"At home, getting ready for bed."

"How soon can you get up here?"

"Well, ...in about an hour and a half, I guess. What's up?"

"Got an idea. Need your input. See you in a bit."

Dr. Fulton dressed and left in haste. He'd been 'on call' around the clock for Nautilus® inventor Arthur Jones for 15 years.

The drive from New Smyrna Beach to Ocala, Florida was tedious but tempered with excitement. Jones always had something up his sleeve.

As soon as he arrived, Arthur had his ear. The discussion involved the MedX® Lumbar Extension machine, now in its final stages of development. Opinions flew as the night dragged on. Finally, not sure of the time, Dr. Fulton suggested some sleep before his busy morning schedule.

He bedded down in the guest cottage behind the house.

Hours later - and it may have been minutes - Fulton was startled by a loud knock at the door followed by an outright intrusion as it flew open.

"I've got it."

Fulton propped himself up enough to catch a sleepy glimpse of his boss in nothing but undershorts, hair scattered skyward like a "mad-scientist."

Jones' solution had strong elements of what Fulton had proposed.

For a guy who believed that one head was better than two, the telephone call alone was bold. Yet, throughout his career in the field of exercise and medicine, Arthur Jones was quick to acknowledge input from other sources.

During the development of a combination Squat/Hip-and-Back machine, Jones went to great lengths to recognize the contribution made by Dan Fogel, a man who planted a seed of progress. "Why don't you prevent the thigh from moving?" suggested Fogel. It set Arthur on a new pattern of thought that eventually led to the completion of one of his more significant conquests - a machine I never saw.

When his equipment first hit the market, Jones offered to give credit to anyone who came up with an additional ingredient for what he called "a perfect form of exercise," and to immediately incorporate the idea into his machines.

He never had to perform that duty.

He also gave credit to many of the people he worked with during the 14 years he spent developing the MedX medical tools. He realized that it took more than one mind to get the job done.

It was obvious throughout that Jones respected the opinion of Dr. Fulton - or wouldn't have called him in the first place. It was equally obvious that once the seed was planted in Jones' fertile mind - regardless of its source - it grew quicker than it would have in whatever other mind. Arthur was plugged into a channel - many channels for that matter - in a way that few were.

The "mad scientist" was wired differently.

Dr. Fulton may not have got the credit he deserved on that occasion, but working alongside Jones for 30 years was reward enough.


# NOVEMBER 26

---

## Compatible Atrophy

There are two kinds of atrophy - disuse and overuse. The first occurs when you don't use something enough; the second, when you use something too much. The first is associated with rust; the second with wear and tear. The third has something to do with love.

I operated a low-back rehabilitation facility within an existing gym for three years. Medical doctors and chiropractors referred patients with chronic back pain based on two things: that the patients were candidates for treatment and that I had the only MedX® Lumbar Extension machine in town.

One day, the 'odd-couple' entered. She was outgoing, pleasant, inquisitive, impeccably dressed and expressed herself with her hands and eyes. He was sloppy, grumpy, non-talkative, introverted, did not want to be there and kept his eyes glued to the floor when they were open.

While he sat waist-deep in a magazine, I tested the fresh strength of the muscles that extended her spine and exercised her to exhaustion with a weight that allowed approximately two minutes of movement. I then followed with a second, post-exercise test of the same muscles to determine what strength remained. The computer reported a small loss in strength - a predominance of slow-twitch muscle fibers. She wasn't strong, but her endurance was above average. On he read.

I went over the results, answered a few questions and ushered her to a series of machines to strengthen adjacent muscle groups.

It was his turn.

I secured him in the machine and followed an identical procedure: a test of fresh strength, exercise to exhaustion and a second strength test to determine the effect of the exercise. It was much the same - little fatigue from one test to the next. I reviewed the results with him and mentioned that, like his wife, he tended to fatigue slowly.

Suddenly, from the back of the room came a high-pitched voice, as sweet as could be, "Honey, isn't it nice to know that we're compatible?"

He turned his head away from his spouse's ear and mumbled a series of unfavorable comments.

Their results *were* similar, but the entire story was yet to be told. Both suffered from disuse atrophy and their tests reflected *less* fatigue than there would have been without atrophy. The reason was clear.

Atrophy affects the fast-twitch (powerful) muscle fibers to a greater degree than the slow-twitch (endurance) fibers. In such a state, the prevalence of less powerful fibers makes muscles appear to have more endurance than they do. As atrophy is overcome by strengthening, the fast-twitch fibers wake up, and their activation on subsequent tests allows the muscle to demonstrate fatigue at a quicker rate. When a muscle has reached its strength potential (normally at 20 weeks on a MedX machine), the same test reveals an *accurate* rate of fatigue and fiber-type.

I exercised the couple using the University of Florida's research protocol for muscles that possess an *average* - rather than slow - rate of fatigue, and re-tested both at 12 weeks - the maximum allowed for treatment. He fatigued at a rate slightly higher than normal. She fatigued at a normal rate.

The two shared more than atrophy.


## NOVEMBER 27

---

### Marketing 101

For a man who quit school in the fourth grade, the thought of lecturing to a group of doctors was not intimidating at all. Nautilus® inventor Arthur Jones had 13 physicians in his immediate family including his father, mother, sisters, brothers and children, and as someone once commented, "He was probably smarter than all of them together."

It showed.

Every day for years, he flew doctors to his home in Ocala, Florida "for educational purposes," and every other Friday lectured at the University of

Florida's Center for Exercise Science "to anyone interested." Unlike his soft-spoken brother (and physician), Edgar, Arthur's passion was butting heads in the spotlight. This Friday's challenge was no different - a group of local physicians, therapists and exercise clinicians, and a contingent from New York City that included a world-renown back specialist.

It didn't matter. Arthur treated everyone the same - and it wasn't always pretty.

He began without fanfare, addressing topics that were new to some. At the end of the presentation - during a question-answer period - a hand went up in the back of the room. A well-dressed man approached the microphone and asked a question that most would have considered relevant.

Not Jones. "When has it ever been shown," he thought, "that the majority was right about anything?"

Arthur subdued his tendency to interrupt and riveted his eyes on the victim. When the man finished, Jones slipped from the podium, locked on his prey and slowly paced the length of the room. In what seemed an eternity, he stationed himself in front of the man as in a pre-fight stare-down. The nearby microphone amplified the message. "Sir, *that* is the *stupidest* question I've *ever* heard. Where the *hell* did you go to medical school?"

The silence was deafening.

World-renown had just met world-renown - and the collision meant another customer down the drain.

The 'why' was clear.

Jones was more passionate about the message than the sale. If you weren't smart enough to buy his product (in this case, the MedX® Lumbar Extension machine), the next guy would. Most physicians owned isokinetic machines and were reluctant to change regardless of how good the 'new' piece proved. It didn't matter to Jones. His enemy was ignorance and he would often demonstrate the inadequacy of their tools (still used in the majority of clinics in the nation) and the stupidity of their choices in minutes. He would have been a nightmare for the Board of Directors he refused to create.

The approach was nothing new to those around him: Jones was a one-man show from the start. Every day his sister came home from school, she found Arthur working on body parts he kept "in the deep freeze." Self-education - "the only form of education" - carried him a long way.

Michael Fulton, M.D., an orthopedic surgeon who worked with Jones for 30 years confirmed the fact. "When he lectures to us (medical doctors)," he said, "he's up there somewhere (pointing skyward) and we're down here. At times, I don't even know what he's talking about."

There was no middle ground with Arthur Jones. You either liked him or you didn't...and he didn't care which.

## NOVEMBER 28

---

### The Low-Back Muscle Surprise

When Arthur Jones set out to isolate muscle function in 1972, he didn't take the easy way out in targeting the front thigh, and later, the muscles that extend the lumbar spine. Both proved all the challenge he could handle. By 1986, his MedX® Lumbar Extension machine was ready.

Among a handful of subjects first tested on the new device was a gym owner named Joe Cirulli who had performed seven years of heavy exercise on a Nautilus® Low Back machine. Joe produced the lower curve in Figure 1. In flexion (right side of chart, normally the strongest position), Cirulli produced 340 foot-pounds of torque, a value that was thought to be an error.

"We had been testing the strength of this same subject's quadriceps muscles for several years," said Jones, "and with both legs working together his fresh strength of the quadriceps muscles was only 400 foot-pounds of torque (which is well above average) ...it did not appear to make any sense that his much smaller lumbar muscles were nearly as strong as the much larger thigh muscles."

Jones re-tested the accuracy of the machine and found an error of less than one tenth of one percent. He believed Cirulli "was probably the strongest man in the world in these muscles" and that his exercise history was responsible for the unexpected result.

The surprise was yet to come.

Figure 2 shows two strength curves. The bottom one, marked "C," is the same as the bottom curve in Figure 1, Cirulli's initial strength. The top curve, marked "N," represents the average strength of males with *no* exercise experience, a standard later established by research at the University of Florida. Instead of being unusually strong, Joe was *below* average in initial strength - and he wasn't alone.

Another early subject, Jim Flanagan (6'4", 250 pounds) produced 381 foot-pounds of torque in flexion despite a similar history of exercise. In extension (left side of chart, normally the weakest position), he registered 31 foot-pounds. Without norms, everyone assumed his curve was outstanding.

It was anything but.

In 1988, I tested the low-back strength of a 92-pound physical therapist in Caracas, Venezuela. She entered looking for work and ended up tightly secured in a MedX machine. Her strength was high for her age and weight; and in extension, she was *more than three times stronger* than Flanagan. If you placed the two side-by-side, you'd bet your house that it couldn't be. I should have hired her on the spot.

The small, weak low-back muscles are linked to a superior leverage system (especially in flexion, bent forward) and are capable of producing high levels of torque. In contrast, the large muscles of the front thigh are plagued by a lousy system of leverage.

A second surprise occurred when the low-back muscles were exercised. The top curve in Figure 1 represents Cirulli's fresh strength measured five months and eight days after the lower curve, results produced by one exercise every 14 days. On the right side of the chart, his increase was 103%; on the left, 450%. Flanagan increased his strength 1,460% in extension. Both results were impossible without atrophy.

Twenty years of hard exercise, seven on the best low-back machine available, had no meaningful effect on the strength of the muscles that extend the lumbar spine...and you can bet your house on that.

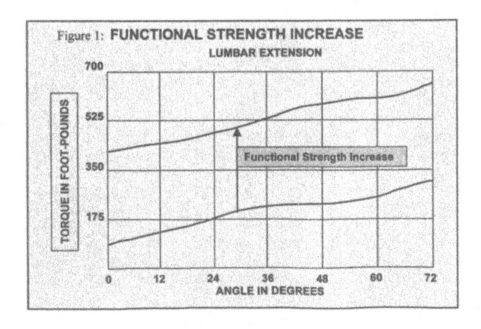

Figure 1: FUNCTIONAL STRENGTH INCREASE
LUMBAR EXTENSION

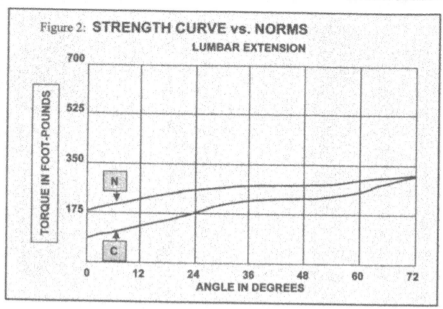

Figure 2: STRENGTH CURVE vs. NORMS
LUMBAR EXTENSION

NOVEMBER 29

_____

### Selective Atrophy

In 1972, Arthur Jones set out to build a machine that isolated muscle function.

"If I say something about a muscle," he declared, "I want it to be 100% of that muscle, nothing less." His estimate of six months and $200,000 slowly turned into 14 years and $88 million. Three thousand prototypes later, he introduced a machine that isolated the muscles that extend the lumbar spine (low back). Eight years later, he ushered in his fifth and (to date) final device - a front- and back-thigh machine that took 22 years to build at a cost of $120 million.

Jones was not easily satisfied. He tested the new tools until he was certain they were accurate and re-tested subjects to ensure their reliability. If you didn't cooperate, Jones knew exactly 'when' and 'where' by the accuracy of the machine, and handled the 'why' by the fact that he always carried a gun, with or without which (your choice) he could motivate.

Among the innovative tests he designed was a non-invasive method of determining muscle fiber-type, a measure of how quickly a muscle fatigues.

He first tested a muscle's fresh strength through a complete range of motion, exercised it to momentary failure with an appropriate weight (a predetermined percentage of its peak force) and then re-tested its remaining level of strength. The difference between fresh and exhausted strength levels determined the immediate *effect* of the exercise.

Most subjects (80% of low back, 72% of front thigh) lost approximately 2% of their fresh strength per repetition. That is, 10 repetitions of exercise reduced their starting strength by 20%. Some, however, lost as much as 50% of their strength per repetition while others *gained* strength regardless of how many repetitions they performed. Muscles that fatigued quickly were presumed to have an abundance of fast-twitch fibers; those that fatigued slowly or not at all, a predominance of slow-twitch fibers.

It was not until Jones began working with injured limbs that he realized another facet of fiber type, one that had created confusion and controversy with traditional muscle biopsies. His three-fold testing procedure revealed that muscle atrophy (weakness due to lack of use) was selective. It reduced the strength of fast-twitch fibers to a much greater degree than slow-twitch fibers.

To prove his point, Jones tested a subject who repeatedly demonstrated a loss of 40% of his fresh strength following 10 repetitions to fatigue with his healthy left leg (a high percentage of fast-twitch muscle fibers). When his injured right leg was tested using the same procedure, its strength was reduced by only 11% after 10 repetitions to fatigue, an *effect* much less than expected (after all, left and right limbs possess similar fatigue rates). Midway through the rehabilitation process, the same exercise reduced fresh strength by 25%. The fast-twitch fibers were making a comeback. At complete recovery, when the strength of both legs was equal in every position throughout the range of motion, the effect of the same exercise was almost equal (40%).

The fast-twitch fibers, dormant by atrophy, made the muscle appear to fatigue slowly. When they finally awoke to the call of exercise, the normal fatigue rate was restored.

Muscle fiber-type is genetic and not subject to change. The apparent disparity with atrophied muscles has led many scientists and practitioners to believe that the rate of muscle fatigue can be varied by using different repetition schemes. Not so.

The only training that affects the fatigue characteristics of muscle is no training at all.

## NOVEMBER 30

---

### Chronic Back Pain - Solved

A phrase used by Arthur Jones to address a group of bodybuilders echoed through my head as I clung face-down to two pegs on a table in the dank basement of a hospital somewhere in Caracas. "When your back is out," said the MedX® inventor, "you won't care how big your arms are."

My back was out - a second crisis following two surgeries - and I remember only one thing about my arms, they shivered.

Dr. Jeckl - white coat and all - jabbed a needle into my lower spine and hit the jackpot, if bone counts. He tried again, then disappeared behind a one-way window that reflected what looked like a spear dangling from a back in a Tarzan movie. The slow tilt of the table in the direction of my head produced an instant headache. When it reversed, it felt as if someone had poured lead into my legs.

CLICK. CLICK. "Steady." (Was there an option?) CLICK.

Jeckl's hide-and-seek tactics continued until he had enough photos, whereupon he invited me to the viewing room for the results.

"What is that L-shaped thing in the middle?" I asked as I peered over his shoulder.

"The needle."

"Is it supposed to be bent like that?"

"Well..." he hesitated with a smile.

I bent the doorknob on the way out.

There was nothing to smile about then, but there's plenty now. What Jones called "specific exercise" on his MedX Lumbar Extension machine took my back from 'sorry' to 'pain-free' in months - a minor miracle considering the small amount of exercise required.

"Specific exercise" is exercise that targets one muscle group. Eighteen years of research at the University of Florida has shown that the only way to target the muscles that extend the lumbar spine is to prevent the pelvis from rotating during torso extension. If the pelvis moves, low-back muscles get zero benefit.

How do you know if the pelvis moves? The MedX machine has a round pad that presses tightly against it. If the pelvis rotates one millimeter, the pad rotates two. If the pad moves at all, the patient is secured until it doesn't.

Low-back muscles require infrequent exercise for best results, and even less for maintenance. I first used the MedX device once a week for two minutes and was pain free in 20 weeks. I've kept that status for 17 years by using it once a month for approximately 90 seconds - not enough to satisfy the needs of other muscles but plenty for the lumbar spine.

How effective is the machine in clinical settings?

Regardless of diagnosis, 80% of patients with chronic low-back pain experience a reduction in pain perception following a 12-week protocol. Thirty to thirty-three percent become pain free.

Miracles are common with the right equipment. So far, the MedX Lumbar Extension machine stands alone as the 'right' tool for strengthening the low back in a meaningful way.

Find one, and rid yourself of more than Jeckl's number.

CLICK.

# DECEMBER

"Only time will tell just how many of my current opinions about exercise turn out to be correct, but I have at least produced something of great value that never existed previously: the tools required for meaningful and accurate measurement of the results of exercise...

...I am arrogant enough to believe that my lifetime of interest in the field of exercise has produced developments that can provide great benefits to millions of other people if my discoveries and developments are not flushed down the toilet of history."

Arthur Jones

## Abnormal Strength Curves - Part 1

Valid strength testing began when MedX® Corporation introduced a line of cervical and lumbar tools in 1986. Valid because testing was specific, accurate, meaningful and safe; valid, because what preceded it was not.

We now know what the shape of a strength curve *should* be throughout the range of motion at any level. The 'ideal' curve for the muscles that extend the lumbar and cervical spines, for example, is a straight line that reflects 40% more strength in flexion than extension. Yet, the curve of most subjects, when first tested, demonstrates the following:

- A below-average level of strength, especially in extension.
- Disproportionate strength throughout the range of motion.
- Anything but a straight line.

Not to fret, the same machine that detects the 'abnormality' can help correct it.

Figure 1 shows three tests of fresh strength taken over a period of 76 days. The bottom curve (#1) represents the initial test of a subject who was 1,000% (not 40%) stronger in flexion than extension (left side of chart). The ideal curve for a subject at this level of strength is indicated by the dotted line adjacent to the curve. Note the two apparent abnormalities - a boat-shaped area to the right, and a triangular area to the left, near extension. Both are indications of functional deficiency and spinal pathology...and they repeat in subsequent tests.

The middle curve (#2) was a similar test taken six weeks later following specific exercise (once every two weeks). The ideal curve at this level is indicated by the nearby dotted line. The boat-shaped area hadn't changed, but the triangle had decreased in size.

By the third test (curve #3) and after 76 days of infrequent exercise, the triangle had disappeared, indicating a deficiency due to muscle atrophy - correctable by exercise. The boat-shaped area, however, remained the same indicating an abnormality unaffected by exercise. A year later, it too disappeared and the subject produced an ideal curve with a relationship from flexion to extension of 1.4:1. More importantly, by the second test, the chronic back pain he suffered for 12 years disappeared and never returned.

Figure 2 demonstrates three strength tests of an elite athlete conducted over a period of 150 days. The middle curve (#1) represents his initial test of fresh strength; the bottom curve (#2), a test of exhausted strength immediately following a hard exercise. Note the similar shape of the curves. The dips at 60° and 36° indicate apparent abnormalities in lumbar function. The ideal curve (dotted line) indicates near-proportionate strength (a flexion-extension ratio of 1.72:1) yet highlights an inadequacy *throughout* the range of motion. His strength level is *below* average, as was the case in Figure 1.

Curve #3 shows a fresh-strength test conducted five months later, following specific exercise (once every three weeks). Besides an overall strength increase of 56.6%, the subject's strength ratio improved to 1.53:1. Four months later, it was close to 1.4:1.

Deviation from the 'ideal' curve is an indication of spinal pathology. But, as MedX inventor Arthur Jones warned, "It must be clearly understood that such test results are not diagnostic, do not tell us the nature of pathology."

A dip at 36°, for example, does not indicate a herniated disc at L4/L5.

Fortunately, 80% of back problems are muscular in nature. And research with the MedX tool indicates that abnormalities associated with muscle atrophy generally correct themselves within 20 weeks.

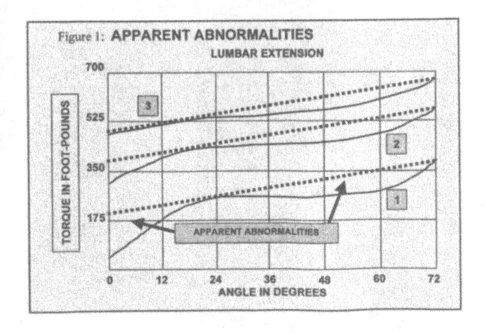

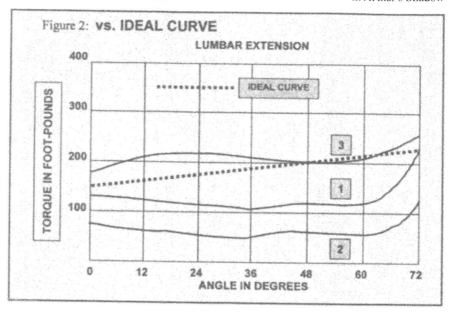

Figure 2: **vs. IDEAL CURVE**

LUMBAR EXTENSION

DECEMBER 2

---

### Abnormal Strength Curves - Part 2

I don't like the term 'normal,' but in the case of the lumbar spine, it's not so bad - and no longer a guess. The determination of true function of the muscles that extend the low back has been established by MedX® inventor, Arthur Jones.

When first tested for the strength of these important muscles (July 11, 1987), I fatigued at a normal rate, was below average in strength and disproportionately weak in full extension despite a long history of exercise.

Figure 1, Curve A shows my fresh level of strength from that test; Curve B, what strength remained immediately after exercise. The difference between A and B is fatigue caused by the exercise (13 reps with 150 ft.lbs.; a strength loss of 20.86%, 1.6% per repetition). Curve C shows the ideal relationship of strength to position. A muscle should be 1.4 times stronger in flexion than extension, and the relationship (1.4:1) should remain linear at all points between, regardless of strength level.

What should occur, however, rarely does. The average person is 2-3 times stronger in flexion than extension (I was 2.56), some as much as 65 times stronger. And backs that are strong in some angles and weak at others are begging for problems.

Figure 2 demonstrates the strength curves of an individual whose lines are anything but straight. The bottom one (A) represents the subject's initial strength test, while the top one (B) represents his strength level three weeks later. Both curves have peaks and valleys in the same relative positions, confirming the validity of the test and subject cooperation. Although his strength increased 50% in extension, the curve did not alter in shape, indicating a problem that is idiopathic in nature and unrelated to muscle atrophy. When atrophy is involved, the curve adopts a shape that eventually mimics the ideal relationship illustrated by Curve C, Figure 1.

The repeating curves in this case indicate a problem (a dip in the curve) at similar angles of movement, but cannot determine the nature of the problem. MedX machines are not diagnostic.

Figure 3 demonstrates the initial strength test of a subject who claimed no history of back problems. Her strength in full flexion (right side of chart) was normal for her height and weight, and above average in full extension. The measure of either position alone would have revealed no abnormality, but the plunge in the mid-range was far from normal or ideal when she moved toward extension. She later admitted having a benign spinal tumor.

Specific muscle testing can reveal risk factors related to lumbar problems - factors that cannot be identified in any other way. Current imaging practices reveal nothing about strength levels (vs. norms or vs. ideal), muscle fiber type (how quickly muscles fatigue), strength distribution throughout the range of motion, or subject cooperation (does a subject have a problem, or only claim to?).

Specific exercise for the muscles of the lumbar spine can change a strength curve quickly if atrophy is involved, as it is in most cases. It restores function and provides protection from injury by increasing: (a) range of motion, (b) overall strength and the distribution of strength throughout the range, and (c) awareness of functional limitations (what subjects can and can't do).

If the response to specific exercise is normal, 6-8 sessions of a couple of minutes each can put most people on the road to *less* or *no* pain.

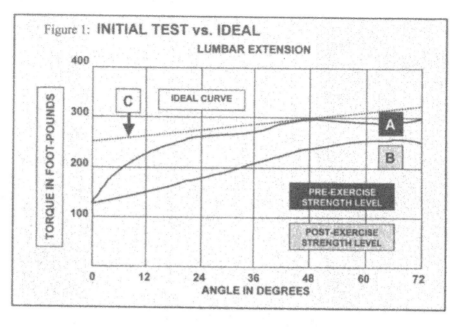

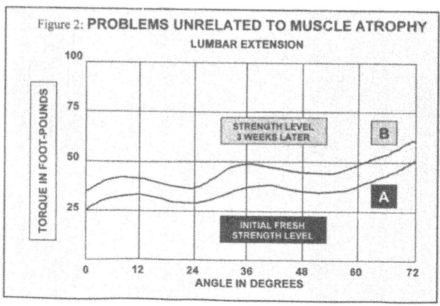

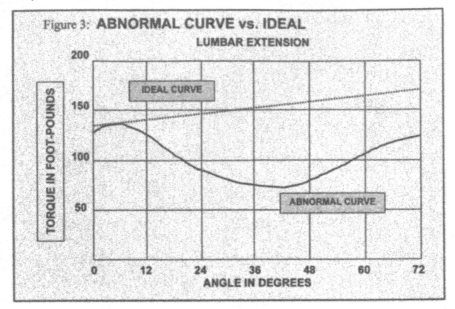

Figure 3: ABNORMAL CURVE vs. IDEAL
LUMBAR EXTENSION

DECEMBER 3

## Bending Strength Curves

"You will become very rigid," said Doug Henning as he ran his hands down the sides of a hypnotized football player. He then placed the man face-up between two chairs and sat on his waist, bouncing up and down. The guy didn't bend or break.

In a similar vein, but with an opposite result, I watched Uri Geller bend a spoon, held in the tip of two fingers, just by staring at it. I was left with the impression that changing the shape of things was in the mind. Things were different in the real world.

Straightening the wood shaft of an antique golf club with linseed oil and heat, and re-shaping a strength curve with an exercise machine took more than mind power.

Unknown to most trainees, the introduction of Nautilus® machines was all about bending strength curves. The change of resistance brought about by the 'cam' filled gaps left by the barbell (generally in flexion or extension, or both) and led to improved muscle mass, strength distribution and protection from injury.

MedX® machines took strength-curve modification to new heights by isolating the muscles that support the most vulnerable areas of the body - the knee, the lumbar spine and the cervical spine - and establishing 'norms' for curve shape and range of motion.

According to MedX inventor Arthur Jones, strength curves change in response to two signals - exercise and lack of exercise - and one of the first things to respond is range of motion. With normal subjects, a restricted range of motion is caused by either mechanical limitation or muscle weakness. And strengthening, not stretching, is the solution.

"Movement of the body produces internal resistance against continued movement;" he said, "when the existing level of muscular strength has produced movement to a point where the co-existing level of internal resistance has been increased to an equal level, then continued movement is impossible. At that point you have equal and opposite forces. But when an initial limited range of movement is produced only by muscular weakness, the range of movement will be increased as strength is increased in response to exercise."

Jones identified the cause of restricted movement by testing the level of functional torque at the end of the range of possible motion. A zero reading indicated a limitation by muscle weakness; more than zero, a mechanical limitation. When a mechanical limitation existed, increasing the range of motion by stretching was contraindicated.

The shape of a strength curve changes where its needs are greatest in response to proper exercise. Most muscles are weakest in full contraction and initial gains are greatest there. But once a muscle can produce a force that matches the ideal curve throughout the range of motion, additional gains in strength will be proportionate from end to end.

A changing strength curve provides information about what has been accomplished, identifies areas that need additional improvement and indicates how much improvement can be expected. Lumbar and cervical extension strength curves are compared to ideal curves, while limb and spinal rotation curves, right and left, compare the 'good' side to the 'bad' to determine whether normal function has been restored. "Abnormal strength curves produced during spinal-rotation testing," says Jones, "are seldom duplicated in both directions of movement."

Abnormal curves that don't bend in response to exercise indicate a 'real' problem. Those that bend indicate that the abnormality was likely caused by muscle atrophy.

And when strength curves bend, things are less prone to break.

## DECEMBER 4

---

### All That Glitters Is Not Gold

Thirty years ago, I was invited to a gym in Miami by world-record holder and water-ski champion, Ana Maria Carrasco. I had a role in the design of her conditioning program in Venezuela and she thought I could salvage a routine from a set of Nautilus® machines abandoned in a corner of her club. Not so.

The equipment was in such poor shape that I was forced to assemble a workout from what remained. One selection was a leg extension device from a group of computerized machines that represented the latest innovation of a reputable manufacturer. It had by far the best 'feel' and, judging from the enthusiasm of its users, was the greatest thing since the barbell.

Following Ana's workout, I stood in line to try a chest-press machine. An instructor guided me through phase one, a strength test. I pushed hard against the movement arm as buttons clicked and lights flashed. The machine then selected a resistance for the exercise phase based upon that effort. I performed as many repetitions as I could and illuminated the entire range-of-motion panel.

The lifting phase felt normal, but lowering felt as if someone sat on the weight stack. Because a 'fresh' muscle is 40% stronger lowering than lifting, I realized that I had just been exposed to some engineer's version of full-range exercise - both up *and* down. It was unique, difficult and had great potential to reduce overall workout time.

In search of more information, I came across an article by Arthur Jones about *dynamic* strength tests (phase one of my ordeal). According to Jones, a test conducted while lifting a weight produced a measure of strength lower than the actual strength of the muscle, while a test conducted lowering weight produced a measure of strength that was higher. The discrepancy was due to the influence of "internal muscle friction" which was affected by speed of movement and level of fatigue.

The accuracy of dynamic testing was further hampered by three factors: insufficient muscle-fiber recruitment at the start of a test; fatigue toward the end of a test; and impact force produced by the acceleration and deceleration of the movement arm. Impact exposes a muscle to high and potentially dangerous levels of force.

To prove his point, Jones hired a Canadian medical doctor/engineer to investigate isokinetic (constant speed-of-movement) exercise and dynamic testing. Dr. Les Organ, an advocate of both, spent 18 months and $3,000,000 to build "the best isokinetic machine possible." After testing, he concluded what

Jones had 20 years before - that isokinetics was "the least productive form of exercise for any purpose."

Dynamic tests with the new device revealed errors of 100-200% in the measurement of force, and errors of 40-60° in the measurement of the angle to which the force corresponded. Dr. Organ called the information an artifact.

Years later, their work revealed more complications. The selection of resistance based on a fixed percentage (usually 70-80%) of a maximum tested force was suitable for an average mix of fibers, but some muscles were not average. According to Jones, "A training routine that is ideal for a slow-twitch (endurance) muscle, can be utterly devastating for a fast-twitch (powerful) muscle." Therefore, even with accurate force measurements, the exercise prescription would fail for 20-30% of trainees.

Design flaws are common in exercise and rehabilitation equipment. Go by how it feels - with one exception. If it's isokinetic, have someone else crank the Edsel®.

## DECEMBER 5

### One Upsmanship

In 1989, I attended a certification program for MedX® technicians at the University of Florida's Center for Exercise Science, a small building east of campus. The Center was established by a $10 million donation from MedX inventor Arthur Jones, and provided an official stamp on the doctrine he long promoted.

One morning around 11:00 o'clock, our classroom was interrupted by a group of Japanese guests led by Jones. Arthur pointed out the purpose of our being and then placed a hand on my shoulder in passing.

"This young man," he said with an Oklahoma drawl and hint of pride, "recently established a MedX facility in Venezuela." I felt huge.

Several Japanese businessmen eventually purchased a MedX Lumbar machine, took it apart and presented their findings at the annual convention in Daytona Beach, Florida, "Spinal Rehabilitation Update '91."

According to Jones, the MedX device counterbalanced the subject's torso weight during exercise. In flexion (seated, knees to chest), gravity worked against the upward extension of the torso. As such, the subject had to overcome the selected weight *and* the effect of gravity to extend the spine. Once the torso moved past a vertical position toward extension, however, the effect was the opposite - gravity assisted the effort. The counterbalance system devised by Jones added or subtracted the exact amount of counterweight to the weight of the torso *throughout* the motion, so that neither *gravity* nor the weight of the torso affected the result.

The Japanese agreed that the weight of the torso could be counterbalanced during the stationary set-up of a subject, but questioned the relationship (torso weight plus or minus gravity vs. counterweight) during movement.

They dismantled the machine, tested the accuracy of the mechanism and reported that the counterbalance system was 98.5% correct at every angle of movement throughout the range of motion. As with many things, Jones was more right than wrong (although he claimed that real learning occurred only through mistakes). It was tough to pull the wool over his eyes.

But it happened, and it happened more than once.

At a medical conference in Ocala, Florida, Jones claimed that it was impossible to swallow a slice of bread in less than 30 seconds. The bread, he said, would absorb the saliva so quickly as to render the act of swallowing impossible. A hand flew up in the back of the room and soon thereafter staff member Walt Anderson took up the challenge. A slice of bread was secured and the timer set.

"Ready, go."

Walt quickly ran to the nearest faucet, wet the bread and consumed it in less than the required time. An argument relating to the rules of the game ensued.

On another occasion, Jones mentioned that he could type at a rate of 80 words per minute. Walt expressed some doubt again, born of a recent typing class and a familiarity with his boss' ancient typewriter and one-finger technique. They went up to Arthur's room for the test. When the smoke cleared, Jones had typed approximately 45 words per minute, still perhaps a single-digit record.

Walt Anderson pushed the envelope a few times with Arthur, but didn't dare make it a habit. He needed a job and his boss was usually right.

## DECEMBER 6

---

### What Does It Take?

For a fleeting moment, I entertained the thought of writing a book like those I scan at the bookstore. After all, I too pretend to know something about exercise.

Yet, anyone can photograph an exercise and list procedures from A to B. Anyone can scan a glossary of movements and include it as part of a success story. Anyone can print or rationalize anything he or she pleases - anyone. So, if I ever stooped to writing it - which I won't - my contribution would be different, as follows:

Deep in the heart of the script, past the legs, chest and arms would lay a series of blank pages - no script, no photos. Chapter 12 on "Strengthening Lower Backs" would be empty. Why? Nothing traditional works - which doesn't mean there isn't a solution.

Figure 1 shows the results of a three-part test of the isolated muscles that extend the lumbar spine - a pre-exercise test, an exercise and a post-exercise test. The top curve (#1) depicts a subject's fresh strength determined by a static test on a MedX® Lumbar Extension machine; the bottom curve (#2), a test of his exhausted strength following an exercise on the same. His fresh strength was reduced an average of 18.4% by the performance of six repetitions.

In contrast, Figure 2 represents the same three-part test with the exercise portion performed on a Nautilus® Low Back machine. The post-exercise test (Curve #2) shows an average increase in strength of 2.5% throughout the range of motion, with the exception of a slight decline in full extension (left side of chart). Eleven repetitions to fatigue had virtually no effect on the status of fresh strength.

Combined, the charts clearly illustrate the effect of specific vs. non-specific exercise. The MedX machine targets low-back muscles by preventing pelvic rotation. The benefits of the Nautilus machine are directed to hip muscles, namely gluteus and hamstrings.

The charts were produced amid manufacturer's claims that commercial low-back tools - copies of the Nautilus machine - and other forms of lumbar exercise using Roman chairs, Swiss Balls and hyperextensions 'worked.'

They were wrong.

In 1997, a research study conducted at the University of Florida examined muscle activation of the erector spinae, gluteus maximus and hamstrings during sub-maximal repetitions of isolated and non-isolated exercise (MedX vs.

Roman-chair extensions and straight-leg dead lifts). The Roman chair elicited the highest activation (recorded by surface electromyography). The investigators then examined the effect of the same non-isolated exercises on isolated lumbar strength and found that only MedX provided increases in full-range isolated lumbar strength. Dead lifts showed a partial effect, in flexion; the Roman chair, little or no effect.

A recent study by Dr. J. Graves (*Archives of Physical Medicine and Rehabilitation*, 1999) concluded that pelvic restraint was *not* required to promote neural drive to the lumbar muscles during sub-maximal work on a MedX machine. Yet, Graves agreed: (1) his was not a training study; (2) neural drive is not necessarily related to training effect (non-specific exercise may elicit notable neural activity without strengthening lumbar muscles); and (3) EMG analysis is not an accurate means of determining adaptation.

In the end, if it ever comes, exercise on a MedX machine will be recognized as the *only* way to stimulate full-range strength in the muscles that extend the spine.

Until then, more blank pages, please.

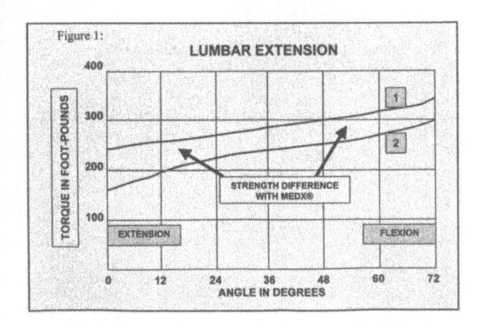

Figure 1:

LUMBAR EXTENSION

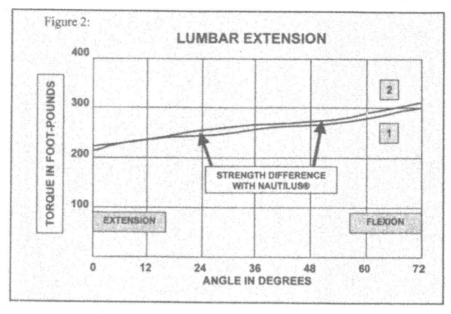

Figure 2:

LUMBAR EXTENSION

DECEMBER 7

### Trunk Extension Dilemma

Gary Reinl and I had three things in common when first tested on the MedX® Lumbar Extension machine: the same first name; muscles that were below average in strength despite a long history of strength training that included low-back exercise; and curiosity. That's where it ended.

While my back muscles were normal, Gary wasn't as lucky. His test - conducted at "The Challenge of the Lumbar Spine" (New York City, 1987) - revealed an abnormal strength curve, a high percentage of fast-twitch muscle fibers and poor recovery ability.

It motivated him to turn it around.

Gary returned home, trained three times a week on a Cybex® Low Back machine and became very strong. Four years later, he visited Florida and re-tested on the MedX device. His low back was 22% weaker with the same abnormal strength curve. He then trained for a year on a Nautilus® Low Back machine, was tested again on the MedX and produced the same result. The next year, he switched to a Nautilus (Second-Generation) Low Back machine and tested again - more deterioration.

Despite progressively heavier weights on each machine, an awareness of his needs and plenty of hard work, the muscles that extended his trunk steadily lost strength for six years. Why? They had never been used. Traditional low-back exercise increases hip and rear-thigh strength, but fails to stimulate the muscles that extend the spine.

"So far," claimed MedX inventor Arthur Jones, "we have found only two exceptions to that general rule: One, so-called 'hyper extension' movements performed on a simple bench called a 'Roman Chair,' and two, water-ski activities; but, in both cases, any resulting increases in lower-back strength are produced only near the fully extended position of the movement."

The reason is lack of isolation and leverage. A maximum resistance for the large hip muscles is not enough to stimulate the muscles of the lumbar spine due to the mechanical advantage provided by its joint system.

"A very similar situation exists in your arm muscles," said Jones. "Your upper-arm muscles move your forearm around the axis of the elbow joint, while your forearm muscles move your hand around the axis of the wrist joint, and since the resistance in a curling or triceps exercise is imposed against the hand, that is to say, beyond the wrist joint, it might appear that exercise for the upper-arm muscles would also develop the forearm muscles, but in fact this does not happen...the wrist joint has an enormous mechanical advantage when compared to the elbow joint...The result being that a maximum level of resistance for upper-arm muscles is not high enough to even be noticed by the forearm muscles because of the mechanical advantage of the wrists."

"Both lumbar muscles and forearm muscles," he concluded, "can be strengthened only with isolated exercise."

Reinl and I strapped a number of potential solutions on our backs, only to discover they didn't work. My 4-year stint on a Nautilus Low Back machine was eventually replaced by an ongoing, 17-year stint with the MedX.

"'Trial and error?' Absolutely," said Jones, "since nothing else works. Design it, build it, strap it on your back and head off down the runway...then it will either fly or it won't; but until you try it you will never know for sure."

Two Garys know. The job can't be done in a gym.

## DECEMBER 8

### Appropriate and Inappropriate Exercise x 2

Trial and error goes a long way in determining what works and, more often, what doesn't in exercise. It also helps justify the radically different paths athletes take to reach what appears to be the same end. Its only drawback is time, which steers many to exercise 'experts' or to research publications - neither a great choice.

The only thing the experts agree upon is that no two people are alike - what works for one may not work for another, which makes the use of identical twins (scarce in research) the only meaningful way to evaluate the effectiveness of an exercise program.

In 1985, Nautilus[®] inventor Arthur Jones conducted a 20-week research project with 12 sets of identical twins in an effort to determine the most effective way to strengthen the quadriceps (front thigh) muscle. He first tested the isolated quadriceps strength of all participants through a complete range-of-motion and then exercised each twin using what he called an 'appropriate' resistance (based upon fresh strength levels) - one that led to momentary failure at 10-12 repetitions. Immediately after the exercise, all subjects were re-tested to determine what strength remained. Some pairs of twins lost more than 40% of their strength after only 3-4 repetitions, while others showed no fatigue after more than 30 reps.

Jones realized that the difference reflected muscle fiber-type - a genetic factor. Excess fatigue from brief exercise indicated a higher than average percentage of 'fast-twitch' (fast-fatigue) fibers. Little or no fatigue from a lot of exercise indicated an abundance of 'slow-twitch' (slow-fatigue) fibers. In prior studies, 70% of a random group of people lost approximately 2% strength per repetition when exercised to failure, an average rate of fatigue.

Following the initial screening, the twins were divided into three groups: fast-twitch, slow-twitch and average. Each group was assigned what was considered an 'appropriate' repetition scheme for their fiber-type. Average subjects performed 8-10 repetitions; slow-twitch, 15-20; and fast-twitch, 3-6.

After that determination, one twin was exercised twice a week for 10 weeks with an 'appropriate' repetition pattern while the other worked with an 'inappropriate' one (for example, high repetitions for a fast-fatigue subject). After 10 weeks, all subjects were carefully tested to determine their progress. As expected, those who exercised with an appropriate number of repetitions produced better results than those who exercised with an inappropriate system.

The siblings then switched programs for another 10 weeks. The twin who changed to an appropriate exercise regimen produced a rapid increase in strength, while the one who switched to an inappropriate scheme lost strength...

... with one exception.

One twin (of a pair of 30-year-old males) who produced an expected result during the first 10 weeks of training continued to produce a result superior to that of his brother, regardless of repetition pattern. Because all sessions were carefully supervised and pushed, the odd result could not have been due to lack of cooperation.

Encountering one of the few surprises in muscle physiology with identical twins, Jones replied, "It happened, but we don't know why."

Unless you have a twin to ask, only you can determine what is 'right' and 'wrong' for you - and that information can best be gained by trial and error.

## DECEMBER 9

### Treatment for Back Pain – A Study

Got a low-back problem? Find a MedX® machine.

Over the years, doctors and therapists have recommended a variety of exercises for the treatment of chronic back pain, yet few have examined their value. Are they effective at all? Are they effective in the long run?

According to Brian Nelson, MD, "the best designed study on the treatment of low back pain with specific back exercises" was conducted at the Rehabilitation Foundation in Helsinki, Finland by Harkapaa, Mellon and others in 1990. The major aim of the study was to determine whether professional intervention using therapeutic back exercises had any long-term effect. The 2½-year study involved 476 blue-collar workers and farmers whose major health problem was back pain. It monitored: the degree of pain; the amount of disability (work days lost); compliance with self-care (performing exercise at home); and physical measurements of strength and flexibility in the hip and lumbar areas.

The subjects were randomly divided into three groups and examined by a rehab doctor and physical therapist. The first group ('inpatients') received three weeks of *daily* treatment that included instruction in the proper execution of exercises from therapists and personal attention from doctors. The patient-to-professional-staff ratio was 7:1. At specified intervals for the remainder of the study, the patients returned for a 'refresher' program of back exercises, relaxation techniques, stretching, strengthening, instruction in proper work-posture, heat, massage, electrotherapy treatments and discussions on back care by a physician.

The second group ('outpatients') took part in a twice-a-week, two-month program that was similar to, but less extensive than the inpatient group. Training took place in local health clubs or at work during hours. Patients were not attended by physicians but were given exercise instruction and brief follow-up visits (at the same interval as inpatients) by physical therapists. Outpatients received no massage, heat or modality treatments, and performed no stretching or strengthening exercises.

The third group ('control') received written and oral instruction on back exercises (including frequency, duration and sequence) but no hands-on practice from doctors or therapists, or professional counseling at any time. Like the others, they were tested five times during the study to collect data on the correct performance of exercise, compliance to frequency, hip and back strength and flexibility, and disability claims.

The use of three groups addressed several questions unanswered by traditional studies. Was daily care effective or necessary? Would constant supervision make a difference? Would less supervision be better than no supervision? Would the therapist/patient rapport matter? If exercises were effective, would they remain so long-term?

**Results**: During the first three months, there was a significant decrease in disability and back pain in both monitored groups. Thereafter, despite the fact that compliance was superior throughout the study in those groups, there was no difference and no perceivable trend. There was also "no demonstrable effect at any time during the study" in regard to strength and flexibility increases - a lot of effort, but no result.

Compare that to my result with the MedX tool: exercise, 90 seconds a month; strength increase, 100+%; flexibility, full-range; pain, none for 17 years; work-days missed, none; therapeutic modalities, none; massages, none; stretching, hardly.

Like the MedX inventor said, "It's like comparing the Concorde® to an ox cart."

## DECEMBER 10

---

### Fear

Arthur Jones often related the story of a Biblical king who wished to build a temple on a mountainside. The task involved the transport of heavy boulders up steep terrain. The man selected to head the project gathered 1,000 laborers and began. That evening, he approached the king.

"Your Highness, the boulders are too heavy. We cannot move them up the mountain."

"Kill half the men," the king replied.

The men were killed; the temple was built.

According to Jones, fear is the greatest motivator - and Arthur could motivate.

During a medical conference he hosted in Ocala, Florida, the MedX® inventor mentioned that one of his research subjects, Scott Leggett, was due at noon to perform a weekly exercise on the lumbar machine. He expected Scott to complete 10 repetitions with a weight that was heavy for a man his size. Leggett appeared on time and removed his coat. Jones supplanted a formal greeting with a concrete stare.

"Scott, I fully expect you to get 10 repetitions with 200 foot-pounds today. Do you understand?"

Scott had no choice; he made 10 - barely.

On another occasion, Jones requested a volunteer to demonstrate muscle fatigue on a leg machine. Of the few hands that rose, he selected one that looked least likely to die. The young man dropped his notepad, rushed up and, between the pressure of performing before a crowd and that of Jones insulting his manhood, produced the expected effort, if not the result. His carcass was dragged back to its notepad.

Only full-out efforts were accurate and meaningful in research. And seeing it live left little doubt - Arthur squeezed *every* statistic from *every* subject.

He took the same approach in the field of medicine where accuracy and accountability were greater issues. There was money at stake, and people lie for money. The accuracy of his tools in measuring the strength of low-back muscles had been well documented through research at the University of Florida. The issue was patient reliability. People could fake a test or memorize an effort that matched expectations.

Jones solved that issue by installing a lie-detection system in the software to identify 'malingering.' If you failed to cooperate, he knew exactly when and where.

It was done in one of two ways:

A. By use of a random test scale (from 100-2,000 foot-pounds) where the same effort (if less than cooperative or memorized) produced a torque shoot on the screen (seen by the patient) that sputtered at one angle and exploded at another. Other than the first of seven test angles, there were no lines on the screen to gauge effort.

B. By use of a standard scale during one test and a different scale on subsequent tests. If a patient memorized his effort by the lines on the screen during a test, and produced his 'normal' strength curve, he was dead in his tracks - the scale had changed.

The information was valuable in the detection of non-cooperative subjects and false injury claims, but too many attorneys screamed. It could have saved insurance companies a lot more than the time and money spent filming disabled back patients on water skis.

Jones was in the film business in the 1950's, but would not have wasted film on that nonsense.

Arthur carried a gun...and could probably find out where you lived.

## DECEMBER 11

### The Appearance of Strength

Dr. Squat (nicknamed 'Didley' for his perceived knowledge of exercise - and called D hereafter) asked to test the strength of his front thigh muscles during the demonstration of a prototype leg machine at MedX® headquarters in Ocala, Florida. At the time, he held the world record for a barbell squat (at or near 1,000 pounds) and was only months away from another attempt. MedX chairman Arthur Jones was curious to see what the champion had.

D gathered himself as the machine's movement arm was set in the first test position. He pressed his lower leg hard against the padded arm to register a force. The exertion - the only sound to eclipse the clash of egos present - could be heard in the adjacent building. With several assistants and computer feedback urging him on, D repeated the process at seven different angles.

His legs, according to Jones, "looked like two barrels in a pair of shorts," and both trembled as he turned a deep red, his efforts in vain. "When are you going to push that damned thing?" prodded Jones. "That's worse than my Grandmother and she's been dead for 40 years." D pressed on with the same result. His strength was less than that of some women Jones had tested, which left observers scratching their heads.

The subject demanded a re-test.

Next morning, a more motivated D produced exactly the same result. Jones then tested his fiber-type on an isokinetic (motorized) machine and concluded that D's thigh muscles consisted primarily of endurance (slow-twitch) fibers - excellent for a marathon runner, lousy for a power-lifter. Arthur offered to test his hamstring and gluteus muscles. The champion refused and left.

"His hamstrings had to be opposite in fiber-type (primarily fast-twitch)," said Jones. "If not, he probably couldn't lift himself out of a chair." But the question remained: "How could a man squat 1,000 pounds with weak thighs?" The 'go-to' muscles in the squat, according to Jones, are the butt and rear thigh. D must have had his power there and minimized the contribution of quadriceps in his lifting style.

Muscle fiber-type is a measure of how quickly muscles fatigue. Seventy to eighty percent of skeletal muscle has an average mix of both slow-twitch (endurance) and fast-twitch (strength) fibers. When exercised, that mix loses approximately 2% of its strength per repetition, making 8-15 an optimal repetition range for best results. A predominantly fast-twitch muscle demonstrates greater than average strength, but fatigues quickly, and responds better to fewer repetitions. A muscle with an abundance of slow-twitch fibers demonstrates a high capacity for endurance, but poor strength, and responds better to a higher repetition scheme. The majority of D's training was typical of power-lifters - heavy weight, few repetitions. To strengthen his front thighs, he should have performed a high number of repetitions.

Muscle fiber-type is genetic and explains, among other factors, how a thin person can lift more than the gym gorilla. Despite the claims of some research studies in muscle physiology, radically different repetition schemes or movement speeds have no effect on altering the fatigue characteristics of a muscle. Athletes are born, not made - and their strength, or lack thereof, is not always apparent.

Dr. Squat broke his own record two months later on quadriceps only a distance runner could appreciate.

DECEMBER 12

---

## The Appearance of Strength – The Aftermath

Arthur Jones liked horses - had a few on his ranch among a bevy of exotic creatures - but didn't like horseplay.

In the winter of 1986, he signed a contract with Joe Weider and Fred Hatfield (Dr. Squat) to publish an unedited article in one of Weider's magazines. "Exercise 1986: The Present State of the Art, Now a Science" revealed, among other discoveries, the effect of muscle fiber-type on exercise. Days later, Jones flew Hatfield to Ocala to attend a seminar on the same. He measured the strength of Hatfield's front thighs and found an abundance of endurance fibers, a fact mentioned by Jones in related articles.

Years later, Hatfield published his version of the story. "No less a personage than Arthur Jones said it (the predominance of endurance fibers in his quadriceps) in one of his never-less-than-incredible diatribes in one of the other muscle mags. Said Mr. Jones, 'Hatfield's quads are the weakest I've ever tested.'...The self-proclaimed greatest exercise physiologist who ever lived did indeed test my quads at his gator-infested airstrip in Ocala. Rather than incite his ire, I submitted to being tested. Hey! What would you have done? And I didn't have the guts to tell Arthur, who was at the time reputed to be packing a concealed revolver. So, I obligingly grimaced and pushed with what appeared to be great effort. Arthur appeared content. Little did I know that the bogus data he collected would find its way into one of his half-baked training theories!" ("The Days of Whines and Poses," *Muscular Development*, July, 1995).

Jones replied: "It was not my idea to test his strength; quite the contrary, he insisted on being tested; then, when the first test indicated a very low level of strength in his quadriceps muscles, he was literally stunned by the results. Then he insisted upon a second test that was conducted about 24 hours after the first. And, guess what?...his second test results were almost identical. At the time I told him...'Look, Fred, if 20 years of hard training has not done it, then 24 hours certainly won't do it.'"

"I have never said that he was 'the weakest subject I ever tested,'" he continued, "but I have tested several women who were stronger than he was, in spite of the fact that they weighed less than half as much as he did. During his visit, in attempts to demonstrate just how smart he was (and how dumb we were), Fred raised several points which he assumed would be new to us. But every time he mentioned one of these factors, I immediately whipped out a copy of an article on that subject that I had published 15 years earlier."

The testing tool Jones used was not perfect, but close. It was equipped with what he called a 'whimpometer' that provided information about effort. "You may be able to fool the person conducting the test," he said, "but you cannot fool the testing machine... Hatfield almost busted a gut in his attempt to produce as high a test result as possible."

About the revolver (which Jones had a permit to carry)? "I look upon a pistol in much the same way that I do a tourniquet: you hope that you will never need one, but if you do then you need it badly, need it quickly, and nothing will take its place."

Jones left an open challenge. "For a cash bet of $10,000.00, I will retest his quadriceps strength in comparison with a man who weighs more than 60 pounds less than he does, and give him another clear example of just how strong quadriceps muscles are capable of being, provided they have the right type of fibers." He concluded by saying, "So...having heard from the other end, you have now heard from the horse's mouth."

Jones' article was never published, and Hatfield has yet to knock on Arthur's door.

## DECEMBER 13

### More Gain, Less Pain, No Brain

We hunch, shuffle and moan. There's no spring in our step, joy in our greeting or future in sight. When our back is 'out,' nothing matters.

We deal with it in different ways. Some are quick to bring it up each time an occasion presents itself; others try to hide the notion that they have a problem at all. Most of us have been there; it's not fun - and neither is the cure.

Exercise has recently come into vogue with the medical community as a treatment alternative for back pain - which doesn't imply that we have left the dark-ages behind. As someone once said, "Much hath been done, but more remains to do."

"How much?", "How often?", "How hard?" and "What kind?" are exercise questions that doctors no longer need to search. In the area of back pain, the groundwork has been laid - and answers provided - by the MedX® inventor.

From the time he started 'weightlifting' in the 1930's, Arthur Jones became a staunch ally of exercise. His research throughout the 1970's and 1980's led him to conclude that, in the case of the muscles that extend the lumbar spine, not just any exercise would do. It had to be specific (isolated), direct, brief, infrequent, intense and progressive.

How did he find out? He built tools to isolate and strengthen the muscles of the spine, discovered the most efficient and effective ways to use them, and spread the word. Some claimed he got lucky along the way: Stronger muscles meant less pain.

It was something Jones expected.

The accompanying graphs show the effect of proper exercise on pain perception.

Figure 1 compares the strength levels of 150 males following a 12-week protocol of exercise on a MedX Lumbar Extension machine. The upper curve represents the average strength level of 46 patients who were subjectively "pain free" (on a pain-perception rating scale). The middle curve shows the average of 78 patients reporting "reduced pain;" and the lower curve, the average of 26 who reported "no change" in pain.

Figure 2 demonstrates the same with 111 females. The upper curve shows the average strength of 23 patients who were "pain free;" the middle curve, the average of 67 with "reduced pain;" and the lower curve, the average of 21 who reported "no change" in pain.

The subjects in the study (150 males and 111 females) were patients of orthopedic surgeon, Dr. Michael Fulton, and represented less than one third of over 900 patients he treated for chronic low-back pain in a two-year period.

A good look at the curves raises some questions. Did the patients represented by the lower and middle curves not reach the same strength level as the "pain-free" group because their pain did not allow them to push with a maximum effort? Perhaps, but it doesn't matter. The charts clearly show that, as back strength increases (whether limited by pain or genetic potential), the likelihood of pain decreases.

The combined group (all 261 patients) produced the following statistics: 26.4% became "pain free;" 55.5% had a reduction in pain perception; and 18% had no improvement - similar to those of other clinical and research studies.

Approximately 80% of people report a reduction in pain perception following a 12-week protocol on the MedX machine; 30-33% become "pain free."

The protocol is heaven as exercise goes: two sessions of two minutes each per week for the first four weeks, followed by one session a week for eight more weeks.

Simple and effective, the chance of improvement is too great to ignore.

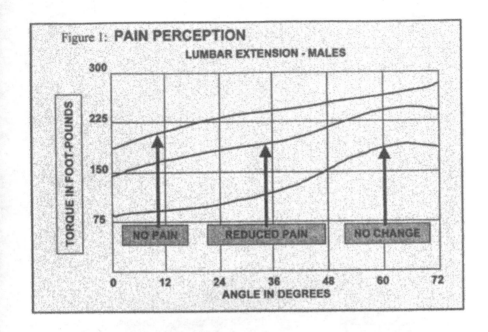

Figure 1: **PAIN PERCEPTION**
LUMBAR EXTENSION - MALES

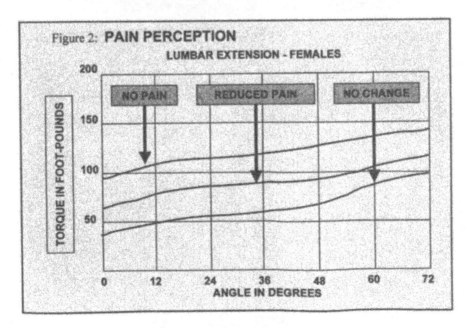

Figure 2: **PAIN PERCEPTION**
LUMBAR EXTENSION - FEMALES

DECEMBER 14

---

## Believe It or Else

"You should try the MedX® machine to strengthen your back," suggested the employee in an apologetic tone. "Once a week for two minutes is all it takes."

"There's no way," responded a man who had spent enough hours performing exercise to know better.

"That's what I did when I had my problem, and it worked."

The reply had the impact of a breeze on a boulder.

"And maintenance is only once a month," he added.

The boulder tripled in size.

Greg Norman's reaction to the exercise protocol on the MedX Lumbar Extension machine was like that of the protocol's inventor, Arthur Jones, in response to a statement that had proved itself true in research: "If you had told me that 20 years ago, it would have been the end of the conversation and the beginning of a fight."

Norman has a problem common among golfers, a bad back. Every week on tour a few players withdraw because of back-related injury. Weeks ago, paramedics whisked an agonizing Hale Irwin from the 2003 US Open in Chicago and there were doubts that Fred Couples would finish. Davis Love, Ernie Els, Larry Mize, Jim Furyk - the list goes on, and yes, Mr. Norman.

Before the above conversation took place (approximately April, 2003), Greg Norman had never heard of the MedX machine, astounding in one way - it has performed near miracles since 1986 - but not in another. The PGA Tour fitness van with its entourage of specialists and trainers has managed to prove what Jones has for the last two decades - that you can't fix a back with the wrong tool.

On November 29, 2002, I performed 86 seconds of exercise on the MedX machine with a resistance of 190 foot-pounds. On January 12, 2003, following six weeks of no back exercise, I performed the same weight for 106 seconds. Twenty seconds (two reps) more under load is not hard to believe. It's been happening for 17 years - one month, a few seconds more; the next month, a few less. The muscles that extend the lumbar spine increase and maintain strength with *infrequent* exercise - a blessing to anyone whose quality of life, if not livelihood depends on a healthy back.

Norman's long-time trainer has written a book about golf fitness, one of many on the market. The section on back strengthening (in all such books) uses a traditional approach despite the fact that it doesn't work. And it is FACT. Traditional exercises fail to target the low-back muscles, fail to provide a meaningful stimulation. If it was my book, the low-back section would be brief to the extreme - one picture and an introduction: "You can't strengthen your back in a gym or at home. You need this tool (see photo)."

Greg Norman has always been a wonderful spokesman for golf - intelligent, articulate, successful and demanding. In his ongoing search for a solution, he has recently hooked up with a group in Pittsburgh that uses a 'special' treatment. I suggested (through an associate of his) that he call Dr. Michael Fulton and hook up with something he likes to do, exercise - specific, isolated exercise on an *appropriate* tool.

"A single experience," said Arthur Jones, "can trigger a thought pattern that leads out of a blind alley...and having emerged into the light, you then have the opportunity to examine the involved factors."

The legendary boat designer and golfer is missing the boat on this one.


# DECEMBER 15

---

## Row, Row, Row Your Boat

I was born and raised near St. Catharines, Ontario, a city steeped in the tradition of competitive rowing. From early morning outings, running and strength training to the grind of competition, there was nothing easy about it, as Ian Hay described in 1909.

"Faster and faster grew the stroke...never had they traveled like this. Six was rowing like a man possessed. Four had ceased to encourage himself, and was plugging automatically with his chest open and his eyes shut. Bow may or may not have been singing: he was certainly rowing. There was a world of rolling and splashing..."

And when they crossed the line, "The eight men let go their oars and tumbled forward on to their stretchers, and listened, with their heads and hearts bursting, to the din that raged on the bank...the Stroke lay doubled up over his oar, with his head right down in the bottom of the boat, oblivious to everything save the blessed fact that he need not row any more...At the other end Bow, with his head clasped between his knees, was croaking half-hysterically to himself." ("Going Head of the River," from *A Man's Man*)

It takes a man to row. The sustained pull from the large muscles of the upper back and the forceful extension of the legs, hips and torso produces a cardiovascular effect that few can fathom, let alone handle. I grew up believing that rowers were conditioned athletes - until Dr. James Graves came along.

In 1994, Dr. Graves performed a study at Syracuse University that examined the isolated strength of the muscles that extend the lumbar spine. He tested 16 *elite* male rowers from the collegiate team on a MedX® Lumbar Extension machine and examined their performance on a rowing ergometer (a 5,000-meter time trial of about 18 minutes).

Graves compared the strength results to norms of untrained men, found them "marginally higher at full extension, but not statistically significant" and concluded, "Rowing does not develop a significant amount of lumbar extension strength."

He then compared the results to performance and found that the strongest rowers did not exhibit the best endurance on the ergometer. In general, stronger muscles fatigued more quickly (and the low back is one of the weak links in the rowing chain).

The study concluded with an electromyographic analysis and comparison of the activation of the paraspinal muscles (those adjacent and parallel to the spine) during rowing vs. exercise on the MedX device. It was no contest.

In a follow-up (1995), Dr. Graves studied the effect of MedX training on strength gains and pain perception in 10 experienced rowers vs. 10 inexperienced rowers. In a 10-week protocol (that included the same ergometer test), inexperienced rowers increased strength by 25%, while experienced rowers showed no increase (a control group of rowers lost 28% strength). Despite that, *all* trained subjects increased their performance and reported a reduction in pain perception. The conclusion: Athletes at all levels benefit from the increased strength provided by the MedX machine.

That experienced rowers gained no strength is not unique. A female patient in Caracas showed a 1% decrease in back strength with 13 weeks of MedX exercise, yet was pain free after 6-8 visits. She was above average in strength to start and had difficulty recovering from the protocol (1X/wk., 2 min.). Less exercise may have been better.

Few activities, if any, recruit the muscles that extend the lumbar spine as effectively as MedX exercise. It may have a positive effect on symptoms, even when it fails to elicit vast gains in strength - which should send a few back theories gently down the stream.

# DECEMBER 16

---

## Ratio of Strength to Muscle Endurance

In his world of muscle testing, Arthur Jones left no room for error. He cared little about the outcome ("Let the chips fall where they may"), was meticulous about the process and demanded one thing from subjects - cooperation.

This guy didn't get the message.

In hundreds of strength/endurance tests, the MedX® inventor found that most people were able to perform approximately 10 repetitions using 80% of their maximum force output. This guy barely made *one*, which triggered accusations that ranged from "lazy" and "uncooperative" to a bevy of expletives. It took several test sessions to realize that the man was doing his best. His results were simply different.

Jones spent decades on the development of tools to isolate muscle function, and routinely measured strength immediately before and after exercise to determine muscle fatigue characteristics and strength/endurance ratios.

The majority of subjects demonstrated the following: if they could lift 100 pounds once, they could perform 10 repetitions with 80 pounds (80% of their maximum), reflecting a strength loss of about 2% per repetition. The strength/endurance ratio remained unaffected by an increase or decrease in strength, which meant that once the strength of a muscle was known, its anaerobic (local muscular) endurance could be determined. Conversely, muscle strength could be predicted from a known performance of muscle endurance (the number of repetitions in a set).

Not all subjects demonstrated the same ratio. One world-class tri-athlete performed 34 repetitions using 80% of her maximum tested strength. She also mentioned that she had an identical twin sister with whom she lived, ate and trained. Months later, Jones tested her twin, and without knowledge of her sister's performance, the twin produced exactly the same result - 34 repetitions with 80% of her maximum tested strength. She also produced the same number of repetitions (as her sibling) using percentage levels other than 80. 'Identical' means just that.

Jones used another method to test the same. He measured the torque output of a first repetition (a maximum effort) and rated subsequent full-out repetitions as percentages of the first using computer technology. In the case of the endurance twins, the first repetition with their right quadriceps (front thigh) produced 100% torque. Their sixth produced 109% (9% more than the first), then remained at a level above 100% for 12 repetitions. Little or no fatigue from prolonged exercise demonstrated a typical slow-twitch (slow-fatigue) response to exercise.

In contrast, another subject demonstrated a loss of 27% from his first three full-out efforts. Excess fatigue from brief exercise reflected a typical fast-twitch (fast-fatigue) response.

After testing more than 10,000 subjects, Jones was stunned by the magnitude of the range of individual differences. The implications for training were clear:

- Fast-twitch subjects showed a higher initial level of strength, but fell off rapidly with fatigue. They couldn't stand much exercise.
- Extreme slow-twitch subjects were weaker but almost immune to fatigue (could tolerate a lot of exercise). Their training had to be unique.

The research helps explain why some people produce extremely good results from strength training and others don't.

## DECEMBER 17

### Lousy Rehab

Some people listen; some don't. Sometimes it doesn't matter one way or the other.

The best time to catch an ear, though it may be selective, is when there's injury. People listen better in rehab centers than gyms; and females listen better than males.

Larry was a case in point. He had the worst form of anyone I'd seen in a gym. My co-workers agreed and threw in the fact that Larry was, as we say in Spanish, "un caso perdido" - a lost cause. He was. Regardless of what I said or how I said it, he continued to exceed the speed limit *during* exercise. It was hard to believe that someone could make a machine move that fast.

What was more difficult to believe, however, was the speed he adopted on the MedX® Lumbar and Cervical Extension machines, rehabilitative exercise for the spine. Larry proceeded at such a slow pace that technicians needed a nudge to remove him when he was done, always on his own time. Larry had his own protocols - four minutes on the Lumbar machine, three and a half on the Cervical - and performed both exercises once a week, though he'd been at it for nearly a decade.

Slow was great - someone must have hammered home the importance of controlled movements for his back and neck - but the protocol was poor. Larry required only one exercise a month on the Lumbar machine and one every two weeks on the Cervical. Money or not, when patients dictate protocols, it's lousy rehab.

Stan was another case. He listened, through no fault of his own, to the wrong instructions from a therapist who was equally not at fault. He was on the wrong equipment with, according to the manufacturer, the right instructions. The therapist just followed. Stan performed set after set of bone-jarring repetitions on an isokinetic leg-extension machine that he was lucky to survive. It was bad equipment, suicidal instruction, lousy rehab...and a habit he carried to the gym.

Figure 1 shows another result, this time of listening and good intent. The patient was on the right equipment, but obtained the wrong instructions.

The three curves represent static tests of quadriceps (front thigh) strength during a program of knee rehabilitation. The top curve (C) represents the fresh strength of the subject's normal leg (which is the standard by which progress of the injured limb is measured). The bottom curve (A) shows the fresh strength of the injured leg at the start of treatment; the middle curve (B), fresh strength of the same injured leg following a period of rehabilitation - lousy rehab.

The injured leg (as represented by Curve B) demonstrates a near total recovery of strength in flexion (right side of chart), but a level of strength far below normal in extension (left side of chart). This selective recovery was due to the performance of exercise restricted to the first 40° of movement, in flexion. Beyond that, the therapist feared increased compression forces on the knee - a false assumption. Compression forces are highest in flexion and lowest (to non-existent) in extension.

To avoid lousy rehab:
- Start with good equipment (broomsticks don't fix backs). Avoid isokinetic tools.
- If the test isn't static, don't take it. Avoid dynamic testing.
- If exercise (or testing) is conducted at high speeds, leave while you can.
- Stick with proven protocols. Don't do more "just to be sure."
- Find a therapist who knows his or her stuff, and then some. Intent matters little.

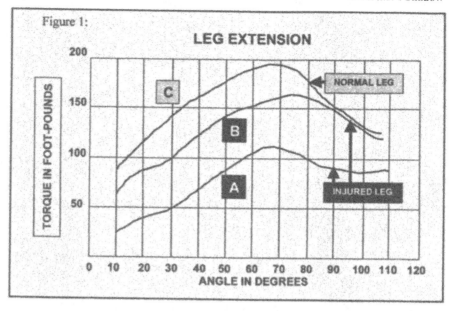

Figure 1:

LEG EXTENSION

DECEMBER 18

## I Miss the Education

I must have asked the wrong question. He edged forward with a deep-furrowed brow, eyes locked on mine. My collar shrunk as my heart thumped on a nearby rib. I was no match as he drew near, his resolution unwavering. A sudden waft of after-shave and nicotine merged with a stream of air from his upturned nostrils and warned that my fate was sealed. Arthur was in my face.

His gentle whisper turned to stone - louder, faster. He snatched my arm and stared me down the way Moby Dick must have Ahab before the final plunge. Five bone-deep fingers tried to raise me off the floor, but I was glued. Two more penetrated my temple as a gruff voice etched its message, "...and if I were to put a gun to your head and fire..." Knowing that he always carried a pistol, it felt like he had just used it.

After he made his point, he withdrew in the same calculated manner. Slowly, the scent, the breath, the grip, the voice, the heat, everything but my elevated physiology and those piercing eyes receded. At a comfortable distance he resumed a whisper, "Now, do you understand?"

Nautilus® inventor Arthur Jones was passionate about everything he did. He thrived on challenge, conflict and controversy, all of which he flew to his home on a daily basis in the form of people who "knew nothing about exercise" - doctors, therapists and anyone interested. His purpose was education, a bold undertaking for a man who quit school in the fourth grade, and who looked more like a janitor than a teacher.

A beady-eyed 5'8", his rounded shoulders generally sported a long-sleeve dress shirt while his belly buoyed a pair of Sansabelt® slacks always tight at the calf. The toes of his black-leather shoes turned up and splayed out like Charlie Chaplin. When he wasn't lecturing, he could be found curling the stub of an unfiltered Camel® in the palm of a discolored hand behind his back - vintage 1940.

In the spotlight, things were different.

Jones was a non-stop barrage of facts, people, numbers and stories aimed at reversing ignorance in the field of exercise. Every word, soft or emphatic, was delivered as if from a master script. Endless facts, intense opinions and ruthless insults flavored with an Oklahoma twang bellowed from the side of his mouth and continued through the five-star lunch he provided. With more facts spewing out than food going in, his genius commanded attention. His eye contact took no break.

Off-stage, the intensity continued. Delighting in the role of tutor, Arthur often sat the inquirer aside and drew a solution using his favorite props, a searched-for pen and napkin. He remained until it was certain you understood, no matter who you were.

Arthur's eccentric lifestyle was one of control and contrast. One moment, he towered over a crowd; the next, he was dwarfed by a hoard of exotic creatures (snakes, elephants, crocodiles, rhinos, gorillas), a fleet of commercial planes and a trail of wives. He made all the decisions, yet found time to write extensive, penetrating articles.

So, it came as a bit of a surprise to hear that he recently sold controlling interest in the company he created (MedX®) and sold off most of his animals. He then announced in the December (1997) issue of *Ironman* magazine, "...this is the last article I will ever write on the subject (of exercise)." Arthur had had enough.

His followers will miss his brilliance, passion for knowledge and brutal honesty. It's what made him loved, hated and special...even if you did ask the wrong question.

DECEMBER 19

---

## A Smart Move

The daylong attempt to move the one-ton beast sprawled in the back of the 10-wheeler had failed; the sun was fast descending. It was now or never. I hailed a passing tow-truck and secured the brute to a large hook. The truck dragged the cargo toward what light remained and steadied it for the final thrust. The driver nudged forward and out swung the monster, like a pendulum, over the dim streets of Caracas.

My first thought, "I just spent $60,000 on an exercise tool that's bobbing over some half-lit street in South America." My last, "Never again." I had also just spent five months dragging my right leg down the same street, the result of a nerve impingement in the low back. The monster represented a last-ditch effort at relief.

As if my condition wasn't bad enough, it took 13 hours to move the contraption to the fifth floor of an old building and four more to put it together next morning. Once in place (and once I had recovered), I performed two-minutes of exercise once a week and was pain-free in 20 weeks.

The MedX® Lumbar Extension machine was worth the effort. It also provided the opportunity to test 800 people and confirm what its inventor Arthur Jones had discovered about muscle fiber-type. Sixty percent of subjects lost approximately 2% of their starting strength per repetition (what he called an average rate of fatigue). Thirty percent fatigued more rapidly (due to a predominance of fast-twitch muscle fibers); and 10% fatigued at a slower rate (due to a predominance of slow-twitch fibers). My results (as a technician) revealed a higher percentage of slow-fatigue subjects for the following reasons:

- I used a single test that skewed results (2-3 tests are needed for reliability).
- I probably did not fatigue subjects as thoroughly as Jones during exercise.
- I lacked the technical skill during the testing protocol and allowed too much time between exercise and post-exercise tests. This made subjects appear to fatigue less than they had.
- I was unaware of the effect of atrophy on the rate of muscle fatigue.

According to Jones, 90% of the subjects he measured were in a state of chronic disuse atrophy - they had never used their lumbar muscles in a meaningful way. He also claimed that atrophy was selective: It affected a muscle's fast-twitch fibers to a greater degree than its slow-twitch fibers. Therefore, the test of an atrophied muscle produced a fatigue rate that was deceptively slow, and one that accelerated when the muscle's fast-twitch fibers were rejuvenated by exercise.

In November of 1989, I tested the fatigue characteristics of the Carrasco sisters, a trio of elite Venezuelan water-skiers. Anna Maria (World Champion, 1988) lost 28% of her strength after 13 repetitions to fatigue, an average rate. Esperanza lost 2.7% of her strength following 10 repetitions to fatigue, a slow rate. Maria Victoria (undefeated World Champion, 1972-1979) fatigued at a rate somewhere between her siblings.

According to Jones, professional water-skiers are the only athletes with above average strength in the low back (at least in extension), a product of their activity. Anna's greater strength and rate of fatigue (compared to that of her sisters) were due, perhaps, to her active status. Her retired siblings had suffered the effects of disuse atrophy (would have demonstrated less of a difference in fiber-type had they been active).

How quickly a muscle fatigues is not subject to change. Yet, the *apparent* variation with exercise continues to forge a debate that only the monster can solve.

## DECEMBER 20

### Who's Kidding Who?

Ed was short (about 5'5") and round (about 260 pounds) and wore an old, greasy baseball cap that was severely curved at the brim and pulled down in front. He must have parked the 18-wheeler in a nearby lot.

As instructed by his doctor, I tested his back strength on a MedX® Lumbar Extension machine. Ed's cautious reaction to the intimidating device was common; his strength was not. It was pitiful - but at the same time, his greatest asset.

"What do you do for a living?" I asked as I peeled him off the machine.

"I was a jockey for 27 years," a statement that required a lot of spine itself.

"Interesting," I thought as I pondered who rode whom. It was only the beginning.

Four weeks later, I surprised him with a test when he was expecting an exercise.

"It's not going to show that I'm better, is it?" he asked.

"I hope so. I think we've made some progress."

"Oh no!" he jumped (to use the term loosely). "My case is coming up in three weeks and I don't want anything to show I'm better." Ed had a fishing trip planned to Canada.

He wasn't alone.

Figure 1 demonstrates the average strength curves of two groups of males following a program of low-back rehabilitation on the same MedX machine. The upper curve shows the strength level of 103 patients not involved in litigation (average age, 43.4 years; treatment time, 129 days). The lower curve represents the strength of 47 patients involved in litigation (average age, 37.7 years; treatment time, 144 days).

Figure 2 demonstrates the same with two groups of female patients. The upper curve shows the average strength of 64 patients not involved in litigation (average age, 46.0 years; treatment time, 117 days). The lower curve represents the strength of 47 patients involved in litigation (average age, 37 years; treatment time, 133 days).

Patients in litigation were weaker throughout the range of motion (with a notable difference in extension, left side of chart) despite the advantage of 7+ years in age (younger) and 15+ days (more) in rehabilitation than those not in litigation.

One of three things occurred. Patients in litigation were: (1) actually weaker than their counterparts; (2) in such pain that they were unable to demonstrate higher levels of strength; or (3) non-cooperative during the tests, did not put forth an honest effort.

If I had to choose, it would be curtain # (3).

Years later, while working in a rehab center in Jupiter (Florida), a Pain Management Team of therapists, doctors and psychologists moved in to share the equipment. Their job was to rate disability and dismiss (with monies paid) patients in the Worker's Compensation system - patients 'in treatment' 6-8 hours a day.

First up was a man named "Lexus" whose effort on a treadmill that was barely alive could best be classified as 'pre-owned.' Next came "Prince" who, at 6'3" and 240 pounds, produced a rhythmic, grunting sound as he attempted to lift a *single* plate on a leg extension machine. "Fingerprints" (we called him) deserved jail for fraud.

Ironically, the only thing the Team did not try was the only thing that might have helped. A brief test on the MedX machine could have quickly determined the sincerity of the efforts and allowed countless others the opportunity to fish.

At a time when you literally can't pay people to do exercise, you can certainly pay them not to.

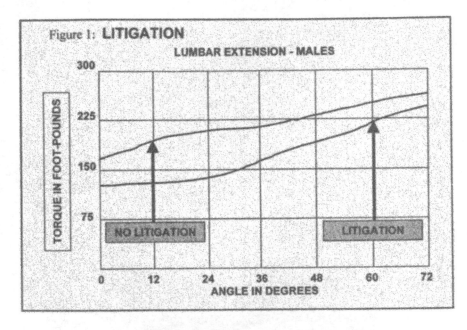

Figure 1: LITIGATION
LUMBAR EXTENSION - MALES

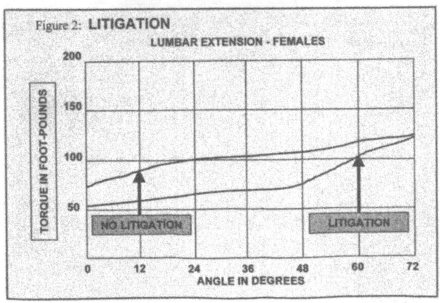

Figure 2: LITIGATION
LUMBAR EXTENSION - FEMALES

## DECEMBER 21

---

### ...*And God Laughs*

There was nothing ordinary about Arthur Jones. He was self-educated, outspoken, flamboyant, brash, opinionated and above all, honest.

The youngest son in a family of doctors, Arthur quit grade school early and spent, according to Ellington Darden, "much of his childhood reading medical books and applying what he read to the animals he caught in the fields and forests near Seminole, Oklahoma." As an adult, he pioneered an airline in South America and later developed an import-export business based upon the capture and sale of wild animals to circuses and zoos. The venture took him around the world and led to a career in the film industry and the production of his own TV series, "Wild Cargo." But his enterprise came to a halt when he was expelled from Rhodesia during political turmoil in 1968.

Down, but not out, Jones embarked on another passion that had intrigued him for years - exercise - specifically, the construction of a device that would directly stimulate his upper-back muscles. He left a trail of such prototypes in foreign jungles.

The machine he eventually built was scientifically sound and the success of Nautilus® - not planned or dreamed - became history. His contributions to the field of exercise stood the test of time, but the best was yet to come. He developed a tool that isolated and measured muscle function in a safe and accurate way - the MedX® Lumbar Extension machine, a 'miracle' in the prevention and treatment of chronic low-back pain.

Jones was a writer and a speaker, but when he retired, he left a void. "Our memory is not perfect," he said. "Sometimes we give ourselves credit for ideas that in fact we learned from somebody else. Which is not a lie but is, instead, an example of a failed memory. In an attempt to avoid that, I have been keeping detailed records of everything that I considered to be significant for more than fifty-five years; and, recently, these records became very useful to me, when I decided to attempt the writing of an autobiography. Throughout the last twenty-odd years several people tried to get me to write an autobiography, but I always refused; refused on the grounds that I do not believe it is now possible to publish the truth in today's 'politically correct' environment."

He must have softened his stance along the way.

"We all make mistakes, and God knows I have made at least my fair share of mistakes, but publishing lies serves no worthwhile purpose while doing a great deal of damage. My forthcoming autobiography, if it is ever published, is primarily an account of my mistakes; is not an attempt on my part to prove how smart I am, instead comes a lot closer to proving just how stupid I have been throughout most of my life. But me being stupid does not make other people smart; might, however, provide them an opportunity to learn from my mistakes without having to make similar mistakes themselves."

Then he warned. "Quite a long list of people will be outraged if and when my autobiography is published, because it is nothing short of being frank; and many people do not want to hear the truth, particularly if it concerns them. So, if it is ever published, you can count on it, there will be a massive outcry of rage from many of the people named therein. So be it, they have published their bullshit stories, now let them read the truth; none of which will help them because such people are beyond help, but might be of value to a lot of other people who are interested in the truth."

*And God Laughs*, the autobiography of Arthur Jones is out. When I read it, I can hopefully fill in the missing blanks - of which there are many - and learn.

## DECEMBER 22

### Impressions

I can forget the name of someone within seconds of an introduction, yet vividly recall encounters with sports figures and the 'famous.' But it was something beyond that when I met Nautilus® inventor, Arthur Jones.

You didn't just meet Jones; he met you, head on, and the impact - positive or negative - stuck. And the nice thing about it was, you didn't have to be there.

"I never had the honor of meeting Mr. Jones," said John Turner of Hamilton, Ontario. "I have had the privilege of speaking with him many times and corresponding with him. I no longer blindly accept anything I'm told or read. This is a gift beyond measure."

Years later, Turner spent a Florida afternoon with Jones, who he called "an amalgam of Howard Hughes, Vince Lombardi and Indiana Jones." When he left, he told Arthur, "No family member, friend, teacher or coach had the impact on my life you have," and added, "I was numb. It had been an honor to inhale that man's secondhand smoke."

Turner was not alone.

Joseph Mullen: "Anyone who has seen Arthur in action knows that he can be intense, demanding, profane, humorous, unsympathetic to bunglers, and possess a temper and tongue that can render an adversary senseless...There is nothing more valuable than a rational mind, capable of deductive logic and the inherent ability to educate others. His ability to perceive abstract concepts and integrate them into useful information is what sets him above his contemporaries."

Ellington Darden (who worked with Jones for 20 years): "The thing I remember most is his authoritative, commanding and powerful voice. He is by far the best speaker and storyteller that I've heard...there is no way I could condense his impact to several paragraphs. Thank you, Arthur, for living life in CAPITAL LETTERS."

Matt Brzycki: "Arthur is legendary for being opinionated, abrasive, rude, boisterous and other assorted adjectives...(yet) Arthur spoke the only language that hardhead party-liners understood. Arthur has probably had more detractors over the years than anyone. Yet, it's difficult to name someone else who has had such a profound impact on strength training. He changed the industry forever. Plain and simple."

Jim Bryan: "What most people don't know is that he has gone FAR out of his way to help people. I have seen him give time to strangers that turned up at Nautilus looking for answers (when it was obvious to me that these people were 'plants' from another exercise company)," and, "He just didn't like bullshit or bullshitters. If you were wasting his time, he would tell you straight out. You always knew where you stood."

Dave Schoffler (about Jones' *Ironman* magazine articles): "His straight forward way of explaining concepts was one of the things that kept me interested in his writings...sometimes a kick in the butt can do more than a pat on the back."

Brian Johnston (president IART): "I became certified with the ISSA, reaching one level in qualifications below Masters. Regardless,...nothing made sense, and there were numerous contradictions. One day I began speaking of speed strength, starting strength, explosive strength, anaerobic strength, etc., thinking that these concepts could be valuable aspects to training. Dr. Kudlak (who owned a MedX® clinic and credited Jones with teaching *him* how to think) looked at me dumbfounded, began to question me on their validity, and I quickly realized how little I (and the ISSA) knew."

Arthur Jones hit audiences like a sledgehammer. Few escaped unscathed.

# DECEMBER 23

---

## Looking Ahead

I once scraped through layers of paint to restore an 1891 scale in the same manner that Arthur Jones sifted through a century of myth in search of the bottom line in exercise - with one difference. What the Nautilus® inventor found wasn't pretty. There were no tools to work with and little interest in the same bottom line.

If you want to know where you're going, you have to know where you've been and where you are - which requires proper tools and renders the strength-testing segment of a fitness evaluation useless. You can't weigh yourself with a toaster.

"True muscular strength can be meaningfully tested in only one way," said Jones. "ONE, you must measure the level of torque produced by the force of muscular contraction; TWO, the muscle being tested must be totally isolated, so that force of contraction from other muscles does not influence the test results; THREE, you must determine the exact position in which a strength test was conducted, because even a slight change in position will either increase or decrease the output of torque; FOUR, you must remove the influence of nonmuscular torque that results from gravity acting upon the mass of the involved body parts; FIVE, you must avoid the influence of nonmuscular torque produced by muscular friction; SIX, you must measure the level of nonmuscular torque produced by stored energy, a very significant level of torque that would be produced even if you were trying to test the strength of a dead man; and having measured it, this level of nonmuscular torque must be added to or subtracted from the measured level of torque."

Jones developed tools (MedX®) that featured all the requirements for proper testing of the lumbar spine, cervical spine and knee. The fact that they were largely ignored leaves us with the current practice of estimating strength from the execution of several repetitions of non-specific exercise. Performing a set of leg presses to determine lower-body strength and chest presses for upper-body strength, for example, reveals about the same as a kindergarten sketch on a refrigerator door. The common result - 'world-class' lower-body and 'pitiful' upper-body strength - casts additional doubt on so-called norms.

Future testing tools must determine range of motion, true strength levels throughout the range (as outlined), specific response to exercise (Type S or Type G), and muscle fatigue and recovery rates. From that, trainers can establish an appropriate repetition scheme, initial resistance and training frequency.

Now, the bottom line. ONE, who has the intelligence to construct the needed tools? Manufacturers are still scratching their heads over the formula Jones handed them for a perfect form of exercise in 1970. TWO, it's a tough sell to a majority that favors tubing, Swiss balls and pulleys over machines; and prefers compound movements and functional training over isolation. THREE, it's a tougher sell to those who could make a difference - scientists and doctors who choose to ignore less educated sources. FOUR, according to one such source (Jones), "It is still not possible to accurately test the strength of all of your muscles, primarily because it is impossible to isolate all of your muscles."

One day, someone will unearth a MedX machine and declare (if they so recognize), "Hey, this culture had a machine to measure strength." Then, they will house it in a local museum instead of where it should have been from the start - in every household.

I hope your grandchildren are good at polishing toasters. The answers to important questions in exercise won't come anytime soon.


## DECEMBER 24

---

### The Great American Tragedy – Part 1

The expiration of patents on MedX® medical machines will soon unleash a flood of copied technology that, for the most part, has been ignored. The good news: 17 years may not be long enough for manufacturers to get it right, having failed to successfully copy Nautilus® machines 30 years ago. The bad: those who should be most interested - industry, government and insurance companies - never realized the value of the old.

Why should they be interested? It would save billions of dollars per year - enough, that if they had adopted inventor Arthur Jones' proposal in 1986, the government alone could have paid for both wars in Iraq 10 times over.

His equipment isolated and screened the muscles of the lumbar spine for potential problems. The test information answered the following questions (among others): How much can a worker lift in different positions? How long would he last in a lifting task? Who is at risk of having back problems? What is an appropriate job for a worker and why? Does a worker really have a back problem, or only claim to?

"Testing for potential lumbar problems," he claimed, "may soon be an insurance requirement for many occupations." And rightfully so. The MedX pre- and post-exercise strength test determined muscle endurance, range of motion, strength, fiber-type, work-capacity, curve shape and subject cooperation.

Figure 1 shows the pre- and post-exercise tests of a subject who Jones described as "at least twice as strong as an average individual." The top curve (A) represents his fresh strength level, before work; the bottom (B), his strength immediately following a low level of work (six reps with 200 ft.lb., 45% of what he was capable of lifting fresh, an exercise Jones described as "the equivalent of a large man doing only two deep knee bends with no resistance.") The exercise, continued to fatigue, reduced his starting strength by 54.9% (9.15% per repetition).

"His high level of strength in the muscles which extend the lumbar spine," he pointed out, "is not a result of great muscular size, is a result of the fiber type in these muscles. He has an abnormally high percentage of so-called fast twitch muscle fibers; a genetic factor which makes him very strong, while increasing the risk of injury...Employed in a position that involved even relatively light lifting on a continuing basis, this man would probably suffer from lower-back problems."

Figure 2 shows an individual at low risk of back problems, despite having only 40% of the former subject's strength. Curve (A) represents fresh strength; curve (B), strength immediately after *hard* exercise with a heavy resistance (six reps with 200 ft.lb., 100% of what he was capable of lifting fresh). Following exercise, he was 10.1% stronger.

Sixteen weeks later, he increased his overall strength by 70% (228% in extension) and range of motion by 8°, and was tested again. Curve (C) represents his fresh strength level; curve (D), strength after exercise - this time, 12.3% stronger. Hard work, no fatigue.

"With the use of proper, specific exercise," stated Jones, "the lower-back strength can be greatly increased in almost any individual; and increasing the strength in the lumbar muscles will reduce the chances of injury. But subjects in the high-risk group will still be likely to suffer from lumbar problems. Exercise will help, but cannot alter a genetic risk factor."

The MedX Lumbar Extension machine provided the information *and* the solution.

Yet, with the estimated annual cost of low-back problems at $120 billion and rising, people are still scratching their heads and waiting for the bad copies.

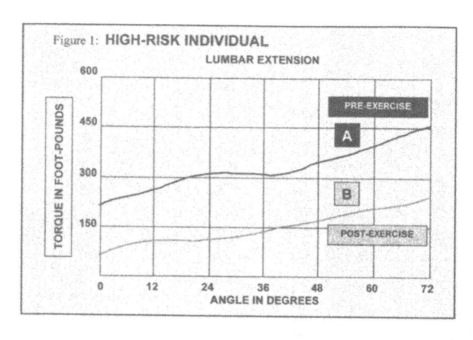

Figure 1: HIGH-RISK INDIVIDUAL

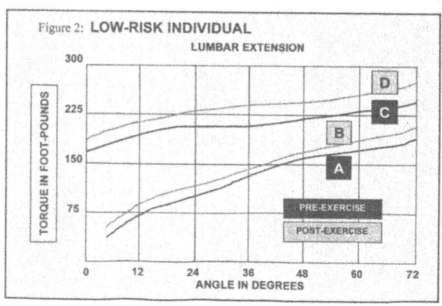

Figure 2: LOW-RISK INDIVIDUAL

# DECEMBER 25

---

## The Great American Tragedy – Part 2

In 1986, MedX® inventor Arthur Jones was convinced that proper, specific exercise for the lumbar spine was close to a 'cure-all' for low-back problems. Yet, its use as preventive medicine had been ignored. It was something he wanted to change.

He first developed a tool to isolate the muscles that extend the lumbar spine, identified risk factors and proposed pre-employment and job-placement screening for industry, insurance companies and government to detect *potential* problems.

The need was great. "Eighteen million annual lumbar tests is a conservative estimate," he said, "the number will probably be far higher; because the savings should run into the billions of dollars, so the tests will be performed...must be performed."

Jones sought to clarify testing and treatment protocols through research conducted at four major centers. "By the end of this year (1987) we should have completed testing of 30,000 subjects, and will test at least another 100,000 during 1988."

Prior to his lumbar machine, all low-back testing failed to weed out the large muscles of the hips and legs, which rendered the tests useless, misleading and dangerous. The muscles had to be isolated.

"Weakness in the large muscles of the buttocks and legs is not the problem;" he said, "on the contrary, the strength of these muscles may be the source of the problem in lower-back injuries. When these larger and far stronger muscles produce a high and dangerous level of force that is then imposed on the much weaker muscles of the lumbar area, then you frequently will have a problem."

When the small spinal muscles were isolated, their lack of exercise was apparent from their response. "Almost anybody," claimed Jones, "can increase the strength of these muscles to a degree, and at a rate, that was previously considered impossible."

Figure 1 shows the results of three specific exercises for the low-back muscles. The bottom curve (A) represents the fresh strength of a stronger-than-average subject; the top curve (B), his strength after three exercise sessions (one set of approximately 10 reps to failure, once per week). His strength increased 36.76%, or 12+% per session.

Figure 2 shows the results of another subject who increased his strength (from curve A to B) by 23.45% in 14 days, almost 12% per week. After 18 weeks, his strength increased 120% (73% in flexion, 300% in extension and 110% midway between).

The subject of Figure 2 (Part 1 of this article) increased his strength by 33% in flexion and 228% in extension, which shows that increases must be correlated with angles. Initial gains are greatest in the weakest positions (usually extension), but from the moment strength is restored throughout the range of motion, further gains are proportionate.

After screening, Jones recommended less than five minutes of exercise once a week. "Exercise will not change their (an industrial worker's) fiber type," he said, "will not remove some people from the high-risk group, but will increase both their functional and structural strength in these muscles, and will probably reduce their chances of injury."

Statistics confirmed his premise. Yet, to everyone's loss - especially those who suffer back pain and those likely to - the availability of specific lumbar testing failed to usher in new thinking. Could no one spare five minutes a week?

Last night, a friend called from Georgia concerning the unsuccessful back operation of his wife. Her neurosurgeon had never heard of MedX or Nautilus®. It's tough to sell pre-employment screening to people who are unaware of exercise.

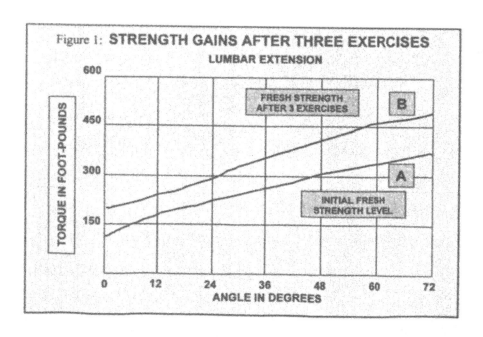

Figure 1: STRENGTH GAINS AFTER THREE EXERCISES
LUMBAR EXTENSION

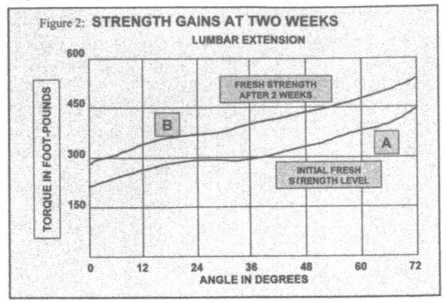

Figure 2: STRENGTH GAINS AT TWO WEEKS
LUMBAR EXTENSION

DECEMBER 26

## "The Challenge of the Lumbar Spine"

The slender, balding Dr. Graves had no cape or phone booth. At 6'2" and 185 pounds, the soft-spoken research professor was not likely to stand out in a crowd or bend steel with his bare hands. Yet, when he took center stage at "The Challenge of the Lumbar Spine," a gathering of the latest research on low-back problems (New York City, 1987), few were prepared for the fireworks.

The man who lit the fuse was Nautilus® inventor Arthur Jones, there to introduce his latest creation, the MedX® Lumbar Extension machine. Jones first tested the low-back strength of Dr. Graves and health-club owner, Joe Cirulli and found Joe nearly twice as strong on seven test angles. Both men then performed the same exercise - six repetitions with 200 foot-pounds of resistance, a weight that was light for Joe (relative to his starting strength) but heavy for Dr. Graves. After 53 and 54 seconds of exercise respectively, they re-tested to determine what strength remained. Joe had lost more than 50% of his starting strength, while Dr. Graves had gained 10% and was now stronger than Joe on five of seven test angles.

Prior to this, Jones had measured both men on numerous occasions. Regardless of the resistance used or the number of repetitions performed, Joe always lost his shirt while nothing short of kryptonite would stop Dr. Graves from gaining strength.

In the winter of 2001, the vacationing professor spent a few days in our fitness center in Jupiter (Florida) where I put together some questions.

"What happened when Jones first put you on the MedX machine?" I asked.

"Arthur tested my strength," said Graves, "and selected a weight he thought would allow 10-15 repetitions of exercise. After about 50 repetitions, his mumbling converted into a cursive blurt, 'Get him off the d - - m machine.' Days later, he performed the same test and got the same result. He was more than perplexed."

"Was there ever a time he tried to see how far you could really go?" I asked.

"Oh, yeah. One day, I knew he was up to something when he said, 'OK, boy, let's see what you can do with this.' The resistance felt heavy but I performed over 100 repetitions and lasted nearly 20 minutes before he threw in the towel and his standard line."

"Did you feel any fatigue?"

"Not a thing."

Dr. Graves is not the kind to brag or boast. He was born with a high percentage of slow-twitch (slow-fatigue) fibers in the muscles that extend his spine. As such, his endurance in that muscle group is superhuman.

Research has determined several things about the rate of muscle fatigue. It is consistent from limb to limb (i.e., right and left biceps fatigue at the same rate) yet differs from muscle to muscle (biceps may fatigue slowly, triceps quickly). It is genetic and cannot be altered by training. And the best news, the fatigue rate (sometimes referred to as muscle fiber-type) can be ascertained by specific testing and the outcome used to optimize results from exercise.

Muscles that fatigue quickly can't stand much exercise and must be stimulated infrequently with few repetitions. Muscles that fatigue at a slow rate can exercise all day, everyday and still improve.

Individuals like Dr. Graves are rare. I've come across only two of 800 subjects in a 5-year span - and neither wore anything that resembled a cape.

## DECEMBER 27

---

### A Blueprint For Change

"Human beings are afraid, unsure, and fearful of change," said Nautilus® inventor, Arthur Jones. "Especially so, if they've been even moderately successful in reaching some goal."

He called it human nature and it explains a lot.

It explains why people are still hesitant to apply the logical strength-training concepts he developed in the early 1970's. Jones compared the reluctance to an old man in the desert digging for gold with his hands. When someone came along and showed him the task could be performed in much less time with a shovel, the old man became angry and threw the shovel away.

"If you returned to that rugged location in the desert a year later," said Jones, "what would you expect to see that old man doing? Would he be using the shovel properly and have holes as big as school buses spread over the immediate and adjacent surroundings? No, absolutely not! Instead, the prospector would be at that same spot - with a somewhat bigger hole - still digging with his even-more-callused fingers. And there, in plain sight, only a few yards away...would be the unused, and now rusty, shovel."

Many hardcore trainees failed to understand the improvements that Nautilus machines brought to the table. The novelty posed a threat that made them retreat to the barbell. Thirty years later, when things should have changed, they haven't - and the reasons are clear.

The breakthrough was bombarded by negative publicity via the powers that controlled the field of bodybuilding, to the point that the majority gave machines only second billing (despite the fact that machines paid most gym bills). More importantly, that ignorance and influence spilled into the next generation, a generation that now has no idea what Nautilus was or is. The only hope is to reach trainees before they are brainwashed - an unlikely occurrence in a market of myths.

How do you tell an athlete that slower in the gym makes him faster on the field? That muscle isolation is essential to reaching strength potential? That more exercise is a step in the wrong direction? That high intensity is vital to best results when he has driven around the parking lot three times to find a spot closer to the door?

Human nature explains why Jones hesitated to publish his autobiography. The politically correct environment strangling the country held him back until his daughter convinced him to do it before someone else got it wrong. "It is not even possible to publish the truth in today's society," he said, "and I have no desire to publish lies."

His book is strong, but a must read. Jones, a brilliant writer, rarely withholds viewpoints. He knew that the content would expose outrage and 'put some people off.' "So be it," he said resolutely. "While it is neither my intention nor my desire to insult anybody, I am not trying to please anybody either."

Human nature explains the greatest tragedy in the legacy of Arthur Jones. The formula for specific testing inherent in his MedX® machines left the leaders of muscle testing in this country reeling from the fact that they did nothing right. When handed the formula, the field that was moderately successful in reaching its financial goals - not those of truth - ignored it and set everyone back another 50 years.

In the same gloom, government, industry and the military have ignored a tool that could save billions of dollars - all in the name of uncertainty and political correctness.

## DECEMBER 28

---

### The Medical Connection

I often marveled at how a man who quit elementary school could lecture to medical doctors in such a relaxed manner. Yet, there he was every morning, armed with a cup of coffee, pacing before the distinguished crowd.

As I came to learn, Arthur Jones had a long history of doctors in his family.

"During the late 1700's, about the time of the American Revolution," he said, "my great-great-grandfather was a doctor; he was followed by my great-grandfather, grandfather, father (and mother), both my brother and sister, several cousins and uncles, and currently my daughter, all of whom were, or are, doctors."

Besides that, the Nautilus® inventor spent 24 years performing what he called "medical research," and an additional 30 involved in the treatment of poisonous-snake bites - mainly his own - during which time he saw many doctors.

"Overall," he said, "my opinion of doctors is favorable." But there was more. "While there certainly are at least a few exceptions, it remains my clear impression that most doctors know nothing about exercise, and that in many cases they hold firm opinions that are nothing short of dangerous." Jones blamed the education system.

"By and large, if they are 'taught' anything about exercise in school," he said, "such supposed teaching consisted almost entirely of filling their heads with a lot of bullshit based on utterly phony research performed with such worthless testing tools as Cybex® machines."

He also recognized that the medical profession was strapped with the burden of a system that required excess administrative paperwork and a "defensive" approach to medicine. That is, doctors were forced to order tests of little or no value and to pay high insurance premiums to protect themselves from lawsuits.

The cure, he believed, was in prevention rather than treatment, with proper exercise at the helm: "The potential benefits of proper exercise are far greater than most people in the medical and scientific communities even suspect, are primarily important for preventing medical problems." Bravo.

At the end of my latest 'physical' exam, the physician commented, "If more people like you come in, we'll be out of business." I once exercised in a gym across the hall from the office of a chiropractor. As young and old shuffled toward his door, the only thing I could think of was, "If they were here, they wouldn't be there." Good genes? Perhaps. I'd like to think it has something to do with 42 years of strength training.

Jones identified two requirements for the widespread application of proper exercise to the field of general health-care: (1) education of the medical and scientific communities about the potential benefits of proper exercise and (2) a definition of 'proper exercise.'

His 'home-school' seminars aided the first; his medical tools, the second.

"Only time will tell," he said, "just how many of my current opinions about exercise turn out to be correct, but I have at least produced something of great value that never existed previously: the tools required for meaningful and accurate measurement of the results of exercise." But there was still concern.

"I am arrogant enough to believe that my lifetime of interest in the field of exercise has produced developments that can provide great benefits to millions of other people if my discoveries and developments are not flushed down the toilet of history."

The current medical community has a large and heavy hand on the crank.

# DECEMBER 29

---

## Arthur Jones – Part 1

A well-dressed Tom Weiskopf approached his ball on the side of a steep, grassy slope, the Canadian Open on the line. "BLEEP this and BLEEP that," he raged. Luckily, no microphones and only a handful of spectators braved the decent. Tom looked at his lie - worse than expected - and hacked it out. The bleeps increased in magnitude and volume. I was only fifteen.

As unfair as it may seem, and as human nature dictates, we often form opinions about people based upon an incident, chance encounter or something said, seen or done. Those notions are reinforced or negated as we observe the same individual in other situations. When we gather enough pieces of the puzzle, we cast our ultimate vote - we like him or we don't.

The same process occurred during my brief encounters with the Nautilus® inventor. Brief, because I couldn't get enough of him or find enough pieces to complete the puzzle; encounters, because no one felt totally comfortable in his presence.

"Arthur Jones is not a relaxing person to be with," said bodybuilder Mike Mentzer. "He does not lightly exchange words. He spews facts, torrents of them, gleaned from his studies and, perhaps more important, from practical application of theory, personal observation and incisive deduction. You don't converse with Arthur Jones; you attend his lectures. He is opinionated, challenging, intense, and blunt."

Jones didn't trust people and retained only a small entourage. He believed that human nature hadn't changed throughout history and that the problems around him were (in his words) "a direct result of the motivations of some of the people now involved in the fields of exercise and diet; in plain English, many of these people are involved in outright fraud, dangerous fraud in some cases, simply foolish fraud in others."

Jones was interested in truth, and had a unique way of expressing its opposite.

"If you are really interested in losing weight fast, and don't care what you lose," he said, "then you might try letting a rattlesnake bite you. About thirty years ago, I lost 28 pounds within a period of 24 hours as a result of a rattlesnake bite; which rate of loss, since the actual loss was primarily fluids, is supposed to kill...and it almost did kill me. And some of the diets that are now on the market are doing much the same sort of thing, except that some of the people using these diets are being killed."

Nutrition wasn't the only outrage he confronted. Fraudulent claims from leaders in the field of exercise about the amount of training required for best results (and from the field of rehabilitation concerning the use of dangerous testing and exercise equipment) stirred his ire.

"You should question the motives of people," he said, "particularly when seeking their advice; and, even when their motives appear to be aboveboard, never forget that advice is really only somebody's opinion. It is my opinion that proper exercise offers benefits of enormous value to almost everybody, but it is also my opinion that the entire field of exercise is neck deep in outright fraud and foolishness. Separating the facts from the foolishness is not always easy, but at least we are making the attempt."

Somebody once said, "Life does not require us to be the biggest or the best, it asks only that we try." Regardless of how Arthur Jones is perceived in the scheme of things, he spent a lifetime sorting chaff from bran with an effort far beyond the call of duty - and a few bleeps of his own along the way.

## DECEMBER 30

### Arthur Jones – Part 2

"Gary is a golfer," said Jack Nicklaus about his son's failure to qualify for the PGA Tour. "He's a great ball striker, got all the shots, but he can't compete with guys hitting a drive and an 8-iron to the par fives." I concurred.

"Walk softly, but carry a big stick," a phrase made famous by President Theodore Roosevelt, is as applicable in strolling fairways as it is in life.

Nautilus® inventor Arthur Jones didn't quite see it that way. He came up with his own version, updated for modern times, "Sneak around quietly and carry a Thompson® submachine gun."

Jones spent a lifetime challenging bodybuilders, athletes, trainers, coaches, therapists and doctors (literally anyone who crossed his path) to think - but there was nothing soft about his walk.

Arthur could 'read' people, size up situations and respond to adversity so quickly and completely that victims were left searching for the exit by a word, question or gesture. He remained a step ahead by using experience, logic, humor, analogy, intimidation and parody as his tools.

"Always a practical observer," said Grant McClaren (*Professional Pilot Magazine,* Nov., 1984), "Jones takes lessons from the less sophisticated predators (he spent years with animals). 'The only ways to control people and advance are by terror and appealing to greed. Of the two, terror is the more effective.'"

Jones was never without a word or comeback, and rarely without the 'right' one. In his youth, someone tried to kill him with an axe. "Yes," he said, "but he didn't know that I had a cross-cut saw - a magnificent weapon."

"Like mice," wrote Ellington Darden, "most trainees follow their favorite Pied Piper to nowhere. Instead of thinking for themselves, they attempt to become carbon copies. Unfortunately, they copy the wrong people doing the wrong things." He, like others, decided to follow the logic and common sense of Jones.

My contact with the Nautilus inventor was limited, but of great impact. The respect and admiration I had for him was best matched by Bernard Darwin's description of James Braid, one of golf's 'Triumvirate:'

"Up to a point it is not difficult for a prominent player of games to inspire personal liking, and it is perhaps easier for golfers than for the heroes of other games, since in the nature of their game they are surrounded and hemmed in by potential admirers, longing to repeat a single word overheard or, still better, to extract one addressed to themselves. To suffer them gladly is one of the tasks to which the Champion must school himself, and he must also learn, if he can, to make some pretense of remembering the man...of whom he has not the faintest recollection. But they (the admirers) remember him vividly, often crediting themselves with a familiarity with the great man which is wholly illusory, and retailing the mildest of small stories of what he said or did." (*James Braid*, 1952)

I was fortunate that Jack Nicklaus and Arthur Jones had a faint recollection.

"Life is a tragedy for those who feel, a comedy for those who think," said Jean de la Bruyere in a quote that precedes the first chapter of Jones' autobiography. It may explain why the man who once called Gordon Liddy a "left-wing pansy" when Liddy said something he didn't like spent a lifetime teaching people to think.

Life deserves more comic relief.

# DECEMBER 31

---

## Arthur Jones – Part 3

Arthur Jones was, and still is, a prolific reader. In retirement, he devours shelves of books each year, which explains why it was so difficult to pull the wool over his eyes. He read just about everything out there and did not limit his palate to exercise.

His favorite essay, "The Hunting of the Slan" written by Edgar Allen Poe and published in *Southern Literary Messenger* in June, 1849, "summed up," according to Joe Mullen, "his view of life." More specifically, it summed up the destiny of others like him:

**"I have sometimes amused myself by endeavoring to fancy what would be the fate of any individual gifted, or rather accursed, with an intellect very far superior to that of his race. Of course, he would be conscious of his superiority nor could he (if otherwise constituted as man is) help manifesting his consciousness. Thus he would make himself enemies at all points. And since his opinions and speculations would likely differ from those of all mankind - that he would be considered a madman, is evident. How horribly painful such a condition! Hell could invent no greater torture than that of being charged with abnormal weakness on account of being abnormally strong.**

**In like manner, nothing can be clearer than that a very generous spirit - truly feeling what all merely profess - must inevitably find itself misconceived on every direction - its motives misinterpreted. Just as extremeness of intelligence would be thought fatuity, so excess of chivalry could not fail to be looked upon as meanness in its last degree - and so with other virtues. This subject is a painful one indeed. That individuals have so soared above the plane of their race is scarcely to be questioned; but, in looking back through history for traces of their existence, we should pass over all biographies of 'the good and the great,' while we search carefully the slight records of wretches who died in prison, in Bedlam, or upon the gallows."**

Jones first mentioned Poe's essay in an article in the 1983 April/May issue of *Nautilus Magazine*. The aftermath was typically Arthur:

"So far, at least...I have managed to avoid both prison and the gallows, and having long since become accustomed to living in a largely mad world, I don't imagine that a madhouse such as Bedlam would be that much of a change; but perhaps there is still hope for me...I haven't died yet, either."

Arthur continued at the helm of Nautilus® until 1986 when he plunged into the medical field with a line of testing tools under the name MedX®. In December of 1997, he wrote his last article on the topic of exercise.

"More recently," he said, "my life has been a series of outrages - outrages brought on by foolish people. I have no use for fools. Yet, I'm constantly subjected to their presence - in every city, in every country. There is no place on the planet left untouched by foolish people. I'm exhausted...I'm tired of it all. But I'm not ready to die, at least not tomorrow, or the next week, or the week after."

The subject of a man imprisoned - and liberated - by his own brilliance is a painful one indeed. Some day, Arthur Jones will collect humanity's debt. Until then, as golf writer Bernard Darwin uttered toward the end of his career, "...the wind is still blowing on the heath."

## DECEMBER 32

### Curtain Call

Three weeks before, I sent a letter and copies of graphs I was requesting permission to re-print in my book. No reply.

I then resorted to a phone number that was passed on to me with little confidence. It proved correct, but the party on the other end was not available; was, at the time, "taking a nap." I left my number, hoping for a return call. Day One. Nothing. Day Two. Nothing. When it finally came - Day Three, November 26, 2004 at 10:15 PM - I was unprepared.

"Hello," I said as I picked up the receiver.

"Arthur Jones," replied an old and broken voice.

I fumbled a little, thanked him for returning my call and began to re-introduce myself. It had been a long time, too long.

"Can you remember me at all, Mr. Jones?" I asked, hoping my preamble had sparked a recollection.

"No, I really can't remember," he said in a matter-of-fact way.

I thanked him for his contribution to my health (via the MedX® Lumbar Extension machine) and, on a broader scale, to the fields of exercise and rehabilitation. He would have nothing of accolades.

"There's still a lot of bullshit out there." He said, "And nowadays, even more."

Arthur couldn't resist a parting swing and promptly granted permission to use the graphs of his writings "in any way that you'd like." I asked about his health.

"Bad," he replied, hesitating a second or two, then continuing in the same firm voice. "My brother died this morning. My wife passed away six months ago. And I'm sitting here waiting to die myself."

I expressed my condolences (I had met his brother, a physician, at a medical conference and studied with his wife at the University of Florida's Center for Exercise Science), thanked him again and wished him well.

He hung up without a formal "Goodbye."

The man who meant so much to so many for so long, who displayed such boundless energy and who rarely backed down from a fight - physical or otherwise - seemed broken, ready to abandon the big fight.

I returned to reading his autobiography that night (something I hadn't completed) and came across a line that may have summed up his feelings. When contemplating the thought of 'doing it all again,' he concluded that, without 20/20 hindsight, he would probably repeat the errors of the past and do things about the same as he had. Then he added, "...so don't try to figure out what is coming, you don't want to know, couldn't stand it if you did."

At that moment, life did not seem fair. Maybe it's not supposed to be. A man who should have been carried out on a pedestal, sits at home like some wretch in prison awaiting his fate - exactly as Edgar Allen Poe described in history's search for those who have "so soared above the plane of their race."

Arthur was right. Someday we'll all look like Sergio.

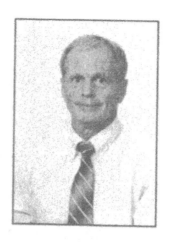

## About the Author

Born in Welland, Ontario, Canada, Gary Bannister attended McMaster University in Hamilton, Ontario where he received Bachelor's Degrees in English (B.A.) and Physical Education (B.P.E.). He then attended The University of North Carolina at Greensboro where he graduated with a Master's Degree in Physical Education (M.Ed.) in 1971.

From there he spent four years (1972-76) teaching and coaching at Averett College in Danville, Virginia followed by four years at Colegio Internacional de Caracas (an American high school) in Caracas, Venezuela. In 1980, he opened the first commercial Nautilus® gym and, in 1988, the first MedX® low-back rehabilitation center in South America. He returned to the United States in 1990 and has since worked in fitness and rehab centers (including his own) in Florida and North Carolina.

The author participated in many sports - hockey, gymnastics, soccer, track and field, distance running and golf - but believed that progressive resistance exercise was the base of physical preparation. He was highly influenced by Arthur Jones and wrote newsletters and fitness articles for local newspapers based upon what the Nautilus inventor called "Proper Strength Training."

An accomplished golfer, Gary currently resides in Tequesta, Florida where he enjoys reading, writing, exercising and two hobbies: collecting antique golf paraphernalia and indulging in the royal and ancient pastime.

*In Arthur's Shadow* is his first book.

978-0-595-48915-2
0-595-48915-X

Made in the USA
Lexington, KY
05 July 2015